HIV and Respiratory Disease

Editors

KRISTINA CROTHERS
LAURENCE HUANG
ALISON MORRIS

CLINICS IN CHEST MEDICINE

www.chestmed.theclinics.com

June 2013 • Volume 34 • Number 2

ELSEVIER

1600 John F. Kennedy Boulevard • Suite 1800 • Philadelphia, Pennsylvania, 19103-2899

http://www.theclinics.com

CLINICS IN CHEST MEDICINE Volume 34, Number 2
June 2013 ISSN 0272-5231, ISBN-13: 978-1-4557-7074-8

Editor: Katie Saunders
Developmental Editor: Donald E. Mumford

Clinics in Chest Medicine (ISSN 0272-5231) is published quarterly by Elsevier Inc., 360 Park Avenue South, New York, NY 10010-1710. Months of issue are March, June, September, and December. Periodicals postage paid at New York, NY and additional mailing offices. Subscription prices are $329.00 per year (domestic individuals), $526.00 per year (domestic institutions), $157.00 per year (domestic students/residents), $361.00 per year (Canadian individuals), $645.00 per year (Canadian institutions), $448.00 per year (international individuals), $645.00 per year (international institutions), and $219.00 per year (international and Canadian students/residents). International air speed delivery is included in all Clinics subscription prices. All prices are subject to change without notice. **POSTMASTER:** Send address changes to Clinics in Chest Medicine, Elsevier Health Sciences Division, Subscription Customer Service, 3251 Riverport Lane, Maryland Heights, MO 63043. **Customer Service: Telephone: 1-800-654-2452** (U.S. and Canada); **1-314-447-8871** (outside U.S. and Canada). **Fax: 1-314-447-8029. E-mail: journalscustomerservice-usa@elsevier.com** (for print support); **journalsonlinesupport-usa@elsevier.com** (for online support).

Reprints. For copies of 100 or more of articles in this publication, please contact the Commercial Reprints Department, Elsevier Inc., 360 Park Avenue South, New York, NY 10010-1710. Tel.: 212-633-3812; Fax: 212-462-1935; E-mail: reprints@elsevier.com.

Clinics in Chest Medicine is covered in *MEDLINE/PubMed (Index Medicus), Current Contents/Clinical Medicine, EMBASE/Excerpta Medica, Science Citation Index,* and *ISI/BIOMED.*

Printed and bound by CPI Group (UK) Ltd, Croydon, CR0 4YY

Transferred to digital print 2013

Contributors

EDITORS

KRISTINA CROTHERS, MD
Associate Professor, Division of Pulmonary and Critical Care Medicine, Department of Medicine, Harborview Medical Center, University of Washington School of Medicine, University of Washington, Seattle, Washington

LAURENCE HUANG, MD
Professor of Medicine, Division of Pulmonary and Critical Care Medicine and HIV/AIDS Division, Department of Medicine, San Francisco General Hospital, University of California San Francisco, San Francisco, California

ALISON MORRIS, MD, MS
Associate Professor, Division of Pulmonary, Allergy, and Critical Care Medicine, Departments of Medicine and Immunology, University of Pittsburgh School of Medicine, Pittsburgh, Pennsylvania

AUTHORS

RONALD ANDERSON, PhD
Medical Research Council Unit for Inflammation and Immunity, Department of Immunology, Faculty of Health Sciences, Tshwane Academic Division of the National Health Laboratory Service, University of Pretoria, South Africa

CHRISTOPHER F. BARNETT, MD, MPH
Assistant Professor of Medicine, Division of Cardiology, Health Sciences Assistant Clinical Professor, San Francisco General Hospital, University of California, San Francisco, San Francisco, California

JAMES M. BECK, MD
Chief, Medicine Service, Veterans Affairs Eastern Colorado Health Care System; Professor, Department of Medicine, University of Colorado School of Medicine, Denver, Colorado

KRISTINE K. BROWNING, PhD
Research Assistant Professor, The Ohio State University College of Nursing and Comprehensive Cancer Center-James Cancer Hospital, Columbus, Ohio

RICHARD E. CHAISSON, MD
Center for Tuberculosis Research, Division of Infectious Diseases, Department of Medicine, Johns Hopkins University School of Medicine, Baltimore, Maryland

KRISTINA CROTHERS, MD
Associate Professor, Division of Pulmonary and Critical Care Medicine, Department of Medicine, Harborview Medical Center, University of Washington School of Medicine, University of Washington, Seattle, Washington

PHILIP DIAZ, MD
Professor, Division of Pulmonary, Allergy, Critical Care, and Sleep Medicine, The Ohio State University College of Medicine, Columbus, Ohio

KERRY L. DIERBERG, MD, MPH
Division of Infectious Diseases, Department of Medicine, Johns Hopkins University School of Medicine, Baltimore, Maryland

SARAH R. DOFFMAN, MB ChB, FRCP
Department of Respiratory Medicine, Royal Sussex County Hospital, Brighton and Sussex University Hospitals NHS Trust, Brighton, United Kingdom

CHARLES FELDMAN, MB BCh, DSc, PhD, FRCP
Professor of Pulmonology, Division of Pulmonology, Department of Internal Medicine, Charlotte Maxeke Johannesburg Academic Hospital, Faculty of Health Sciences, University of the Witwatersrand, Johannesburg, South Africa

AMY K. FERKETICH, PhD
Associate Professor, Division of Epidemiology, The Ohio State University College of Public Health, Columbus, Ohio

MEGHAN FITZPATRICK, MD
Department of Medicine, University of Pittsburgh, Pittsburgh, Pennsylvania

ANURADHA GANESAN, MBBS, MPH
Assistant Professor, Department of Preventive Medicine and Biometrics, Uniformed Services University of the Health Sciences, Infectious Disease Clinical Research Program, Walter Reed National Military Medical Center, Bethesda, Maryland

MATTHEW R. GINGO, MD, MS
Assistant Professor, Division of Pulmonary, Allergy, and Critical Care Medicine, Department of Medicine, University of Pittsburgh School of Medicine, Pittsburgh, Pennsylvania

PRISCILLA Y. HSUE, MD
Associate Professor of Medicine, Division of Cardiology, Associate Professor in Residence, San Francisco General Hospital, University of California, San Francisco, San Francisco, California

LAURENCE HUANG, MD
Professor of Medicine, Division of Pulmonary and Critical Care Medicine and HIV/AIDS Division, Department of Medicine, San Francisco General Hospital, University of California San Francisco, San Francisco, California

GREGORY D. KIRK, MD, MPH, PhD
Associate Professor, Departments of Medicine and Epidemiology, Johns Hopkins University, Baltimore, Maryland

KENNETH S. KNOX, MD
Associate Professor of Medicine and Immunobiology Murray and Clara Walker Memorial Endowed Research, Section of Pulmonary, Allergy, Critical Care and Sleep Medicine, University of Arizona, Tucson, Arizona

ALLISON A. LAMBERT, MD
Fellow, Department of Medicine, Johns Hopkins University, Baltimore, Maryland

ANDREW H. LIMPER, MD
Division of Pulmonary and Critical Care, Department of Internal Medicine, Annenberg Professor of Pulmonary Medicine, Mayo Clinic College of Medicine, Mayo Clinic, Rochester, Minnesota

HENRY MASUR, MD
Chief, Critical Care Medicine Department, NIH Clinical Center, Bethesda, Maryland

CHRISTIAN A. MERLO, MD, MPH
Assistant Professor, Departments of Medicine and Epidemiology, Johns Hopkins University, Baltimore, Maryland

ROBERT F. MILLER, MBBS, FRCP
Research Department of Infection and Population Health, University College London, London, United Kingdom

ALISON MORRIS, MD, MS
Associate Professor, Division of Pulmonary, Allergy, and Critical Care Medicine, Departments of Medicine and Immunology, University of Pittsburgh School of Medicine, Pittsburgh, Pennsylvania

JOHN F. MURRAY, MD, FRCP
Professor Emeritus of Medicine, Pulmonary, San Francisco General Hospital, University of California San Francisco, San Francisco, California

JAKRAPUN PUPAIBOOL, MD
Division of Infectious Diseases, Fellow in Infectious Diseases, Mayo Clinic College of Medicine, Rochester, Minnesota

SOFYA TOKMAN, MD
Division of Pulmonary and Critical Care, Department of Internal Medicine, University of California San Francisco, San Francisco, California

HOMER L. TWIGG III, MD
Associate Professor of Medicine, Division of Pulmonary and Critical Care Medicine, Indiana University Medical Center, Indianapolis, Indiana

PETER D. WALZER, MD, MSc
Division of Infectious Diseases, Department of Internal Medicine, University of Cincinnati College of Medicine, Cincinnati, Ohio

MARY ELLEN WEWERS, PhD, MPH
Professor, Division of Health Behavior and Health Promotion, The Ohio State University College of Public Health, Columbus, Ohio

Contents

Abnormalities in Host Defense Associated with HIV Infection   143

James M. Beck

> The broad variety of pulmonary infections encountered in human immunodeficiency virus (HIV)-infected individuals demonstrates that the host defense network is impaired. An improved understanding of these events in the lung can lead to specific interventions aimed at restoration of deficient function. This review summarizes the pulmonary host defense deficits in HIV-infected individuals, focusing on lymphocytes, alveolar macrophages, and neutrophils.

Impact of Antiretroviral Therapy on Lung Immunology and Inflammation   155

Homer L. Twigg III and Kenneth S. Knox

> Human immunodeficiency virus (HIV) infection causes profound changes in the lung compartment characterized by macrophage and lymphocyte activation, secretion of proinflammatory cytokines and chemokines, and accumulation of CD8 T cells in the alveolar space, leading to lymphocytic alveolitis. Because many of the changes seen in the lung can be attributed to the direct effect of HIV on immune cells, therapy to reduce the HIV burden should have significant beneficial effects. Indeed, antiretroviral therapy rapidly reduces the viral burden in the lung, number of CD8 T cells in the alveolar space, and amount of proinflammatory cytokines and chemokines in bronchoalveolar lavage.

Epidemiology of Human Immunodeficiency Virus–Associated Pulmonary Disease   165

John F. Murray

> HIV/AIDS was initially characterized as a progressively worsening disorder of cellular immunosuppression. In 1996, HIV/AIDS was separated into 2 diagnostic, management, prognostic categories: high-income and low-income groups. High-income people with HIV have had access to antiretroviral therapeutic agents, which have transformed HIV from a lethal to an indolent disease, with life expectancy comparable with other chronic conditions. About 50% of low-income people with HIV who are candidates for antiretroviral therapy actually receive it. Since 1996, the principal HIV-associated pulmonary disease in high-income countries has changed from Pneumocystis pneumonia to community-acquired pneumonia; tuberculosis has predominated in low-income countries as long as HIV has prevailed.

Tobacco Use and Cessation in HIV-Infected Individuals   181

Kristine K. Browning, Mary Ellen Wewers, Amy K. Ferketich, and Philip Diaz

> Smoking prevalence estimates among HIV-infected individuals range from 40% to 84%, much higher than the overall US adult prevalence. To date, few tobacco dependence treatment trials have been conducted among HIV-infected smokers. Recommendations for future research include examining underlying factors that contribute to persistent smoking and barriers to abstinence, identifying ways to increase motivation for quit attempts, increasing the number of multicentered

2-arm tobacco dependence treatment trials, and using highly efficacious first-line pharmacotherapy in tobacco dependence treatment intervention studies. Addressing these research gaps will help to reduce the tobacco-related disease burden of HIV-infected individuals in the future.

diagnostic test to diagnose PCP. Use of adjunctive biomarkers for diagnosis requires further evaluation. Trimethoprim-sulfamethoxazole remains the preferred first-line treatment regimen. In the era of ART, mortality from PCP is approximately 10% to 12%. The optimal time to start ART in a patient with PCP remains uncertain.

The incidence, mortality, and epidemiology of human immunodeficiency virus (HIV)-associated pulmonary infections have changed as a result of effective antiretroviral and prophylaxis antimicrobial therapy. The clinical presentation, radiographic abnormalities, and treatment of pneumonia from various uncommon pathogens in patients with AIDS can be different from those in immunocompetent patients. Advances in invasive and noninvasive testing and molecular biological techniques have improved the diagnosis and prognosis of pulmonary infections in patients infected with HIV. This review focuses on pulmonary infections from nontuberculosis mycobacteria, cytomegalovirus, fungi (aspergillosis, cryptococcosis, endemic fungi), and parasites (toxoplasmosis), and uncommon bacterial pneumonia (nocardiosis, rhodococcosis) in these patients.

This review of lung malignancies in human immunodeficiency virus (HIV) briefly highlights key epidemiologic and clinical features in the pulmonary involvement of AIDS-defining malignancies of Kaposi sarcoma and non-Hodgkin lymphoma. Then, focusing on non-AIDS defining lung cancer, the epidemiology and mechanisms, clinical presentation, pathology, treatment and outcomes, and prevention of HIV-associated lung cancer are discussed. Finally, the important knowledge gaps and future directions for research related to HIV-associated lung malignancies are highlighted.

In the era of effective antiretroviral therapy (ART), epidemiologic studies have found that persons infected with human immunodeficiency virus (HIV) have a higher prevalence and incidence of chronic obstructive pulmonary disease than HIV-uninfected persons. In comparison with HIV-uninfected persons and those with well-controlled HIV disease, HIV-infected persons with poor viral control or lower CD4 cell count have more airflow obstruction, a greater decline in lung function, and possibly more severe diffusing impairment. This article reviews the evidence linking HIV infection to obstructive lung disease, and discusses management issues related to the treatment of obstructive lung disease in HIV-infected patients.

Antiretroviral therapy has greatly increased longevity for individuals with human immunodeficiency virus (HIV) infection. About 0.5% of patients with HIV infection develop moderate to severe pulmonary arterial hypertension, which is several thousand times higher than the incidence of idiopathic pulmonary arterial hypertension. As more than 30 million individuals are chronically infected, HIV infection could soon become one of the most common causes of pulmonary arterial hypertension world-wide. Pulmonary arterial hypertension is a relentlessly progressive disease leading to right heart failure and death. In this article the available data on epidemiology, hemodynamics, mechanisms, and therapeutic strategies for HIV-associated pulmonary arterial hypertension are reviewed.

A spectrum of noninfectious, nonmalignant lymphocytic infiltrative disorders, including nonspecific interstitial pneumonitis and lymphocytic interstitial pneumonitis, was frequently described in HIV-infected adults in the precombination antiretroviral therapy (ART) era. With the advent of ART, these conditions are less commonly encountered when caring for HIV-infected adults, possibly as a consequence of the effects of HIV treatment on pulmonary immunology. By contrast, reports of sarcoidosis among HIV-infected persons were uncommon in the pre-ART era, but sarcoidosis is increasingly recognized since the introduction of ART and may represent an immune reconstitution phenomenon. Other causes of interstitial pneumonitis are infrequently encountered among HIV-infected persons.

Antiretroviral therapy (ART) has transformed the prognosis for patients infected with the human immunodeficiency virus (HIV). With effective ART, these individuals can expect to live almost as long as their HIV-negative counterparts. Given that more than a million people infected with HIV currently live in the United States, the likelihood that the practicing intensivist will manage a patient infected with HIV is high. This review discusses the challenges associated with management of critically ill patients infected with HIV, including the immune reconstitution inflammatory syndrome (a complication associated with ART initiation), ART-related toxicities, and the management of some common opportunistic infections.

Chronic lung diseases, including chronic obstructive pulmonary disease (COPD) and pulmonary hypertension (PH), are unusually prevalent among persons infected with human immunodeficiency virus (HIV). Often these disease states are identified at younger ages than would be expected in the general population. Recent epidemiologic, basic scientific, and cross-sectional clinical data have implicated immune dysfunction and cellular senescence as potential drivers of advanced presentations of age-related diseases in HIV-infected persons. This article describes how HIV-associated COPD and PH may fit into a paradigm of immunosenescence, and outlines the hypothesized associations among chronic HIV infection, immune dysfunction and senescence, and cardiopulmonary outcomes.

CLINICS IN CHEST MEDICINE

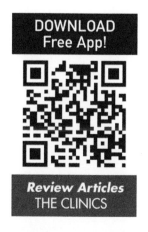

CLINICS IN CHEST MEDICINE

FORTHCOMING ISSUES

September 2013
Interventional Pulmonology
Ali Musani, MD, Editor

December 2013
COPD
Peter Barnes, MD, Editor

March 2014
PAH
Terence Trow, MD, Editor

RECENT ISSUES

March 2013
Pleural Disease
Jonathan Puchalski, MD, MEd, Editor

December 2012
Occupational Pulmonology
Carrie A. Redlich, MD, MPH,
Paul D. Blanc, MD, MSPH,
Mridu Gulati, MD, MPH, and
Ware G. Kuschner, MD, Editors

September 2012
Asthma
Pascal Chanez, MD, PhD, Editor

June 2012
Bronchiectasis
Mark L. Metersky, MD, Editor

Preface

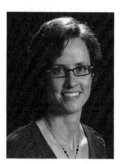 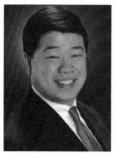 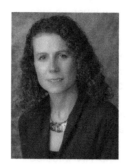

Kristina Crothers, MD   Laurence Huang, MD   Alison Morris, MD, MS

Editors

Recent global estimates indicate that approximately 34 million people are living with HIV infection. A disproportionate number live in low and middle income countries. Many HIV-infected persons residing in these resource-limited regions experience serious or fatal lung complications. HIV-associated lung complications are also frequent causes of illness and death in industrialized, higher income nations, where the greatly improved prognosis due to more widespread availability and access to combination antiretroviral therapy (ART) has turned HIV infection into a chronic disease. Among persons on ART, growing numbers are surviving longer and are developing comorbid diseases that significantly impact mortality, with serious "non-AIDS" conditions accounting for the majority of deaths in the current era. Emerging evidence suggests that chronic lung diseases should be considered among these serious non-AIDS conditions.

This issue is the first *Clinics in Chest Medicine* devoted entirely to topics on pulmonary and critical care complications of HIV infection. The issue begins with 2 articles focused on understanding the impact of HIV infection on host defense within the respiratory tract and on the impact of ART on the immunologic and inflammatory milieu in the lung. HIV-infected persons experience a gradual, but persistent loss of host immunity following infection that results in a syndrome of immune deregulation, dysfunction, and deficiency and depletion of CD4+ lymphocytes, conferring substantially increased risk for opportunistic infections and other complications over the course of HIV infection. While immunologic abnormalities are most marked in those who do not use ART, inflammation and immunodeficiency may persist even in those on ART, and appear to be important risk factors for the premature development of comorbidities.

The next 2 articles consider the worldwide epidemiology of lung complications associated with HIV infection from the beginning of the epidemic to the present, and the prevalence and complications associated with cigarette smoking and strategies for smoking cessation in HIV-infected populations. The high prevalence of cigarette smoking in this population deserves special emphasis, as smoking is a major modifiable risk factor associated with nearly all of the pulmonary complications of HIV infection. Interventions to increase rates of smoking cessation among HIV-infected persons are urgently needed.

As the spectrum of lung complications associated with HIV is broad, the next article considers the general diagnostic approach to HIV-infected patients with respiratory disease. Subsequent articles in this issue are each devoted to specific pulmonary and critical care complications of HIV infection. These include diseases that are AIDS-defining or HIV-associated (such as bacterial pneumonia, tuberculosis, *Pneumocystis*

Clin Chest Med 34 (2013) xiii–xiv
http://dx.doi.org/10.1016/j.ccm.2013.04.009
0272-5231/13/$ – see front matter © 2013 Published by Elsevier Inc.

pneumonia, and other pneumonias); disorders that are not classified as AIDS-defining, but are more common in those with HIV infection (such as lung cancer and other malignancies, chronic obstructive lung disease, and pulmonary arterial hypertension); and conditions whose association with HIV is inconclusive or purely coincidental (such as interstitial lung diseases and sarcoidosis). Because the intensive care of HIV-infected persons can be complex in relation to presenting illness, drug-drug interactions, and management, we include an article on critical illness in HIV-infected individuals. Finally, as the HIV-infected population is aging with successful ART, the concluding article considers the impact of aging and premature cellular senescence associated with HIV infection on the spectrum and pathogenesis of lung complications.

We have recruited leaders in the field for each of these articles and are pleased to present to the reader the first, comprehensive issue of *Clinics in Chest Medicine* devoted to HIV-related pulmonary and critical illness. Given the marked changes in the HIV epidemic, its treatment, and complications, this issue is a timely summary of the current state of knowledge, and we hope it will be a useful review for readers. We wish to thank all of the authors as well as Katie Saunders and the other staff at Elsevier for their contributions.

Kristina Crothers, MD
Division of Pulmonary and Critical Care Medicine
Department of Medicine
Harborview Medical Center
University of Washington School of Medicine
University of Washington
325 Ninth Avenue, Box 359762
Seattle, WA 98104, USA

Laurence Huang, MD
Division of Pulmonary and Critical Care Medicine
and HIV/AIDS Division
Department of Medicine
San Francisco General Hospital
University of California San Francisco
995 Potrero Avenue
San Francisco, CA 94110, USA

Alison Morris, MD, MS
Division of Pulmonary, Allergy
and Critical Care Medicine
Departments of Medicine and Immunology
University of Pittsburgh School of Medicine
3459 Fifth Avenue, 628 NW MUH
Pittsburgh, PA 15213, USA

E-mail addresses:
kcrothers@medicine.washington.edu (K.Crothers)
lhuang@php.ucsf.edu (L.Huang)
morrisa@upmc.edu (A.Morris)

Abnormalities in Host Defense Associated with HIV Infection

James M. Beck, MD[a,b,*]

KEYWORDS

- HIV infections • Lung diseases • Macrophages, alveolar • T-lymphocytes • B-lymphocytes
- Bronchoalveolar lavage

KEY POINTS

- Human immunodeficiency virus (HIV) infects lung lymphocytes and alveolar macrophages, and tropic strains infect lung lymphocytes and alveolar macrophages using distinct chemokine coreceptors.
- Lung CD4[+] T cells are reduced in number but demonstrate impaired proliferative and cytokine responses despite expression of activation signals. Lung CD8[+] T cells are increased in number and cause lymphocytic alveolitis but do not lyse target cells appropriately.
- Specific antibody responses and opsonization of microorganisms are impaired.
- Alveolar macrophages demonstrate intact phagocytosis and killing, enhanced antigen presentation, and increased tumor necrosis factor (TNF) elaboration. Despite these findings, pulmonary infections in vivo may result from impaired activation signaling from T cells.
- Further investigation is needed to clarify discrepant results regarding the capacities of pulmonary neutrophils for chemotaxis and phagocytosis.

INTRODUCTION

Since the early era of widespread HIV infection, the variety of pulmonary infections encountered in the infected population demonstrated that HIV severely impairs lung host defenses.[1] Although most investigations focus on HIV's effects on systemic immunity, an increasing body of literature examines pulmonary immune and inflammatory mechanisms during HIV infection.[2] As impairments in pulmonary host defense are better understood, strategies to correct these defects may be developed for treatment and prophylaxis of pulmonary infections.[3]

The advent of highly active antiretroviral therapy has decreased the incidence of pulmonary infections in HIV-infected individuals dramatically, but this population remains at risk for infection. This review focuses on immune and inflammatory deficits in HIV-infected individuals who are naive to HIV treatment; the effects of ART on pulmonary host defense are summarized comprehensively in the subsequent review.

Several mechanisms have been postulated to explain susceptibility to pulmonary infections.[4] First, HIV can directly infect and kill cells directed against specific pathogens, leaving decreased numbers of cells available to participate in host defense. Second, HIV can impair the metabolic or secretory functions of effector cells. Third, HIV-infected cells may shift their repertoires from elaboration of immunostimulating to immunosuppressive products, such as a shift from Th1 to

Supported by: NIH U01 HL98961.

Conflict of interest: the author has nothing to disclose.

[a] Medicine Service, Veterans Affairs Eastern Colorado Health Care System, 1055 Clermont Street (111), Denver, CO 80220, USA; [b] Department of Medicine, University of Colorado School of Medicine, 12631 East 17th Avenue, Campus Box B178, Aurora, CO 80045, USA

* Medicine Service, Veterans Affairs Eastern Colorado Health Care System, 1055 Clermont Street (111), Denver, CO 80220.

E-mail address: james.beck@ucdenver.edu

chestmed.theclinics.com

Th2 cytokine production. Fourth, HIV infection may interfere with the ability of circulating immune cells to migrate into the lungs and clear pathogens from the alveolar spaces. Finally, coinfection by a second pathogen may contribute to impaired host defense. In all likelihood, all the mechanisms contribute to some extent to deficits in defense.

Although much useful knowledge has been generated by examination of systemic immunity, caution must be exercised in interpreting studies of systemic host defense and applying them to the pulmonary compartment. Many investigations have extrapolated data obtained from peripheral blood cells to reach conclusions about lung immunity. For example, monocyte-derived macrophages (peripheral blood mononuclear cells that are cultured and develop phenotypic characteristics of macrophages) yield important results, but these data may not be directly applicable to alveolar or other tissue macrophages. It is worth noting that the alveolar milieu has significant influence on cellular function in the lung. Therefore, interpretation of in vitro studies may be somewhat limited. The accessibility of lung cells for study by bronchoalveolar lavage (BAL) provides an opportunity to study the direct effects of HIV on lung host defenses.

Considering the function of lung cells, and not just their numbers, is also of importance. Because of the difficulty in studying functional capabilities of lung cells, current clinical practice often depends on measuring numbers of cells rather than their function. For example, the most recent US Public Health Service recommendations suggest that providers should discontinue primary and secondary *Pneumocystis jirovecii* prophylaxis for sustained increases in CD4$^+$ T-cell counts of greater than 200 cells/μL for at least 3 months.[5] No other tests are available clinically to predict risk of *Pneumocystis* pneumonia, but it is reasonable to assume that the functional abilities of these CD4$^+$ T cells are at least as important as their numbers. HIV-infected individuals with weak peripheral blood lymphocyte proliferation to *Pneumocystis* antigens are at significantly higher risk of infection than individuals whose lymphocytes proliferate vigorously.[6] As another example, antibody responses to *Pneumocystis* major surface glycoprotein recombinant fragment C1 distinguish HIV-infected individuals with and without clinical pneumonia.[7] When followed prospectively, lack of immunoglobulin G (IgG) response to the *Pneumocystis* antigen KEX1 predicts individuals who develop *Pneumocystis* pneumonia versus other AIDS-defining illnesses.[8] Although these tests are not available for clinical use, they emphasize the need for further functional investigation.

HIV INFECTION OF LUNG CELLS
HIV Tropism

HIV strains differ in their tropism for lymphocytes or monocytes/macrophages (**Fig. 1**).[9] The CD4 molecule, present on lymphocytes and monocytes/macrophages, serves as the primary cellular receptor for HIV-1. In the lung, CD4 serves as the primary receptor for HIV on alveolar macrophages.[10] Coreceptors are also needed for HIV entry into cells, and these cellular coreceptors define the tropism of HIV strains. Lymphocyte-tropic (T-tropic, X4) strains interact with the chemokine receptor CXCR4 (fusin) to control entry into target cells. Infection can be blocked by the CXC chemokine SDF-1, which is a CXCR4 ligand. Conversely, monocyte-tropic (M-tropic) strains interact with the chemokine receptor CCR5 to control entry into target cells. HIV infection of human alveolar macrophages is preferentially mediated by the CCR5 receptor, although alveolar macrophages also express CXCR4.[11] Infection of macrophages can be blocked with the CC chemokines regulated and normal T cell expressed and secreted (RANTES), macrophage inflammatory protein (MIP)-1α and MIP-1β, which are CCR5 ligands.

As HIV infection progresses, T-tropic virus strains replace M-tropic virus strains, and this change is accompanied by more rapid immunologic decline. Minor chemokine receptors have now been shown to influence progression to AIDS, as well as susceptibility to specific pathogens. For example, variation in CCRL2, which is closely related to CCR5, has been shown to increase progression to AIDS and risk of *Pneumocystis* pneumonia.[12]

HIV Replication

Cytokines and chemokines modulate HIV expression and replication, but conflicts in reported

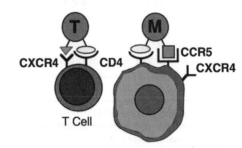

Fig. 1. HIV tropism for T cells and alveolar macrophages. T-tropic HIV strains interact with CD4 and CXCR4 (fusin) on T cells for entry. In contrast, M-tropic HIV strains interact with CD4 and CCR5 on alveolar macrophages, although CXCR4 is also present.

literature probably reflect differences in experimental design. In general, proinflammatory cytokines such as TNF-α, interleukin (IL)-6, and granulocyte monocyte colony-stimulating factor induce HIV transcription. Immunosuppressive cytokines (IL-4, IL-10) have dichotomous effects, and chemokines (MIP-1α, RANTES, and stromal cell–derived factor [SDF]-1) generally decrease transcription.[9]

In the lung, HIV replication occurs in pulmonary lymphocytes and in alveolar macrophages, and infection can be identified in cells sampled by BAL. Alveolar macrophages are likely to be the primary reservoir of HIV in the lung. HIV reverse transcriptase can be detected in alveolar macrophages obtained by lavage from AIDS patients, and alveolar macrophages can be infected with HIV in vitro.[13] Alveolar macrophages from smokers are more susceptible to HIV infection in vitro than alveolar macrophages from nonsmokers.[14] CD8[+] T cells in blood[15] and lung[16] can be infected with HIV and are likely to serve as additional reservoirs.

Reports comparing the HIV burden of alveolar macrophages and peripheral blood monocytes are discrepant. The relative importance of in situ HIV replication in the lung, compared with influx of previously infected cells from bone marrow and blood, is unclear. The percentages of alveolar macrophages expressing HIV antigens have varied considerably among different laboratories.[17] Detection of HIV by polymerase chain reaction suggests that HIV infection of alveolar macrophages is common,[18] and alveolar macrophages become infected with increasing frequency as HIV infection progresses.[19] Direct comparison of alveolar macrophages and peripheral blood monocytes suggests that viral burden is equivalent.[20] The frequency of HIV-specific CD4[+] and CD8[+] T cells has been compared in blood, gut (terminal ileum biopsies), and lung (BAL) in treatment-naive, HIV-infected individuals. Compared with the gut, the lung contained much higher frequencies of HIV-specific CD4[+] and CD8[+] T cells.[21]

Pulmonary infections increase the rate of HIV replication in the lung.[22] For example, BAL from lung segments involved by *Mycobacterium tuberculosis* contains higher viral loads than uninvolved lung segments in the same individual, suggesting increased local replication of HIV.[23] One mechanism leading to increased HIV replication is the ability of *M. tuberculosis* infection to increase surface expression of CCR5 by alveolar macrophages (see **Fig. 1**).[24] Similarly, *Mycobacterium avium* infection activates nuclear factor (NF)-κB in macrophages, leading to increased CCR5 and TNF expression and increased susceptibility to

HIV infection.[25] Patients with *Pneumocystis* pneumonia have increased viral loads in BAL compared with asymptomatic, HIV-infected individuals.[26] One mechanism of increased HIV replication may be increased production of TNF and IL-6, accompanied by decreased production of IL-10.[27]

The effects of ART on HIV infection of lung cells, and on replication, are discussed in the following review.

ALTERATIONS IN LUNG LYMPHOCYTES
Cell Numbers

Data from the early period of the HIV epidemic indicated that lymphocyte percentages or concentrations[28] are increased in BALs from HIV-infected individuals, compared with uninfected individuals. However, most of these data were obtained during bronchoscopies performed during episodes of clinical pulmonary infections. Examination of BAL lymphocyte subsets from AIDS patients shows decreases in the levels of CD4[+] T cells and increases in the levels of CD8[+] T cells. Therefore, CD4 to CD8 ratios in BAL specimens may be even lower than the ratios in peripheral blood.[29] During HIV infection, BALs from smokers demonstrate decreased CD4 to CD8 ratios compared with nonsmokers, suggesting that cigarette smoke further suppresses lung defense.[30] As in peripheral blood, most T cells in the lung bear $\alpha\beta$ T-cell receptors on their surfaces, but a minority expresses $\gamma\delta$ T-cell receptors. Numbers of $\gamma\delta$ T cells are reported to be decreased[31] or increased in HIV-infected patients with opportunistic infections.[32] Recent work demonstrates that most pulmonary CD4[+] T cells are effector memory cells with increased expression of activation markers, at least during episodes of respiratory infection.[33]

CD4[+] T Cells

Decreased numbers of CD4[+] T cells in BALs from HIV-infected individuals undergoing bronchoscopy to diagnose pulmonary infections predict mortality.[34] Low numbers of CD4[+] T cells in BAL from asymptomatic, HIV-infected individuals are an independent predictor of mortality.[35] In addition to accelerated destruction of CD4[+] T cells by HIV infection, underproduction of T cells also occurs. Underproduction can occur from infection-mediated death of progenitor cells and destruction of the hematopoietic stroma.[36] Furthermore, proliferative responses are impaired. Peripheral blood T cells from AIDS patients do not proliferate normally in response to mitogens.[37] Even in AIDS patients showing serologic evidence of prior infection with cytomegalovirus or herpes simplex virus, lymphocytes fail to proliferate normally in response to these viral antigens.[38]

Failure to proliferate may be caused in part by impaired elaboration of IL-2. Peripheral blood T cells from AIDS patients have impaired IL-2 secretion in response to a variety of stimuli.[39] In vitro, recombinant IL-2 can restore some mitogenic responses of blood lymphocytes from AIDS patients.[40] Clinical trials of IL-2 for HIV infection demonstrate that IL-2 increases CD4$^+$ T-cell counts in recipients without increasing HIV replication, particularly when given intermittently.[41] Although this therapy initially seemed to be promising, IL-2 may increase risk of bacterial pneumonia when administered frequently.[42]

A major defect in T-cell host defense during HIV infection is impaired production of interferon (IFN)$-\gamma$ in response to mitogens[37] or antigens.[43] The relative ability of peripheral lymphocytes to elaborate IFN$-\gamma$ correlates with clinical status and CD4$^+$ T-cell count[44] and predicts progression to AIDS.[45] A clinical example of this impairment occurs in the interpretation of IFN$-\gamma$ release assays for tuberculosis. For example, the performance of commercial assays is negatively influenced in M. tuberculosis culture–positive patients with HIV infection and low CD4 counts.[46]

Experimental work suggests that progression from asymptomatic HIV infection to AIDS is accompanied by a switch from Th1-like lymphocyte responses to Th2-like lymphocyte responses.[47] Prevention of this switch in lymphocyte responses could prevent progression to AIDS. IL-12, a cytokine that favors Th1 development and inhibits Th2 development, has been shown to restore cell-mediated immunity in lymphocytes obtained from HIV-infected individuals.[48] Few data exist on the function of lung CD4$^+$ cells, but activation status differs in BAL and blood from HIV-infected and uninfected subjects, and responses to infectious antigens are impaired in BAL CD4$^+$ T cells.[49]

CD8$^+$ T Cells

CD8$^+$ T-cell alveolitis occurs during HIV infection. Some HIV-infected individuals may manifest pulmonary symptoms as a result of CD8$^+$ T-cell influx into the lung, clinically diagnosed as lymphoid interstitial pneumonitis.[50] The functional capabilities of these cells (and their intended targets) require further investigation.

The alveolitis is a result, in part, of CD8$^+$ T cells directed against HIV antigens, as subpopulations of CD8$^+$ T cells are cytotoxic for macrophages or B-cell lines expressing HIV antigens.[51] The intensity of CD8$^+$ alveolitis correlates with the HIV viral load, and the poor prognosis associated with alveolitis may be a result of the elevated viral burden.[52] One mechanism of alveolitis is overproduction of IL-15, a cytokine with IL-2-like effects, by alveolar macrophages. Alveolar macrophages from HIV-infected individuals produce large quantities of IL-15, which enhances antigen presentation by alveolar macrophages and causes proliferation of lung CD8$^+$ T cells.[53]

CD8$^+$ T cells obtained from the lungs of HIV-infected individuals do not lyse appropriate targets in vitro.[54] For example, CD8$^+$ T-cell-mediated cytotoxicity for influenza virus is decreased in HIV-infected individuals.[55] Late in the course of HIV infection, the numbers of CD8$^+$ T cells decline. Depletion of CD8$^+$ T cells may be associated with the development of disseminated cytomegalovirus and M. avium infections.[56]

Phenotypically, CD8$^+$ T cells from AIDS patients express activation markers,[57] and increased percentages of activated cells predict progression of HIV-related disease.[58] Peripheral CD8$^+$ T cells in HIV-infected individuals may be poor effectors because they lack required maturation signals.[59] Unlike the periphery, local concentrations of IL-2 and IFN$-\gamma$ may be increased in the lung during HIV infection because of activation of CD8$^+$ T cells.[60] Functionally, however, CD8$^+$ responses may be deficient because of lack of local CD4$^+$ T-cell help. CD4$^+$ T cells are needed for priming, maintenance of memory, and functional activation in CD8$^+$ T cells.[61]

In theory, modulation of CD8$^+$ T-cell populations directed against HIV-infected cells could provide a novel method to augment host defense. Studies have attempted to exploit this finding by infusion of CD8$^+$ T cells into HIV-infected individuals.[62] CD8$^+$ T cells, expanded in vitro and infused into the donor, result in increased killing of HIV-infected target cells.[63] These infused CD8$^+$ T cells accumulate in the lung, but their eventual benefit as a therapeutic modality is uncertain.

Natural Killer Cells

Increased numbers of natural killer (NK) cells in BAL have been observed in HIV-infected individuals, but with progressive HIV disease, they lose functional capabilities. As with CD8$^+$ T cells, NK cells may be impaired during HIV infection because they depend on signals from CD4$^+$ T cells for optimal function.[64] Biologic response modifiers such as recombinant IL-2 restore lytic ability in vitro,[65] and IFN$-\gamma$ may augment NK cell activity in the early stages of HIV infection.[66] The combination of IL-12 and IL-15 is effective in restoring the expression of cytolytic molecules in NK cells from HIV-infected individuals.[67]

B Cells and Immunoglobulins

The polyclonal activation of B cells that occurs systemically during HIV infection has been appreciated since the early era of the epidemic. Compared with uninfected individuals, measurement of immunoglobulins in BAL from AIDS patients with pulmonary symptoms shows increases in the total amounts of IgG, IgM, and IgA.[29] Local immunoglobulin synthesis may occur in the lung, shown by increased numbers of IgG-, IgM-, and IgA-secreting cells.[68] In contrast to results obtained during episodes of clinical infection, BAL from asymptomatic HIV-infected individuals contains decreased concentrations of IgG compared with uninfected controls.[69]

Although generalized gammopathy occurs, antibody responses to specific antigens are impaired in HIV-infected individuals. B-cell abnormalities begin early in HIV infection, with failure to produce antibody in response to mitogen at the time of HIV seroconversion, before T-cell function is affected.[70] B cells from AIDS patients show impaired proliferation in response to mitogens and do not initiate normal antibody synthesis in response to newly encountered antigens.[71] Altered IgG concentrations in the lung may be a result of the impaired ability of alveolar macrophages to induce IgG secretion from B cells, likely as a result of transforming growth factor-β secretion.[69] Functionally, BAL and serum IgG from HIV-infected individuals demonstrate decreased opsonic activity against Streptococcus pneumoniae than IgG from uninfected controls.[72]

Recent studies examining the utility of antibodies in detection of Pneumocystis are presented in the Introduction.

ALTERATIONS IN ALVEOLAR MACROPHAGES
Cell Numbers

Macrophage numbers in BALs from AIDS patients are probably normal,[28] but percentages are decreased by influx of other cells. As discussed earlier, HIV infection of alveolar macrophages establishes these cells as reservoirs of infection without depletion of their numbers.

Chemotaxis, Phagocytosis, and Killing

Elimination of pathogens by alveolar macrophages depends on an orderly sequence of chemotaxis, phagocytosis, and killing. Peripheral blood monocytes from AIDS patients are reported to be defective in chemotaxis to several chemoattractants,[73] but other investigators find unimpaired chemotaxis.[74] Alveolar macrophages from asymptomatic, HIV-infected subjects demonstrate enhanced phagocytosis for Staphylococcus aureus.[75] In contrast, binding of Pneumocystis to macrophages depends on a variety of mediators, including mannose receptors.[76] Alveolar macrophages from HIV-infected individuals demonstrate decreased binding and phagocytosis of Pneumocystis in vitro, and this defect correlates with the downregulation of mannose receptors.[77] Phagocytic activity is decreased in alveolar macrophages from HIV-infected individuals who smoke.[78]

The magnitude of the respiratory burst of alveolar macrophages from AIDS patients in vitro is not different from that of uninfected controls, and IFN−γ enhances the response in cells from both groups equivalently.[43] Alveolar macrophages and monocyte-derived macrophages do not kill Toxoplasma gondii or Chlamydia psittaci, whether obtained from AIDS patients or from uninfected individuals.[43] When exposed in vitro to IFN−γ, however, alveolar macrophages obtained from AIDS patients increase their killing of these organisms in a manner equivalent to uninfected individuals' cells.[43,79] These data support the theory that suboptimal activation of alveolar macrophages in vivo is a result of impaired signaling from T cells.

Antigen Presentation

During HIV infection, blood monocytes do not present antigens to T cells normally.[80] Alveolar macrophages are poor antigen-presenting cells, in comparison to blood monocytes, but alveolar macrophages from HIV-infected patients demonstrate enhanced ability to present antigen.[81] To explain the pulmonary infectious complications that occur in HIV-infected individuals despite enhanced antigen presentation, the role of dendritic cells must be considered. Dendritic cells may perform most of the antigen presentation in the lung. HIV infection of dendritic cells is cytopathic for these cells, and the numbers of dendritic cells are decreased in asymptomatic HIV-infected individuals and in AIDS patients.[82] Dendritic cells from HIV-infected individuals exhibit defective antigen presentation and may facilitate HIV infection of T cells.[83]

TNF Elaboration

The data regarding TNF production during HIV infection are discrepant. Some AIDS patients are reported to have elevated serum levels of TNF.[84] When peripheral blood monocytes are examined, they are reported to have either high spontaneous release of TNF[85] or suboptimal release after appropriate stimulation.[86] Paradoxically, some investigators have found that HIV infection of monocytes or monocyte-derived macrophages in vitro does not induce TNF release.[87]

Alveolar macrophages from asymptomatic, HIV-seropositive individuals demonstrate increased spontaneous TNF release, which correlates with the extent of HIV expression.[88] BAL cells from smokers release less TNF than BAL cells from nonsmokers, suggesting that smoking and HIV infection interact to suppress macrophage function.[30] Work examining responses of alveolar macrophages to *Salmonella typhimurium* demonstrates no differences in phagocytosis or killing between cells from HIV-infected individuals and controls, but TNF elaboration is increased significantly in cells from HIV-infected individuals.[89] The literature does not reach consensus, however, and there are experimental examples of impaired TNF release as well. Some of this discrepancy may be explained by the stimuli used to provoke TNF elaboration. For example, when stimulated with lipopolysaccharide, alveolar macrophages show decreased TNF release via a toll-like receptor (TLR) 4-dependent mechanism.[90] Conversely, it has been demonstrated that TNF release from alveolar macrophages in response to HIV-1 single-stranded RNA depends on TLR8 signaling.[91]

TNF may have beneficial and detrimental effects during *Pneumocystis* pneumonia. *Pneumocystis* infection stimulates production of TNF by macrophages,[92] and alveolar macrophages from HIV-infected individuals with *Pneumocystis* pneumonia elaborate increased amounts of TNF.[93] Expression of TNF by human alveolar macrophages during *Pneumocystis* pneumonia correlates with decreased arterial oxygenation, suggesting that TNF-induced inflammation is detrimental.[94] Part of the beneficial effect of corticosteroid therapy during *Pneumocystis* pneumonia may be to inhibit TNF elaboration.[95]

ALTERATIONS IN LUNG NEUTROPHILS
Cell Numbers

Several BAL series have reported increases in the concentrations[96] or in the percentages of neutrophils[28] obtained from AIDS patients, compared with uninfected controls. Although AIDS patients may have increased numbers of neutrophils at the time of BAL, little is known about the host defense capabilities of these cells.

Chemotaxis and Phagocytosis

Peripheral neutrophils from some AIDS patients with frequent localized infections show decreased chemotaxis in vitro.[74] Neutrophils from HIV-infected individuals have decreased expression of CD88, the ligand for complement factor 5a, which could contribute to increased susceptibility to bacterial infections.[97] The phagocytic capacity of neutrophils during HIV infection is controversial. Individuals with early HIV infection demonstrate enhanced phagocytosis.[98] Phagocytosis of opsonized *S. aureus* is decreased in some, but not all, AIDS patients' peripheral blood neutrophils.[99] The defect in phagocytosis can be corrected by in vivo administration of granulocyte colony-stimulating factor.[100] Neutrophils from individuals with HIV infection express decreased IgG Fc-γ receptor 1 expression compared with those from uninfected volunteers.[101]

Considering *Pneumocystis* pneumonia, increased numbers of neutrophils in BAL fluid from patients with HIV infection and *Pneumocystis* pneumonia correlate with impaired oxygenation,[102] poor outcome,[103] and increases in mechanical ventilation and mortality.[104] Neutrophils obtained from non–HIV-infected donors are able to ingest and kill *Pneumocystis* organisms and generate superoxide when challenged by organisms.[105] Anti-*Pneumocystis* IgG and complement are required to opsonize the organism and increase the respiratory burst of neutrophils.[106] In vivo, BAL IL-8 concentrations during *Pneumocystis* pneumonia correlate with clinical severity and mortality.[107]

SUMMARY

Although depletion of CD4[+] T cells is a major immunologic manifestation of HIV infection, multiple components of the host defense network are impaired. CD4[+] T cells demonstrate impaired proliferative and cytokine responses, despite expression of activation signals. Lung CD8[+] T cells are increased in number and cause lymphocytic alveolitis but do not lyse target cells appropriately. Specific antibody responses and opsonization of microorganisms are impaired. Alveolar macrophages demonstrate intact phagocytosis and killing, enhanced antigen presentation, and increased TNF elaboration. Despite these findings, pulmonary infections in vivo may result from impaired activation signaling from T cells. Further investigation is needed to clarify discrepant results regarding pulmonary neutrophils' capacities for chemotaxis and phagocytosis. In the future, improved understanding of these impairments in the lung could lead to specific interventions aimed at prevention of lung infection.

REFERENCES

1. Beck JM. The immunocompromised host: HIV infection. Proc Am Thorac Soc 2005;2:423–7.

2. Agostini C, Zambello R, Trentin L, et al. HIV and pulmonary immune responses. Immunol Today 1996;17:359–64.

3. Beck JM, Rosen MJ, Peavy HH. Pulmonary complications of HIV infection: report of the fourth NHLBI workshop. Am J Respir Crit Care Med 2001;164:2120–6.

4. White NC, Agostini C, Israël-Biet D, et al. The growth and the control of human immunodeficiency virus in the lung: implications for highly active antiretroviral therapy. Eur J Clin Invest 1999;29:964–72.

5. Centers for Disease Control and Prevention. Guidelines for prevention and treatment of opportunistic infections in HIV-infected adults and adolescents. MMWR 2009;58:1–207.

6. Atzori C, Clerici M, Trabattoni D, et al. Assessment of immune reconstitution to *Pneumocystis carinii* in HIV-1 patients under different highly active antiretroviral therapy regimens. J Antimicrob Chemother 2003;52:276–81.

7. Djawe K, Huang L, Daly KR, et al. Serum antibody levels to the *Pneumocystis jirovecii* major surface glycoprotein in the diagnosis of *P. jirovecii* pneumonia in HIV+ patients. PLoS One 2010;5:e14259.

8. Gingo MR, Lucht L, Daly KR, et al. Serologic responses to *Pneumocystis* proteins in HIV patients with and without *Pneumocystis jirovecii* pneumonia. J Acquir Immune Defic Syndr 2011;57:190–6.

9. Benfield TL, Lundgren JD, Masur H. HIV-1, cytokines, and the lung. In: Nelson S, Martin TR, editors. Cytokines in pulmonary disease: infection and inflammation. New York: Marcel Dekker; 2000. p. 331–64.

10. Guay LA, Sierra-Madero JG, Finegan CK, et al. Mediation of entry of human immunodeficiency virus-1 into alveolar macrophages by CD4 without facilitation by surfactant-associated protein-A. Am J Respir Cell Mol Biol 1997;16:421–8.

11. Park IW, Koziel H, Hatch W, et al. CD4 receptor-dependent entry of human immunodeficiency virus type-1 env-pseudotypes into CCR5-, CCR3-, and CXCR4-expressing human alveolar macrophages is preferentially mediated by the CCR5 coreceptor. Am J Respir Cell Mol Biol 1999;20:864–71.

12. An P, Li R, Wang JM, et al. Role of exonic variation in chemokine receptor genes on AIDS: CCRL2 F167Y association with *Pneumocystis* pneumonia. PLoS Genet 2011;7:e1002328.

13. Salahuddin SZ, Rose RM, Groopman JE, et al. Human T lymphotropic virus type III infection of human alveolar macrophages. Blood 1986;68:281–4.

14. Abbud RA, Finegan CK, Guay LA, et al. Enhanced production of human immunodeficiency virus type 1 by in vitro-infected alveolar macrophages from otherwise healthy cigarette smokers. J Infect Dis 1995;172:859–63.

15. De Maria A, Pantaleo G, Schnittman SM, et al. Infection of CD8+ lymphocytes: requirement for interaction with infected CD4+ cells and induction of infectious virus from chronically infected CD8+ cells. J Immunol 1991;146:2220–6.

16. Semenzato G, Agostini C, Ometto L, et al. CD8+ T lymphocytes in the lung of acquired immunodeficiency syndrome patients harbor human immunodeficiency virus type 1. Blood 1995;85:2308–14.

17. Agostini C, Trentin L, Zambello R, et al. HIV-1 and the lung: infectivity, pathogenic mechanisms and cellular immune responses taking place in the lower respiratory tract. Am Rev Respir Dis 1993;147:1038–49.

18. Rose RM, Krivine A, Pinkston P, et al. Frequent identification of HIV-1 DNA in bronchoalveolar lavage cells obtained from individuals with the acquired immunodeficiency syndrome. Am Rev Respir Dis 1991;143:850–4.

19. Sierra-Madero JG, Toossi Z, Hom DL, et al. Relationship between load of virus in alveolar macrophages from human immunodeficiency virus type 1-infected persons, production of cytokines, and clinical status. J Infect Dis 1994;169:18–27.

20. Lewin SR, Kirihara J, Sonza S, et al. HIV-1 DNA and mRNA concentrations are similar in peripheral blood monocytes and alveolar macrophages in HIV-1-infected individuals. AIDS 1998;12:719–27.

21. Brenchley JM, Knox KS, Asher AI, et al. High frequencies of polyfunctional HIV-specific T cells are associated with preservation of mucosal CD4 T cells in bronchoalveolar lavage. Mucosal Immunol 2008;1:49–58.

22. Orenstein JM, Fox C, Wahl SM. Macrophages as a source of HIV during opportunistic infections. Science 1997;276:1857–61.

23. Nakata K, Rom WN, Honda Y, et al. *Mycobacterium tuberculosis* enhances human immunodeficiency virus-1 replication in the lung. Am J Respir Crit Care Med 1997;155:996–1003.

24. Fraziano M, Cappelli G, Santucci M, et al. Expression of CCR5 is increased in human monocyte-derived macrophages and alveolar macrophages in the course of in vivo and in vitro *Mycobacterium tuberculosis* infection. AIDS Res Hum Retroviruses 1999;15:869–74.

25. Wahl SM, Greenwell-Wild T, Hale-Donze H, et al. Permissive factors for HIV-1 infection of macrophages. J Leukoc Biol 2000;68:303–10.

26. Koziel H, Kim S, Reardon C, et al. Enhanced in vivo human immunodeficiency virus-1 replication in the lungs of human immunodeficiency virus-infected persons with *Pneumocystis carinii* pneumonia. Am J Respir Crit Care Med 1999;160:2048–55.

27. Israël-Biet D, Esvant H, Laval AM, et al. Impairment of beta chemokine and cytokine production in patients with HIV related *Pneumocystis jiroveci* pneumonia. Thorax 2004;59:247–51.

28. White DA, Gellene RA, Gupta S, et al. Pulmonary cell populations in the immunosuppressed patient: bronchoalveolar lavage findings during episodes of pneumonitis. Chest 1985;88:352–9.

29. Young KR Jr, Rankin JA, Naegel GP, et al. Bronchoalveolar lavage cells and proteins in patients with the acquired immunodeficiency syndrome: an immunologic analysis. Ann Intern Med 1985;103:522–33.

30. Wewers MD, Diaz PT, Wewers ME, et al. Cigarette smoking in HIV infection induces a suppressive inflammatory environment in the lung. Am J Respir Crit Care Med 1998;158:1543–9.

31. Hermier F, Comby E, Delaunay A, et al. Decreased blood TcRγδ+ lymphocytes in AIDS and *p24*-antigenemic HIV-1-infected patients. Clin Immunol Immunopathol 1993;69:248–50.

32. Kägi MK, Fierz W, Grob PJ, et al. High proportion of gamma-delta T cell receptor positive T cells in bronchoalveolar lavage and peripheral blood of HIV-infected patients with *Pneumocystis carinii* pneumonias. Respiration 1993;60:170–7.

33. Rubbo PA, Tuaillon E, Balloré K, et al. The potential impact of CD4+ T cell activation and enhanced Th1/Th2 cytokine ratio on HIV-1 secretion in the lungs of individuals with advanced AIDS and active pulmonary infection. Clin Immunol 2011;139:142–54.

34. Agostini C, Adami F, Poulter LW, et al. Role of bronchoalveolar lavage in predicting survival of patients with human immunodeficiency virus infection. Am J Respir Crit Care Med 1997;156:1501–7.

35. Day RB, Wang Y, Knox KS, et al. Alveolar macrophages from HIV-infected subjects are resistant to *Mycobacterium tuberculosis in vitro*. Am J Respir Cell Mol Biol 2004;30:403–10.

36. McCune JM. The dynamics of CD4+ T-cell depletion in HIV disease. Nature 2001;410:974–9.

37. Rudy T, Opelz G, Gerlack R, et al. Correlation of *in vitro* immune defects with impaired gamma interferon response in human-immunodeficiency-virus-infected individuals. Vox Sang 1988;54:92–5.

38. Krowka J, Stites D, Mills J, et al. Effects of interleukin 2 and large envelope glycoprotein (gp120) of human immunodeficiency virus (HIV) on lymphocyte proliferative responses to cytomegalovirus. Clin Exp Immunol 1988;72:179–85.

39. Alcocer-Varela J, Alarcon-Segovia D, Abud-Mendoza C. Immunoregulatory circuits in the acquired immune deficiency syndrome and related complex. Production of and response to interleukins 1 and 2, NK function and its enhancement by interleukin-2 and kinetics of the autologous mixed lymphocyte reaction. Clin Exp Immunol 1985;60:31–8.

40. Sheridan JF, Aurelian L, Donnenberg AD, et al. Cell-mediated immunity to cytomegalovirus (CMV) and herpes simplex virus (HSV) antigens in the acquired immune deficiency syndrome: interleukin-1 and interleukin-2 modify *in vitro* responses. J Clin Immunol 1984;4:304–11.

41. Sereti I, Lane HC. Immunopathogenesis of human immunodeficiency virus: implications for immune-based therapies. Clin Infect Dis 2001;32:1738–55.

42. INSIGHT-ESPRIT Study Group. Predictors of bacterial pneumonia in evaluation of subcutaneous interleukin-2 in a randomized international trial (ESPRIT). HIV Med 2010;12:219–27.

43. Murray HW, Gellene RA, Libby DM, et al. Activation of tissue macrophages from AIDS patients: in vitro response of AIDS alveolar macrophages to lymphokines and interferon-γ. J Immunol 1985;135:2374–7.

44. Murray HW, Scavuzzo DA, Kelly CD, et al. T4+ cell production of interferon gamma and the clinical spectrum of patients at risk for and with acquired immunodeficiency syndrome. Arch Intern Med 1988;148:1613–6.

45. Murray HW, Hillman JK, Rubin BY, et al. Patients at risk for AIDS-related opportunistic infections: clinical manifestations and impaired gamma interferon production. N Engl J Med 1985;313:1504–10.

46. Aabye MG, Ravn P, PrayGod G, et al. The impact of HIV infection and CD4 cell count on the performance of an interferon gamma release assay in patients with pulmonary tuberculosis. PLoS One 2009;4:e4220.

47. Clerici M, Shearer GM. A TH1→TH2 switch is a critical step in the etiology of HIV infection. Immunol Today 1993;14:107–11.

48. Clerici M, Lucey DR, Berzofsky JA, et al. Restoration of HIV-specific cell-mediated immune responses by interleukin-12 in vitro. Science 1993;262:1721–4.

49. Jambo KC, Sepako E, Fullerton DG, et al. Bronchoalveolar CD4+ T cell responses to respiratory antigens are impaired in HIV-infected adults. Thorax 2011;66:375–82.

50. Autran B, Sadat-Sowti B, Hadida F, et al. HIV-specific cytotoxic T lymphocytes against alveolar macrophages: specificities and downregulation. Res Virol 1991;142:113–8.

51. Autran B, Plata F, Guillon JM, et al. HIV-specific cytotoxic T lymphocytes directed against alveolar macrophages in HIV-infected patients. Res Virol 1990;141:131–6.

52. Twigg HL, Soliman DM, Day RB, et al. Lymphocytic alveolitis, bronchoalveolar lavage viral load, and outcome in human immunodeficiency virus infection. Am J Respir Crit Care Med 1999;159:1439–44.

53. Agostini C, Zambello R, Facco M, et al. CD8 T-cell infiltration in extravascular tissues of patients with human immunodeficiency virus infection: interleukin-15 upmodulates costimulatory pathways involved in the antigen-presenting cells-T-cell interaction. Blood 1999;93:1277–86.

54. Semenzato G. Immunology of interstitial lung diseases: cellular events taking place in the lung of sarcoidosis, hypersensitivity pneumonitis and HIV infection. Eur Respir J 1991;4:94–102.

55. Shearer GM, Bernstein DC, Tung KS, et al. A model for the selective loss of major histocompatibility complex self-restricted T cell immune response during the development of acquired immune deficiency syndrome (AIDS). J Immunol 1986;137:2514–21.

56. Fiala M, Herman V, Gornbein J. Role of CD8+ in late opportunistic infections of patients with AIDS. Res Immunol 1992;143:903–7.

57. Barry SM, Johnson MA, Janossy G. Increased proportions of activated and proliferating memory CD8+ T lymphocytes in both blood and lung are associated with blood HIV viral load. J Acquir Immune Defic Syndr 2003;34:351–7.

58. Levacher M, Hulstaert F, Tallet S, et al. The significance of activation markers on CD8 lymphocytes in human immunodeficiency syndrome: staging and prognostic value. Clin Exp Immunol 1992;90:376–82.

59. Lieberman J, Shankar P, Manjanath N, et al. Dressed to kill? A review of why antiviral CD8 T lymphocytes fail to prevent progressive immunodeficiency in HIV-1 infection. Blood 2001;98:1667–77.

60. Twigg HL 3rd, Spain BA, Soliman DM, et al. Production of interferon-gamma by lung lymphocytes in HIV-infected individuals. Am J Physiol 1999;276:L256–62.

61. McMichael AJ, Rowland-Jones SL. Cellular immune responses to HIV. Nature 2001;410:980–7.

62. Herberman RB. Adoptive therapy with purified CD8 cells in HIV infection. Semin Hematol 1992;29:35–40.

63. Ho M, Armstrong J, McMahon D, et al. A phase 1 study of adoptive transfer of autologous CD8+ T lymphocytes in patients with acquired immunodeficiency syndrome (AIDS)-related complex or AIDS. Blood 1993;81:2093–101.

64. Agostini C, Poletti V, Zambello R, et al. Phenotypical and functional analysis of bronchoalveolar lavage lymphocytes in patients with HIV infection. Am Rev Respir Dis 1988;138:1609–15.

65. Agostini C, Zambello R, Trentin L, et al. Cytotoxic events taking place in the lung of patients with HIV-1 infection: evidence of an intrinsic defect of the major histocompatibility complex-unrestricted killing partially restored by the incubation with rIL-2. Am Rev Respir Dis 1990;142:516–22.

66. Poli G, Introna M, Zanaboni F, et al. Natural killer cells in intravenous drug abusers with lymphadenopathy syndrome. Clin Exp Immunol 1985;62:128–35.

67. Rao PV, Ramanavelan S, Rajasekaran S, et al. Natural-killer cell-derived cytolytic molecules in HIV-associated pulmonary tuberculosis - role of exogenous interleukins. J Clin Immunol 2010;30:393–401.

68. Rankin JA, Walzer PD, Dwyer JM, et al. Immunologic alterations in bronchoalveolar lavage fluid in the acquired immunodeficiency syndrome (AIDS). Am Rev Respir Dis 1983;128:189–94.

69. Twigg HL 3rd, Spain BA, Soliman DM, et al. Impaired IgG production in the lungs of HIV-infected individuals. Cell Immunol 1996;170:127–33.

70. Breen EC, Rezai AR, Nakajima K, et al. Infection with HIV is associated with elevated IL-6 levels and production. J Immunol 1990;144:480–4.

71. Lane HC, Masur H, Edgar LC, et al. Abnormalities of B-cell activation and immunoregulation in patients with the acquired immunodeficiency syndrome. N Engl J Med 1983;309:453–8.

72. Eagan R, Twigg HL, French N, et al. Lung fluid immunoglobulin from HIV-infected subjects has impaired opsonic function against pneumococci. Clin Infect Dis 2007;44:1632–8.

73. Poli G, Bottazzi B, Acero R, et al. Monocyte function in intravenous drug abusers with lymphadenopathy syndrome and in patients with acquired immunodeficiency syndrome: selective impairment of chemotaxis. Clin Exp Immunol 1985;62:136–42.

74. Nielsen H, Kharazmi A, Faber V. Blood monocyte and neutrophil functions in the acquired immune deficiency syndrome. Scand J Immunol 1986;24:291–6.

75. Musher DM, Watson DA, Nickeson D, et al. The effect of HIV infection on phagocytosis and killing of Staphylococcus aureus by human pulmonary alveolar macrophages. Am J Med 1990;299:158–63.

76. Ezekowitz RA, Williams DJ, Koziel H, et al. Uptake of Pneumocystis carinii mediated by the macrophage mannose receptor. Nature 1991;351:155–8.

77. Koziel H, Eichbaum Q, Kruskal BA, et al. Reduced binding and phagocytosis of Pneumocystis carinii by alveolar macrophages from persons infected with HIV-1 correlates with mannose receptor downregulation. J Clin Invest 1998;102:1332–44.

78. Elssner A, Carter JE, Yunger TM, et al. HIV-1 infection does not impair human alveolar macrophage phagocytic function unless combined with cigarette smoking. Chest 2004;125:1071–6.

79. Murray HW, Rubin BY, Masur H, et al. Impaired production of lymphokines and immune (gamma)

interferon in the acquired immunodeficiency syndrome. N Engl J Med 1984;310:883–9.

80. Rich EA, Toossi Z, Fujiwara H, et al. Defective accessory function of monocytes in human immunodeficiency virus-related disease syndromes. J Lab Clin Med 1988;112:174–81.

81. Twigg HL 3rd, Lipscomb MF, Yoffe B, et al. Enhanced accessory cell function by alveolar macrophages from patients infected with the human immunodeficiency virus: potential role for depletion of CD4+ cells in the lung. Am J Respir Cell Mol Biol 1989;1:391–400.

82. Macatonia SE, Lau R, Patterson S, et al. Dendritic cell infection, depletion and dysfunction in HIV-infected individuals. Immunology 1990;71: 38–45.

83. Macatonia SE, Taylor PM, Knight SC, et al. Primary stimulation by dendritic cells induces antiviral proliferative and cytotoxic T cell responses in vitro. J Exp Med 1989;169:1255–64.

84. Lähdevirta J, Maury CP, Teppo AM, et al. Elevated levels of circulating cachectin/tumor necrosis factor in patients with acquired immunodeficiency syndrome. Am J Med 1988;85:289–91.

85. Wright SC, Jewett A, Mitsuyasu R, et al. Spontaneous cytotoxicity and tumor necrosis factor production by peripheral blood monocytes from AIDS patients. J Immunol 1988;141:99–104.

86. Ammann AJ, Palladino MA, Volberding P, et al. Tumor necrosis factor alpha and beta in acquired immunodeficiency syndrome (AIDS) and AIDS-related complex. J Clin Immunol 1987;7:481–5.

87. Molina JM, Scaden DT, Amirault C, et al. Human immunodeficiency virus does not induce interleukin-1, interleukin-6, or tumor necrosis factor in mononuclear cells. J Virol 1990;64:2901–6.

88. Israël-Biet D, Cadranel J, Beldjord K, et al. Tumor necrosis factor production in HIV-seropositive subjects: relationship with lung opportunistic infections and HIV expression in alveolar macrophages. J Immunol 1991;147:490–4.

89. Gordon MA, Gordon S, Musaya L, et al. Primary macrophages from HIV-infected adults show dysregulated cytokine responses to Salmonella, but normal internalization and killing. AIDS 2007;21: 2399–408.

90. Tachado SD, Zhang J, Zhu J, et al. HIV impairs TNF-alpha release in response to toll-like receptor 4 stimulation in human macrophages in vitro. Am J Respir Cell Mol Biol 2005;33:610–21.

91. Han H, Li X, Yue SC, et al. Epigenetic regulation of tumor necrosis factor α (TNFα) release in human macrophages by HIV-1 single-stranded RNA (ssRNA) is dependent on TLR8 signaling. J Biol Chem 2012;287:13778–86.

92. Tamburrini E, De Luca A, Ventura G, et al. Pneumocystis carinii stimulates in vitro production of tumor necrosis factor-alpha by human macrophages. Med Microbiol Immunol 1991;180:15–20.

93. Krishnan VL, Meager A, Mitchell DM, et al. Alveolar macrophages in AIDS patients: Increased spontaneous tumour necrosis factor-alpha production in Pneumocystis carinii pneumonia. Clin Exp Immunol 1990;80:156–60.

94. Rayment N, Miller RF, Ali N, et al. Synthesis of tumor necrosis factor-alpha mRNA in bronchoalveolar lavage cells from human immunodeficiency virus-infected persons with Pneumocystis carinii pneumonia. J Infect Dis 1996;174:654–9.

95. Huang ZB, Eden E. Effect of corticosteroids on IL1 beta and TNF alpha release by alveolar macrophages from patients with AIDS and Pneumocystis carinii pneumonia. Chest 1993;104:751–5.

96. Wallace JM, Barbers RG, Oishi JS, et al. Cellular and T-lymphocyte subpopulation profiles in bronchoalveolar lavage fluid from patients with acquired immunodeficiency syndrome and pneumonitis. Am Rev Respir Dis 1984;130:786–90.

97. Meddows-Taylor S, Pendle S, Tiemessen CT. Altered expression of CD88 and associated impairment of complement 5a-induced neutrophil responses in human immunodeficiency virus type 1-infected patients with and without pulmonary tuberculosis. J Infect Dis 2001;183:662–5.

98. Bandres JC, Trial J, Musher DM, et al. Increased phagocytosis and generation of reactive oxygen products by neutrophils and monocytes of men with stage 1 human immunodeficiency virus infections. J Infect Dis 1993;168:75–83.

99. Baldwin GC, Gasson JC, Quan SG, et al. Granulocyte-macrophage colony-stimulating factor enhances neutrophil function in acquired immunodeficiency syndrome patients. Proc Natl Acad Sci U S A 1988; 85:2763–6.

100. Roilides E, Walsh TJ, Pizzo PA, et al. Granulocyte colony-stimulating factor enhances the phagocytic and bactericidal activity of normal and defective human neutrophils. J Infect Dis 1991; 163:579–83.

101. Armbruster C, Krugluger W, Huber M, et al. Immunoglobulin G Fc(gamma) receptor expression on polymorphonuclear cells in bronchoalveolar lavage fluid of HIV-infected and HIV-seronegative patients with bacterial pneumonia. Clin Chem Lab Med 2004;42:192–7.

102. Limper AH, Offord KP, Smith TF, et al. Pneumocystis carinii pneumonia: differences in lung parasite number and inflammation in patients with and without AIDS. Am Rev Respir Dis 1989;140:1204–9.

103. Mason GR, Hashimoto CH, Dickman PS, et al. Prognostic implications of bronchoalveolar lavage neutrophilia in patients with Pneumocystis carinii pneumonia and AIDS. Am Rev Respir Dis 1989; 139:1336–42.

104. Azoulay E, Parrot A, Flahault A, et al. AIDS-related *Pneumocystis carinii* pneumonia in the era of adjunctive steroids: implication of BAL neutrophilia. Am J Respir Crit Care Med 1999;160: 493–9.

105. Laursen AL, Obel N, Rungby J, et al. Phagocytosis and stimulation of the respiratory burst in neutrophils by *Pneumocystis carinii*. J Infect Dis 1993; 168:1466–71.

106. Laursen AL, Obel NS, Holmskov U, et al. Activation of the respiratory burst by *Pneumocystis carinii*. Efficiency of different antibody isotypes, complement, lung surfactant protein D, and mannan-binding lectin. APMIS 2003;111:405–15.

107. Benfield TL, Vestbo J, Junge J, et al. Prognostic value of interleukin-8 in AIDS-associated *Pneumocystis carinii* pneumonia. Am J Respir Crit Care Med 1995;151:1058–62.

Impact of Antiretroviral Therapy on Lung Immunology and Inflammation

Homer L. Twigg III, MD[a],*, Kenneth S. Knox, MD[b]

KEYWORDS

- HIV • Antiretroviral therapy (ART) • Pulmonary immune reconstitution

KEY POINTS

- The lung alveolar compartment in human immunodeficiency virus (HIV) infection is characterized by the presence of HIV in alveolar fluid, accumulation of HIV-specific CD8 memory T cells, and a generalized increase in inflammatory cytokines and chemokines.
- Antiretroviral therapy (ART) decreases the lung HIV load, reduces the number of CD8 T cells in the alveolar space, and decreases alveolar cytokine and chemokine levels, thereby returning the alveolar milieu toward the normal homeostatic baseline.
- ART decreases the infectious complications of HIV but may play a role in newly recognized pulmonary complications including pulmonary hypertension, emphysema, and immune reconstitution inflammatory syndromes (IRIS).
- IRIS is a paradoxic deterioration in clinical status despite virologic and immunologic improvement during ART. IRIS most often is due to an appropriate immune response against residual pathogens because host immunity improves on ART.
- New asymptomatic pulmonary abnormalities are commonly noted on computed tomographic (CT) scans in the first 4 weeks of ART but most often resolve spontaneously on radiographic follow-up.

INTRODUCTION

In its 2010 report, the World Health Organization estimates that 34 million people worldwide are living with HIV.[1] Lung disease is a major source of morbidity and mortality in these patients and can be directly linked to progressive loss of pulmonary immunity. Typically, infectious complications occur in an orderly manner, with increased susceptibility to common pathogens occurring early in HIV infection and susceptibility to opportunistic pathogens appearing later after substantial losses of CD4+ T cells (**Fig. 1**). The immunologic correlate of this progression is the loss of antigen-specific immune responses early in HIV infection, followed by the loss of alloantigen and finally mitogen responses. However, the development of combination antiretroviral therapy (ART) has greatly influenced the morbidity and mortality of HIV infection. This influence has generally been attributed to improvements in immunologic function, either by preventing the progressive loss of immunity in HIV infection or by actually promoting immune reconstitution. The effects of ART are well described in the vascular compartment, whereas their effects at the tissue level, including the lung,

Supported by NHLBI RO1 HL083468 (PI: K.S.Knox); NHLBI RO1 HL59834 (PI: H.L.Twigg); NIAID UO1 AI-25859 (PI: Mitchell Goldman); NIAID Adult ACTG Protocol 723 (PI: H.L.T.).
Conflict of Interest: The author has nothing to disclose.
[a] Division of Pulmonary and Critical Care Medicine, Indiana University Medical Center, 541 Clinical Drive, CL 260A, Indianapolis, IN 46202, USA; [b] Section of Pulmonary, Allergy, Critical Care and Sleep Medicine, University of Arizona, 1501 N Campbell Avenue, Tucson, AZ 85724, USA
* Corresponding author. Indiana University Medical Center, 541 Clinical Drive, CL 260A, Indianapolis, IN 46202, USA.
E-mail address: htwig@iupui.edu

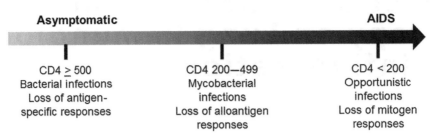

Fig. 1. Progression of cellular immunodeficiency in HIV infection. There is early loss of antigen-specific immune responses and increased susceptibility to bacterial infections. Over time, there is progressive CD4+ T-cell depletion, progressive loss of T-cell responsiveness, and ultimately an increased risk of opportunistic infections.

are just beginning to be understood. This review describes how ART has greatly improved the lung immunologic and inflammatory milieu in HIV-infected subjects. The consequences of this improvement will be discussed extensively in the rest of this issue of *Clinics in Chest Medicine*.

EFFECT OF HIV ON PULMONARY IMMUNE RESPONSES

The respiratory tract from the oropharynx to the alveoli serves as an interface between the host and the environment. Thus, pulmonary immune responses are thought to represent a form of mucosal immunity. Pulmonary immunity can be divided into innate and acquired responses. Most pathogens gaining access to the respiratory tract are phagocytized by alveolar macrophages (AMs), the principal arm of innate immunity. Importantly, phagocytosis of most foreign material gaining access to the alveolar space does not result in an inflammatory response because of the general immunosuppressive properties of AMs.[2] This absence of response results in a generalized paucity of lung inflammation under normal conditions, allowing gas exchange to occur unimpeded. Failure of innate host defenses leads to persistence of antigen in the respiratory tract and initiation of specific acquired immune responses. This process, which typically occurs in regional lung lymphoid tissue, results in the production of antigen-specific effector T and B cells that traffic back to the site of initial challenge, in this case the alveolar space, under the control of local chemokine production in the lung.[3] During the initial antigenic response, memory B and T cells are also created that allow the host to respond more rapidly on reexposure to the same antigen. Importantly, memory cells make up the predominant resident lymphocyte population in the normal lung.[4]

HIV infection affects all components of the pulmonary immune response and has been addressed in a prior article in this issue of *Clinics in Chest Medicine*. Specifically, the alveolar environment in HIV infection is characterized by

- Generalized AM activation.[5,6]
- Generalized CD4 T-cell and CD8 T-cell activation.[7,8]
- Preserved AM phagocytic function.[6,9,10]
- Increased concentrations of most macrophage and lymphocyte cytokines studied to date.[11]
- Mild decrease in absolute CD4 T-cell counts and a large decrease in CD4:CD8 T-cell ratio in the alveolar space.[12,13]
- Early preferential loss of antigen-specific memory CD4 T cells.[14–16]
- Increase in the number and percentage of CD8+ cells resulting in lymphocytic alveolitis.[17]
- High immunoglobulin concentrations[18,19] but poor opsonic activity.[20,21]

The end result of these changes is a generalized state of cellular activation and accumulation of immune cells and proinflammatory mediators in the alveolar space (**Fig. 2**A). Because HIV is easily detectable in the lungs of HIV-infected individuals not on ART,[22] it is reasonable to speculate that the virus itself can drive this response. In fact, very early studies recognized that HIV-infected individuals had an increase in numbers of lung CD8+ T cells consisting of HIV-specific cytotoxic T lymphocytes (CTL),[17] a finding confirmed by later investigators.[13] However, despite this apparent appropriate anti-HIV response and background "inflammatory" state, defects in specific immunity are clearly present as demonstrated by the increase in opportunistic infections. The challenge, and hope, of effective ART is to return the alveolar compartment to a more "normal" state.

EFFECTS OF ART ON PULMONARY IMMUNITY

There is extensive literature on the effects of ART in controlling plasma viral load and improving immune responsiveness of peripheral blood mononuclear cells (PBMCs), whereas there is a paucity of data describing the effect of ART in tissue compartments, especially the lung. Much

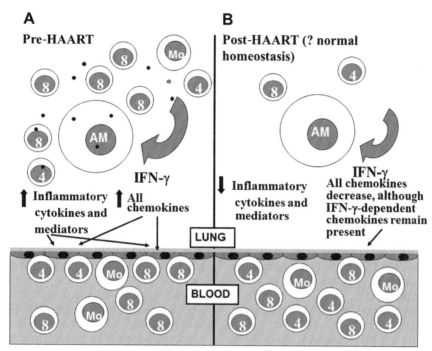

Fig. 2. Effect of ART on the alveolar environment in HIV infection. (*A*) In untreated patients, there is persistent HIV antigen in the lung leading to generalized cellular activation and augmented cytokine and chemokine secretion in response to pathogens and other particulate antigens. This response leads to further cellular activation and promotes influx of inflammatory cells to the alveolar space in a nonspecific manner, including B cells that are producing nonspecific antibody. (*B*) With ART, the pulmonary viral load decreases, reducing the antigenic load driving the nonspecific inflammatory pulmonary response. Less cellular activation is seen, and nonspecific cytokine secretion resolves. Low levels of IFN-γ and IFN-γ-inducible chemokine production continue, leading to the normal trafficking of memory cells into the alveolar space rather than a massive influx of nonspecific inflammatory cells.

of the existing data on lung immunologic changes after starting ART pertain to IRIS, which is a clinically recognized disease discussed later in this article. Less understood is the effect of ART on lung immune function and inflammation in individuals who are otherwise doing well after starting treatment. This type of analysis requires participation of HIV-infected individuals on ART in research protocols in which studies such as bronchoscopy and chest imaging are performed in the absence of clinical symptoms. The existing literature on these types of studies is described here.

Effects on Lung HIV Viral Load

If, as speculated above, the presence of HIV antigens in the lung drives the development of CD8+ lymphocytic alveolitis and induces generalized cellular activation in the pulmonary microenvironment, then control of the pulmonary viral load should return alveolar constituents toward a normal state. Thus, the first question to be addressed is whether ART can reduce the lung viral load. Cross-sectional studies had suggested that

individuals on ART had decreased detection of HIV in bronchoalveolar lavage (BAL) compared with lavages obtained from individuals not on treatment.[22] To address this question prospectively, a longitudinal study was conducted under the auspices of the Adult AIDS Clinical Trials Group in which blood and BAL were obtained from HIV-infected individuals starting ART and again after 4 and 24 weeks.[23]

At each time point, free virus (in plasma and acellular BAL fluid) as well as cellular HIV RNA and DNA (in PBMCs and alveolar cells) were measured. As expected, ART was associated with a significant decline in plasma viral load and a delayed but significant decrease in the cellular viral load in peripheral blood cells. However, the decline in the lung viral load, both in the acellular compartment as well as in alveolar cells, was much more rapid and dramatic. At baseline, the ability to detect HIV in the lung and vascular compartments was similar. After 4 weeks of ART, the ability to detect HIV in BAL was significantly lower than the ability to detect HIV in plasma. After 6 months of therapy, the ability to detect HIV RNA in lung cells was significantly less than the ability to detect HIV RNA in PBMCs. Thus, the lung seems to respond to ART as well as, if not better, than the vascular compartment.[23]

Effects on BAL Cell Counts and Activation

If HIV is the antigen driving the CD8+ cytotoxic T-cell response in untreated patients, then control of the antigenic load through ART therapy should theoretically decrease the lymphocytic alveolitis seen in these subjects. Indeed, ART was associated with a delayed but significant decrease in the absolute number and percentage of alveolar lymphocytes. This decline was due exclusively to decreased numbers of CD8+ lymphocytes in the alveolar space.[23] As a result of the decline in CD8+ cells, the CD4:CD8 ratio in the lung returned toward normal much more rapidly than in the vascular compartment.[23]

When analyzed in more detail, ART was associated with increases in CD8+ naïve and central memory T cells and decreases in CD8+ effector memory T cells in the lung, suggesting that the lung was repopulating its CD8+ lymphocyte pool from the peripheral circulation.[24] The number of CD4+ lung lymphocytes was not changed, suggesting that longer therapy courses may be necessary to cause changes in this population. Indeed, in another longitudinal cohort, it was shown that after 1 month of ART there was a slight but significant increase in lung CD4+ T cells and that this increase was significantly greater after 1 year of therapy.[25]

Furthermore, the increase in CD4+ T cells at 1 month after starting therapy was associated with expression of the proliferation marker Ki67, suggesting that the increase in the lung CD4+ T-cell population was in part occurring through local expansion.[25] Given our understanding of how antigen-specific T cells populate the lung under normal circumstances,[3] it is likely that both recruitment of new T cells and local expansion of resident T cells contribute to the increase in lung CD4+ lymphocytes after starting ART.

In addition to causing changes in lung lymphocyte subsets, ART also significantly affects the activation status of alveolar cells. ART has been shown to reduce the activation state of peripheral blood lymphocytes.[26] Similarly, ART was associated with a significant decline in lung T cell expression of the activation markers CD38 and HLA-DR, most notably in the CD8+ T cell population.[24] Interestingly, this decline was limited to subjects who had demonstrable control of the lung HIV viral load (Fig. 3A).[24] Other work has shown that lung lymphocytes from HIV-infected individuals display polyfunctional responses as determined by intracellular cytokine production when stimulated with mitogens or HIV peptides.[13] As part of a second longitudinal cohort study on lung immunity before and after starting ART, the authors analyzed lung T-cell responses to mitogenic stimulation with the superantigen staphylococcal enterotoxin B (SEB). ART was associated with a significant decline in CD4+ and CD8+ T-cell intracellular cytokine production (tumor necrosis factor-β,

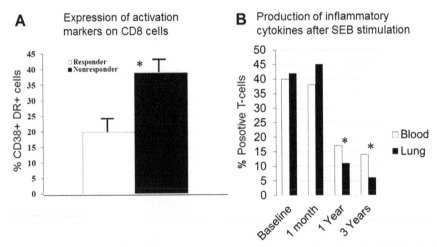

Fig. 3. ART decreases activation of alveolar CD8+ T cells. (A) Alveolar T cells were stained with the lymphocyte activation markers CD38 and HLA-DR. After 6 months of ART, the percentage of dual-positive cells were significantly lower in HIV-infected individuals with a good virologic response in the lung. (B) Alveolar T cells were stimulated with staphylococcal enterotoxin B. Levels of intracellular interferon, tumor necrosis factor-β, and interleukin-2 were measured. The percentage of CD8+ T cells expressing any of these cytokines decreased significantly with time on ART. The asterisk indicates "P<.05".

interferon [IFN]-γ, interleukin [IL]-2) in response to SEB, again most notably in the CD8+ T-cell population (see **Fig. 3**B).

Effects on Lung Cytokine and Chemokine Concentrations

It has long been appreciated that infection of macrophages with HIV leads to their activation and secretion of proinflammatory cytokines and chemokines.[11] If true, then treatment of HIV-infected subjects should result in a decline in lung inflammatory mediators. The authors have examined the change in BAL cytokine and chemokine levels in HIV-infected subjects starting ART. ART induces a significant decline in BAL concentrations of IFN-γ and IL-6.[27–29] Even more striking, ART induces a dramatic decline in BAL concentrations of proinflammatory chemokines, especially the IFN-γ-inducible ones,[27–29] which may have significant implications for recruitment of inflammatory cells to the lung. Despite these decreases, both IFN-γ and the IFN-γ-inducible chemokines (inducible protein [IP]-10, monokine induced by IFN-γ [MIG]) remained easily detectable in both HIV-infected subjects and normal volunteers. These chemokines contribute to the recruitment of memory cells to the lung.[30] Furthermore, there is a correlation between the number of lymphocytes

in the alveolar space and the concentration of IP-10 and MIG but not other chemokines such as IL-8 or RANTES (regulated and normal T cell expressed and secreted). This correlation was weak in untreated subjects but strengthened markedly with time with ART (**Fig. 4**).[27–29]

Model of Pulmonary Immune Reconstitution in HIV-Infected Individuals on ART

In summary, ART is associated with the following changes in the alveolar immunologic and inflammatory milieu:

- Significant decrease in the alveolar HIV load
- Significant decrease in alveolar CD8 T cells, returning the CD4:CD8 ratio toward normal.
- Mild increase in alveolar CD4 T cells resulting from recruitment of cells from the vascular space and in situ proliferation.
- Significant decrease in lymphocyte and macrophage activation.
- Significant decrease in inflammatory cytokines and chemokines but persistence of detectable IFN-γ and the IFN-γ-detectable chemokines.

Based on the above findings, we can propose the following model concerning HIV in the lung

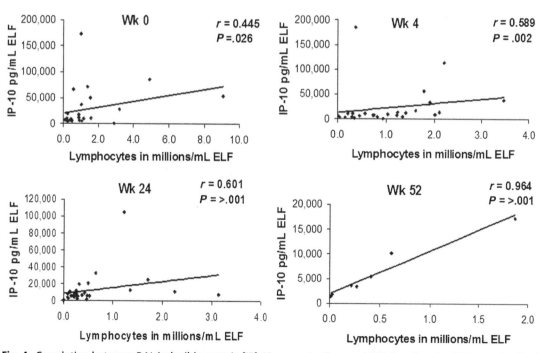

Fig. 4. Correlation between BAL inducible protein [IP]-10 concentrations and BAL lymphocytes. BAL was obtained from HIV-infected individuals before starting ART and again at 4 weeks, 6 months, and 1 year after starting therapy. The number of BAL lymphocytes was plotted against the BAL concentration of the T-cell chemokine IP-10. With time on ART, there is a progressive increase in the correlation between these 2 variables. ELF, Epithelial lining fluid.

and the effect of ART on these changes (see **Fig. 2**). In untreated patients (see **Fig. 2**A), there is persistent HIV antigen in the lung leading to generalized cellular activation and augmented cytokine and chemokine secretion in response to pathogens and other particulate antigens, including those that would not induce an inflammatory response under normal circumstances. This response not only leads to further cellular activation but also promotes influx of inflammatory cells to the alveolar space in a nonspecific manner, including B cells that are producing nonspecific antibody. HIV-specific CTL are also present in the alveolar space and are a rich source of IFN-γ, further leading to even higher concentrations. The large amount of nonspecific cytokine and chemokine secretion leads to a relatively poor correlation between lung lymphocyte numbers and chemokine concentrations. With ART (see **Fig. 2**B), the pulmonary viral load decreases, reducing the antigenic load driving the nonspecific inflammatory pulmonary response. Less cellular activation is seen, and nonspecific cytokine secretion resolves. Persistent low level IFN-γ production from resident memory cells that inhabit the lung remains,[4] which in turn maintains the BAL concentration of IFN-γ-inducible chemokines, leading to the normal trafficking of these cells into the alveolar space rather than a massive influx of nonspecific inflammatory cells. This change results in a much tighter relationship between chemokine concentrations in the lung and lung lymphocyte numbers. In summary, ART therapy is able to return the pulmonary environment toward normal, with normal cellular composition, reduced cellular activation, and normal inflammatory mediator concentrations.

CLINICAL IMPLICATIONS OF ART ON PULMONARY DISEASE IN HIV INFECTION

Although ART is clearly associated with a significant decrease in alveolar inflammation and return of the immunologic environment toward normal, it is not yet clear whether this translates into immunologic recovery. In this regard, there are 3 broad implications of the immunologic and inflammatory changes observed in HIV-infected subjects on ART that may affect patient care.

Change in the Spectrum of Lung Disease in the ART Era

One would posit that the immunologic changes described should result in an enhanced ability to respond appropriately to infectious challenges. In the lung, ART has been associated with decreased opportunistic infections,[31] decreased mycobacterial infections,[32] and decreased incidence of bacterial pneumonia.[33] This improved immunologic milieu has led to the development of guidelines on when primary and secondary prophylaxis against opportunistic pathogens can be discontinued.[34]

With the decrease in pulmonary infections in HIV-infected subjects on ART, other pulmonary complications have become more frequently recognized, leading to a dramatic change in the spectrum of pulmonary disease in HIV infection. These complications include pulmonary hypertension,[35] emphysema,[36,37] and a variety of malignancies.[38] HIV-related chronic obstructive pulmonary disease in particular is becoming more frequently recognized. A discussion of lung complications in the ART era is covered extensively in this issue of *Clinics in Chest Medicine*.

Immune Reconstitution Inflammatory Syndrome

IRIS is perhaps the most intriguing complication in patients on ART because it is likely being mediated by the very immunologic improvements we seek when treating patients. IRIS is best defined as "a paradoxic deterioration in clinical status attributable to the recovery of the immune status during ART."[39] At present, it is estimated that between 10% and 25% of patients who begin ART will experience IRIS of varying intensity and severity.[40]

IRIS can be categorized as either infectious or noninfectious. Infectious IRIS has been described for many different pathogens with a wide array of symptoms depending on the organ systems involved and pathogens identified.[38,41] This condition occurs when subclinical or a partially treated infection persists before initiation of ART and provides the antigenic substrate necessary for an immunopathologic inflammatory response. Infectious IRIS can occur very rapidly (ie, days after starting ART) and usually occurs within the first 3 months after initiating therapy.[42] Pulmonary IRIS is most often due to an ongoing or partially treated tuberculosis[43,44] or atypical mycobacterial (ie, *Mycobacterium avium*) infection. The inflammatory response to these mycobacterial antigens can present as infiltrate or mediastinal lymphadenopathy and is responsible for about one-third of IRIS cases reported.[45] In the lung, early infectious IRIS occurs at a time when antigen-specific memory cells arrive at the alveolar space. One can picture a scenario in which antigen-specific memory cells against mycobacteria are released from lymph nodes after initiating ART. These cells traffic back to the lung where they encounter pre-existing mycobacterial antigens, leading to the inflammatory response characteristic of IRIS.

Interestingly, when examining the cytokine milieu in subjects before and after starting ART, there is an initial slight increase in IFN-γ in BAL after 4 weeks of therapy before it starts to decline.[27] One could speculate that this increase represents antigen-specific memory cells encountering their targets as they traffic back to the lung.

Noninfectious IRIS is increasingly described and frequently occurs after 6 months of successful therapy. Late pulmonary IRIS may manifest as sarcoidosis (up to 3 years) after ART initiation.[46] In the few studies that examined cell phenotype during sarcoid IRIS, CD4+ alveolitis was seen, and in one study, a significant percentage of CD25+ cells were noted.[47,48] Both HIV and sarcoidosis exhibit a state of peripheral lymphopenia, setting the stage for memory cell expansion by homeostatic proliferation.[49] The role of the thymus and naïve cells in IRIS of any type is not defined.

The exact incidence of pulmonary IRIS is not known. To address this question, the authors recently completed a longitudinal study in which chest CT was performed before starting ART and at 4 weeks, 6 months, and 1 year after starting therapy. The incidence of asymptomatic radiographic abnormalities that could be consistent with IRIS (ie, new or increasing infiltrates and new or increasing adenopathy) 4 weeks after starting ART was 10%.[50] These changes were stable or had resolved by 6 to 12 months after starting therapy, always without intervention. Because the current clinical definition of IRIS requires "a paradoxic deterioration in clinical status," one could argue that none of these subjects had IRIS as it is currently defined. However, these studies suggest that there is frequently some level of subclinical lung IRIS that occurs in HIV-infected individuals who start ART and that in the absence of symptoms they can be safely observed without undergoing extensive evaluation.

Predictors of IRIS are for the most part limited to peripheral blood characteristics such as a low CD4+ cell nadir, CD4+ T cell increases after 1 month of therapy, decrease in HIV RNA levels, decreased CD8+ T cell numbers at baseline, and previous opportunistic infections.[43,51–53] A recent investigation found that IRIS was associated with higher frequencies of blood effector memory cells, higher levels of markers of blood CD4+ lymphocyte activation, and higher serum IFN-γ concentrations.[54] There are very few studies of tissue predictors of IRIS, including in the lung. Preliminary data suggest that the influx of CCR5 memory cells into the alveolar space may predict radiographic IRIS.[50] One of the most common settings of IRIS is seen in patients with tuberculosis, and studies have shown that the incidence of pulmonary IRIS is actually higher and more severe if ART is started around the same time as tuberculosis treatment rather than waiting to start HARRT till after the initial intensive phase of tuberculosis treatment.[55] Interestingly, the potential deleterious effect of early ART does not seem to be present in nontuberculous opportunistic infections.[56]

Timing of Antiretroviral Therapy

As discussed at the beginning of this article, antigen-specific responses are lost very early in HIV infection (see **Fig. 1**).[14–16] Furthermore, memory T cells are more susceptible to HIV infection than other T-cell subsets.[57] Thus, one could argue that the loss of antigen-specific memory T cells is the major contributor to many of the infectious diseases seen in HIV-infected individuals. This loss may be particularly important in *Mycobacterium tuberculosis* infection, in which there is clearly an increased incidence of disease relatively early in HIV infection despite the preserved ability of AMs to ingest and kill the organism.[6]

There is evidence that (1) CD4 lymphopenia is not the sole mechanism of immune dysfunction, (2) a low CD4+ T-cell nadir is a marker for suboptimal immunologic recovery after starting ART, and (3) increases in CD4+ T cells during ART do not predict successful restoration of immunologic responses to antigens.[58–60] When one considers that antigen-specific CD4+ T cells are lost early in HIV subjects, they can only be repleted after treatment if the few remaining cells undergo proliferative expansion or if new antigen-specific T cells are generated through stimulation of naïve T cells, an option that is less available as we grow older and the thymus undergoes involution. These speculations suggest that there is a CD4+ T cell-threshold below which immune reconstitution after starting ART becomes suboptimal.

In support of this hypothesis, we previously demonstrated that while antigen-specific responses were decreased in HIV-infected individuals, enrichment for CD4+ T cells was able to "restore" the proliferative response to recall antigens in some individuals.[61] However, in HIV-infected individuals with low CD4+ T-cell counts, proliferative responses to recall antigen remained poor even after CD4+ T cells were enriched to correct for low CD4+ counts. Furthermore, antigen-specific responses were gradually lost in vitro after repeated stimulation by the same antigen in the presence of HIV, whereas in the absence of HIV, the proliferative response just became more robust as a secondary immune response was generated. Taken together, these studies suggest that T-cell immune dysfunction cannot be solely ascribed to loss of CD4 T-cell number and implicate deletion of antigen-specific T cells as an important mechanism of loss of T-cell responses. Because lung CD4 T cells are mostly memory T cells, the timing of ART therapy may be especially important when considering optimal pulmonary immune reconstitution.

SUMMARY

HIV infection causes profound changes in the lung compartment characterized by macrophage and lymphocyte activation, secretion of proinflammatory cytokines and chemokines, and accumulation of CD8 T cells in the alveolar space, leading to lymphocytic alveolitis. These changes affect pulmonary immunity, leading to a progressive loss in the ability to respond to pathogenic organisms, starting with a decreased ability to respond to common bacteria and mycobacteria and progressing to susceptibility to opportunistic pathogens once profound immunologic defects occur. Most of the changes seen in the lung can be attributed to a direct effect of HIV on immune cells. As such, therapy to reduce the HIV burden should have significant beneficial effects. Indeed, ART rapidly reduces the viral burden in the lung, reduces the number of CD8+ T cells in the alveolar space, and reduces the amount of proinflammatory cytokines and chemokines in BAL, thus returning the alveolar microenvironment toward normal. While these effects clearly have had the expected clinical benefit of reducing susceptibility to pulmonary infections, new complications have been discovered. The IRIS in particular is likely a direct effect of improved immunologic responsiveness, occurring when a recovering pulmonary immune system encounters residual pathogenic antigens still present in the lung. Consideration must also be given to the timing of initiation of ART, striving to control the lung viral load and promote immunologic recovery before irreversible immune defects have occurred. Thus, although the clinical outlook for HIV-infected individuals has greatly improved in the ART era, one still has to be vigilant for potential pulmonary complications.

REFERENCES

1. UNAIDS/WHO. Global HIV/AIDS response: epidemic update and health sector progress towards universal access; Progress Report 2011.
2. Thepen T, Van Rooijen N, Kraal G. Alveolar macrophage elimination in vivo is associated with an increase in pulmonary immune response in mice. J Exp Med 1989;170(2):499–509.
3. D'Ambrosio D, Mariani M, Panina-Bordignon P, et al. Chemokines and their receptors guiding T lymphocyte recruitment in lung inflammation. Am J Respir Crit Care Med 2001;164(7):1266–75.
4. Saltini C, Kirby M, Trapnell BC, et al. Biased accumulation of T lymphocytes with "memory"-type CD45 leukocyte common antigen gene expression on the epithelial surface of the human lung. J Exp Med 1990;171(4):1123–40.
5. Buhl R, Jaffe HA, Holroyd KJ, et al. Activation of alveolar macrophages in asymptomatic HIV-infected individuals. J Immunol 1993;150(3):1019–28.
6. Day RB, Wang Y, Knox KS, et al. Alveolar macrophages from HIV-infected subjects are resistant to Mycobacterium tuberculosis in vitro. Am J Respir Cell Mol Biol 2004;30(3):403–10.
7. Barry SM, Johnson MA, Janossy G. Increased proportions of activated and proliferating memory CD8+ T lymphocytes in both blood and lung are associated with blood HIV viral load. J Acquir Immune Defic Syndr 2003;34(4):351–7.
8. Franchini M, Walker C, Henrard DR, et al. Accumulation of activated CD4+ lymphocytes in the lung of individuals infected with HIV accompanied by increased virus production in patients with secondary infections. Clin Exp Immunol 1995;102(2):231–7.
9. Cameron ML, Granger DL, Matthews TJ, et al. Human immunodeficiency virus (HIV)-infected human blood monocytes and peritoneal macrophages have reduced anticryptococcal activity whereas HIV-infected alveolar macrophages retain normal activity. J Infect Dis 1994;170(1):60–7.
10. Gordon SB, Molyneux ME, Boeree MJ, et al. Opsonic phagocytosis of Streptococcus pneumoniae by alveolar macrophages is not impaired in human immunodeficiency virus-infected Malawian adults. J Infect Dis 2001;184(10):1345–9.
11. Twigg HL 3rd. Bronchoalveolar lavage fluid in HIV-infected patients. "Cytokine soup". Chest 1993; 104(3):659–61.
12. Agostini C, Poletti V, Zambello R, et al. Phenotypical and functional analysis of bronchoalveolar lavage lymphocytes in patients with HIV infection. Am Rev Respir Dis 1988;138(6):1609–15.
13. Brenchley JM, Knox KS, Asher AI, et al. High frequencies of polyfunctional HIV-specific T cells are associated with preservation of mucosal CD4 T cells in bronchoalveolar lavage. Mucosal Immunol 2008;1(1):49–58.
14. Jambo KC, Sepako E, Fullerton DG, et al. Bronchoalveolar CD4+ T cell responses to respiratory antigens are impaired in HIV-infected adults. Thorax 2011;66(5):375–82.
15. Tardif MR, Tremblay MJ. LFA-1 is a key determinant for preferential infection of memory CD4+ T cells by human immunodeficiency virus type 1. J Virol 2005; 79(21):13714–24.

16. Kalsdorf B, Scriba TJ, Wood K, et al. HIV-1 infection impairs the bronchoalveolar T-cell response to mycobacteria. Am J Respir Crit Care Med 2009; 180(12):1262–70.

17. Plata F, Autran B, Martins LP, et al. AIDS virus-specific cytotoxic T lymphocytes in lung disorders. Nature 1987;328(6128):348–51.

18. Fahy RJ, Diaz PT, Hart J, et al. BAL and serum IgG levels in healthy asymptomatic HIV-infected patients. Chest 2001;119(1):196–203.

19. Gordon SB, Miller DE, Day RB, et al. Pulmonary immunoglobulin responses to Streptococcus pneumoniae are altered but not reduced in human immunodeficiency virus-infected Malawian adults. J Infect Dis 2003;188(5):666–70.

20. Eagan R, Twigg HL 3rd, French N, et al. Lung fluid immunoglobulin from HIV-infected subjects has impaired opsonic function against pneumococci. Clin Infect Dis 2007;44(12):1632–8.

21. Takahashi H, Oishi K, Yoshimine H, et al. Decreased serum opsonic activity against Streptococcus pneumoniae in human immunodeficiency virus-infected Ugandan adults. Clin Infect Dis 2003;37(11):1534–40.

22. Wood KL, Chaiyarit P, Day RB, et al. Measurements of HIV viral loads from different levels of the respiratory tract. Chest 2003;124(2):536–42.

23. Twigg HL III, Weiden M, Valentine F, et al. Effect of highly active antiretroviral therapy on viral burden in the lungs of HIV-infected subjects. J Infect Dis 2008;197:109–16.

24. Twigg HLI, Day RB, Schnizlein-Bick CT, et al. Effect of highly active antiretroviral therapy (HAART) on pulmonary lymphocyte phenotype. Am J Respir Crit Care Med 2006;173:A476.

25. Knox KS, Vinton C, Hage CA, et al. Reconstitution of CD4 T cells in bronchoalveolar lavage fluid after initiation of highly active antiretroviral therapy. J Virol 2010;84(18):9010–8.

26. Hazenberg MD, Stuart JW, Otto SA, et al. T-cell division in human immunodeficiency virus (HIV)-1 infection is mainly due to immune activation: a longitudinal analysis in patients before and during highly active antiretroviral therapy (HAART). Blood 2000; 95(1):249–55.

27. Twigg HLI, Day RB, Smith PA, et al. Highly active antiretroviral therapy (HAART) markedly decreases bronchoalveolar lavage (BAL) chemokine concentrations. Am J Respir Cell Mol Biol 2007;175:248A.

28. Morris A, Crothers K, Beck JM, et al. An official ATS workshop report: emerging issues and current controversies in HIV-associated pulmonary diseases. Proc Am Thorac Soc 2011;8(1):17–26.

29. Twigg HL 3rd, Knox KS. HIV-related lung disorders. Drug Discov Today Dis Mech 2007;4(2):95–101.

30. Charo IF, Ransohoff RM. The many roles of chemokines and chemokine receptors in inflammation. N Engl J Med 2006;354(6):610–21.

31. Torres RA, Barr M. Impact of combination therapy for HIV infection on inpatient census. N Engl J Med 1997;336(21):1531–2.

32. Kirk O, Gatell JM, Mocroft A, et al. Infections with Mycobacterium tuberculosis and Mycobacterium avium among HIV-infected patients after the introduction of highly active antiretroviral therapy. Euro-SIDA Study Group JD. Am J Respir Crit Care Med 2000;162(3 Pt 1):865–72.

33. Sullivan JH, Moore RD, Keruly JC, et al. Effect of antiretroviral therapy on the incidence of bacterial pneumonia in patients with advanced HIV infection. Am J Respir Crit Care Med 2000;162(1):64–7.

34. Kaplan JE, Masur H, Holmes KK. Guidelines for preventing opportunistic infections among HIV-infected persons–2002. Recommendations of the U.S. Public Health Service and the Infectious Diseases Society of America. MMWR Recomm Rep 2002;51(RR-8): 1–52.

35. Mehta NJ, Khan IA, Mehta RN, et al. HIV-related pulmonary hypertension: analytic review of 131 cases. Chest 2000;118(4):1133–41.

36. Diaz PT, King MA, Pacht ER, et al. Increased susceptibility to pulmonary emphysema among HIV-seropositive smokers. Ann Intern Med 2000; 132(5):369–72.

37. Crothers K, Griffith TA, McGinnis KA, et al. The impact of cigarette smoking on mortality, quality of life, and comorbid illness among HIV-positive veterans. J Gen Intern Med 2005;20(12):1142–5.

38. Grubb JR, Moorman AC, Baker RK, et al. The changing spectrum of pulmonary disease in patients with HIV infection on antiretroviral therapy. AIDS 2006;20(8):1095–107.

39. Shelburne SA 3rd, Hamill RJ, Rodriguez-Barradas MC, et al. Immune reconstitution inflammatory syndrome: emergence of a unique syndrome during highly active antiretroviral therapy. Medicine 2002;81(3):213–27.

40. French MA, Lenzo N, John M, et al. Immune restoration disease after the treatment of immunodeficient HIV-infected patients with highly active antiretroviral therapy. HIV Med 2000;1(2):107–15.

41. French MA, Price P, Stone SF. Immune restoration disease after antiretroviral therapy. AIDS 2004; 18(12):1615–27.

42. Narita M, Ashkin D, Hollender ES, et al. Paradoxical worsening of tuberculosis following antiretroviral therapy in patients with AIDS. Am J Respir Crit Care Med 1998;158(1):157–61.

43. Lawn SD, Myer L, Bekker LG, et al. Tuberculosis-associated immune reconstitution disease: incidence, risk factors and impact in an antiretroviral treatment service in South Africa. AIDS 2007;21(3): 335–41.

44. Murdoch DM, Venter WD, Van Rie A, et al. Immune reconstitution inflammatory syndrome (IRIS): review

of common infectious manifestations and treatment options. AIDS Res Ther 2007;4:9.

45. Cheng VC, Yuen KY, Chan WM, et al. Immunorestitution disease involving the innate and adaptive response. Clin Infect Dis 2000;30(6):882–92.

46. Morris DG, Jasmer RM, Huang L, et al. Sarcoidosis following HIV infection: evidence for CD4+ lymphocyte dependence. Chest 2003;124(3):929–35.

47. Foulon G, Wislez M, Naccache JM, et al. Sarcoidosis in HIV-infected patients in the era of highly active antiretroviral therapy. Clin Infect Dis 2004;38(3): 418–25.

48. Naccache JM, Antoine M, Wislez M, et al. Sarcoid-like pulmonary disorder in human immunodeficiency virus-infected patients receiving antiretroviral therapy. Am J Respir Crit Care Med 1999;159(6): 2009–13.

49. Theofilopoulos AN, Dummer W, Kono DH. T cell homeostasis and systemic autoimmunity. J Clin Invest 2001;108(3):335–40.

50. Hage CA, Teague S, Twigg HL, et al. Cytometric analysis of blood and lung CD4 lymphocyte subsets correlates with CT scan abnormalities after 1 month of highly active antiretroviral therapy. Am J Respir Crit Care Med 2011;183:4372A.

51. Breton G, Duval X, Estellat C, et al. Determinants of immune reconstitution inflammatory syndrome in HIV type 1-infected patients with tuberculosis after initiation of antiretroviral therapy. Clin Infect Dis 2004;39(11):1709–12.

52. Robertson J, Meier M, Wall J, et al. Immune reconstitution syndrome in HIV: validating a case definition and identifying clinical predictors in persons initiating antiretroviral therapy. Clin Infect Dis 2006; 42(11):1639–46.

53. Shelburne SA, Montes M, Hamill RJ. Immune reconstitution inflammatory syndrome: more answers, more questions. J Antimicrob Chemother 2006; 57(2):167–70.

54. Antonelli LR, Mahnke Y, Hodge JN, et al. Elevated frequencies of highly activated CD4+ T cells in HIV+ patients developing immune reconstitution inflammatory syndrome. Blood 2010;116(19):3818–27.

55. Naidoo K, Yende-Zuma N, Padayatchi N, et al. The immune reconstitution inflammatory syndrome after antiretroviral therapy initiation in patients with tuberculosis: findings from the SAPiT trial. Ann Intern Med 2012;157(5):313–24.

56. Grant PM, Komarow L, Andersen J, et al. Risk factor analyses for immune reconstitution inflammatory syndrome in a randomized study of early vs. deferred ART during an opportunistic infection. PLoS One 2010;5(7):e11416.

57. Hellerstein MK, Hoh RA, Hanley MB, et al. Subpopulations of long-lived and short-lived T cells in advanced HIV-1 infection. J Clin Invest 2003; 112(6):956–66.

58. D'Amico R, Yang Y, Mildvan D, et al. Lower CD4+ T lymphocyte nadirs may indicate limited immune reconstitution in HIV-1 infected individuals on potent antiretroviral therapy: analysis of immunophenotypic marker results of AACTG 5067. J Clin Immunol 2005; 25(2):106–15.

59. Elrefaei M, McElroy MD, Preas CP, et al. Central memory CD4+ T cell responses in chronic HIV infection are not restored by antiretroviral therapy. J Immunol 2004;173(3):2184–9.

60. Valdez H, Connick E, Smith KY, et al. Limited immune restoration after 3 years' suppression of HIV-1 replication in patients with moderately advanced disease. AIDS 2002;16(14):1859–66.

61. Knox KS, Day RB, Kohli LM, et al. Functional impairment of CD4 T cells despite normalization of T cell number in HIV. Cell Immunol 2006;242(1):46–51.

Epidemiology of Human Immunodeficiency Virus–Associated Pulmonary Disease

John F. Murray, MD, FRCP*

KEYWORDS

- Community-acquired pneumonia • Human immunodeficiency virus • *Pneumocystis* pneumonia
- Pulmonary disease • Tuberculosis

KEY POINTS

- The epidemiology of HIV-associated pulmonary disease has changed dramatically since the pandemic started in 1981, from a short-course uniformly lethal infection to a chronic disease.
- Since 1996, the availability of potent combination antiretroviral therapy has totally transformed life expectancy in HIV infected people who have access to and take their medications properly.
- In the early years of the HIV/AIDS pandemic, pneumocystis pneumonia was the most prevalent disease in high-income countries; now that has changed to community-acquired bacterial pneumonia.
- Since the beginning of the HIV/AIDS pandemic in low-income countries, tuberculosis has been and remains the most prevalent cause of morbidity and mortality.

INTRODUCTION

Epidemiology comprises the study of the distribution and determinants of health-related activities in well-characterized populations. Based on this generalization, the purpose of this review is to address the epidemiology of human immunodeficiency virus (HIV)–associated pulmonary disease. So far so good, but this simple working definition lacks precision; it keeps falling behind important epidemiologic events and constantly requires updating. The 2 principal categories of countries that separate the world need to be identified: first, those countries traditionally defined as high-income or industrialized, and second, those characterized as low-income or resource-limited. Basically, rich versus poor. Both high-income and low-income countries can be further differentiated according to the prevailing prevalences, which occur over time, of the various kinds of pulmonary diseases that are found in the 2 income-related settings, and when these evolving epidemiologic changes took place and are still taking place (**Table 1**). The emphasis today in high-income countries is on long-term maintenance therapy using powerful antiretroviral regimens to preserve immunologic competence and to prevent intercurrent complications. By contrast, low-income countries remain in desperate need of further use of cost-conserving antiretroviral agents and scaling up to life-saving regimens. Both of these ongoing but different advances affect our current understanding of the epidemiology of HIV-associated pulmonary disease.

EPIDEMIOLOGIC EVOLUTION OF HIV-ASSOCIATED PULMONARY DISEASE
Early Days

The epidemiologic silence that shattered the soon-to-be declared HIV/AIDS pandemic was announced on 5 June 1981 by a report in *Morbidity*

Pulmonary, San Francisco General Hospital, University of California San Francisco, Box 0841, San Francisco, CA 94134-0841, USA
* International Union Against Tuberculosis and Lung Disease, 68, Boulevard Saint Michel, Paris 75006, France.
E-mail address: johnfmurr4@aol.com

Clin Chest Med 34 (2013) 165–179
http://dx.doi.org/10.1016/j.ccm.2013.02.004
0272-5231/13/$ – see front matter © 2013 Elsevier Inc. All rights reserved.

Table 1
Epidemiologic trends in HIV infection and principal pathogens[a]

High-Income Countries	Low-Income Countries
1981 to 1995	1981 to 2000
Increasing PCP and KS	HIV-associated tuberculosis
Antimicrobial prophylaxis	Antimicrobial prophylaxis
Progressive immune deficiency	Progressive immune deficiency
Inexorable mortality	Inexorable mortality
Pneumocystis jirovecii[a]	*Mycobacterium tuberculosis*[a]
1996 to 2012	2001 to 2012
Universal HIV treatment	Cotrimoxazole prophylaxis
Universal ART	Increasing ART
Stepped-up HIV surveillance	Improved prognosis
Community-acquired pneumonia[a]	*M tuberculosis*[a]

[a] Indicates a principal pathogen.

and Mortality Weekly Report (MMWR) concerning a most unusual cluster of 5 previously healthy homosexual men in Los Angeles, CA, who were found to have biopsy-confirmed *Pneumocystis carinii* pneumonia (PCP) as well as both previous or current cytomegalovirus (CMV) and candidal mucosal infections.[1] Two of the patients had already died. These observations suggested the presence of some sort of cellular-immune dysfunction induced by opportunistic infections, such as *Pneumocystis* and *Candida*. One month later, a new MMWR report included the eye-catching citation of 26 cases of Kaposi sarcoma (KS), a rare malignancy, in young male homosexuals, 20 in New York and 6 in San Francisco; 7 KS patients also had PCP, CMV, and other opportunistic infectious complications.[2] Furthermore, in the July MMWR report, 10 additional cases of *Pneumocystis* pneumonia (without KS) were identified, making 22 in all. Something terrifying and never before characterized seemed to be rapidly unfolding.

By the end of 1981, the 2 initial MMWR reports of previously healthy patients with PCP and KS had multiplied into an extensive description of KS in the *Lancet*[3] plus 3 original articles[4–6] and an editorial[7] in the *New England Journal of Medicine*. During this time, more and more patients with opportunistic infections and coexisting cellular-immune deficiencies in different cities with varying manifestations kept coming to light as clusters of new cases were added, including women, Haitians, and hemophiliacs. The name acquired immunodeficiency syndrome (AIDS) was first defined in 1982 and was then widely used by the Centers for Disease Control (CDC) thereafter.

In 1983, a single strain of the supposed causative retrovirus was identified by a French research team led by Luc Montagnier[8]; more than 1 year later, Robert Gallo and colleagues[9] from the National Institutes of Health (NIH) found what was subsequently proved to be the same retrovirus as well as critical ways to enhance its growth. Antibodies for clinical testing of the AIDS virus quickly became commercially available. Both Montagnier and Gallo used different names for their identical viruses, which created considerable patriotic-based confusion. In 1986, a simple and straightforward new name was agreed and officially adopted: the human immunodeficiency virus (HIV). Additional cases of HIV/AIDS were rapidly identified; different kinds of opportunistic infections showed up among enlarging risk groups, and the mortality rate, which was already high, was steadily increasing. By the end of 1986, 38,401 cases of AIDS had been notified by the World Health Organization (WHO): 31,741 from the United States, 3858 from Europe, 2323 from Africa, 395 from Oceana, and 395 from Asia.[10] And this was just the beginning.

Prehistory

Long after it was presumed to have actually happened, the pandemic now known as HIV/AIDS is believed to have included a significant worldwide and largely unwritten prehistory that involved hundreds of thousands of undetected victims. As Jonathan Mann declared,[11] "[b]y 1980, HIV had spread to at least five continents (North America, South America, Europe, Africa, and Australia). During this period of silence, spread was unchecked by awareness or any preventive action and approximately 100,000–300,000 persons may have been infected."

High-Income Countries, 1981 to 1995

Cell-mediated immunologic dysfunction caused by HIV-mediated CD4-T-cell depletion underlay the ever-broadening constellation of clinical manifestations that characterized AIDS. At the outset, PCP and KS were the signature diseases that first attracted the attention of investigators, but many other pathologic conditions, alone or in partnership, were soon playing an increasing disease role. By 1984, as shown in **Table 2**, early collaborative studies under the auspices of the National Heart, Lung, and Blood Institute (NHLBI), which were carried out between November 1980 (actually a few months before the definitive MMRW reports in 1981) and July 1983, cataloged and analyzed the types and frequency of pulmonary diseases in 441 patients with AIDS.[12]

In 1987, a second NHLBI Workshop Summary updated and modified important recent information about the pulmonary complications of HIV infection that considerably enriched what had already been published.[13] Furthermore, significant progress between 1988 and 2005 saw the number of AIDS cases, according to major transmission categories, reach a peak in 1992 and start to decline, as shown in **Fig. 1**.[14] Brief highlights of the chief epidemiologic trends in HIV/AIDS during the first period of clinical and research accomplishments from 1980 to 1995 are itemized here. This period ends with increasing use of new and powerful combination antiretroviral agents that transformed the treatment and prognosis of HIV/AIDS.

- The first decade of the HIV/AIDS pandemic in high-income countries was dominated by increasing numbers of patients diagnosed with PCP. For those with typical diffuse bilateral radiographic infiltrations, fiber-optic bronchoscopy with only bronchoalveolar lavage (BAL) emerged as the procedure of choice, with 90% to 98% sensitivity.[15] Patients showing unilateral, coarse nodular, or other atypical abnormalities warranted transbronchial biopsies in addition to BAL. Chest radiographs were read as normal in 15% to 25% of patients diagnosed with PCP.
- The treatment of choice for PCP has long been trimethoprim-sulfamethoxazole (TMP-SMX or cotrimoxazole), except when contraindicated by known allergy; pentamidine, first intravenously then aerosolized, was the sole alternative agent for cotrimoxazole for allergy, toxicity, or clinical failure. Subsequently, other drugs such as clindamycin-pyrimethamine, trimethoprim-dapsone, and atovaquone were shown to be effective for either treatment or prophylaxis of PCP as assessed by the CDC-NIH-Infectious Diseases Society of America (IDSA).[16]

Table 2	
Types and frequency of pulmonary disorders in 441 patients with AIDS tabulated from November 1980 to July 1983	
Pulmonary Diseases	**No. of Patients**
Pneumocystis carinii pneumonia	373
Without coexisting infection	255
With coexisting infection	118
Cytomegalovirus	50
Mycobacterium avium-intracellulare	37
Mycobacterium tuberculosis	15
Legionella	9
Cryptococcus	8
Other	3
Other pulmonary infections	93
M avium-intracellulare	37
Cytomegalovirus	18
Cytomegalovirus/*M avium-intracellulare*	5
Cytomegalovirus/ Cryptococcus	1
Pyogenic bacteria	11
Legionella	10
Fungi	6
M tuberculosis	4
Herpes simplex	2
Toxoplasmosis	1
Kaposi sarcoma	36

From Murray JF, Felton CP, Garay SM, et al. Pulmonary complications of the acquired immunodeficiency syndrome. Report of a National Heart, Lung, and Blood Institute Workshop. N Engl J Med 1984;310:1682–8; with permission.

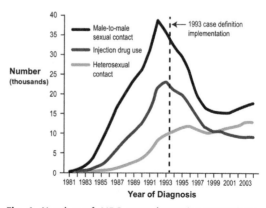

Fig. 1. Number of AIDS cases, by major transmission category and year of diagnosis in the United States from 1981 to 2004. The number of AIDS cases increased rapidly in the 1980s and peaked in 1992, before stabilizing in 1998. (*Modified from* Centers for Disease Control. Epidemiology of HIV/AIDS United States, 1981–2005. MMWR Morb Mortal Wkly Rep 2006;55(21):589–92.)

- By the time the Second NHLBI Workshop results were published in 1987, an additional 27 patients with AIDS from Florida were diagnosed with tuberculosis (TB), of whom 19 had extrapulmonary disease.[17] It soon became apparent that both the clinical and radiographic presentations of TB were profoundly affected by AIDS and those at risk of AIDS and the number of patients began to increase.
- In 1990, a consensus guideline was issued by an NIH-University of California Expert Panel for the use of corticosteroids as adjunctive therapy for PCP.[18] When indicated, corticosteroid therapy should be started within 24 to 72 hours of initial anti-PCP therapy for moderate or severe hypoxia defined as follows: an arterial P_{O_2} of less than 70 mm Hg or an alveolar-arterial P_{O_2} difference of greater than 35 mm Hg. The treatment regimen consists of oral prednisone, 40 mg twice daily, on days 1 to 5; then 40 mg daily on days 6 to 10; followed by 20 mg daily on days 11 to 21.

High-Income Countries, 1996–2012

The HIV/AIDS epidemic took off with vigor in 1981; thereafter, the census of patients with newly diagnosed HIV infections in high-income countries continued to increase up to about 1992 and then began to stabilize. Improved treatment and prophylactic regimens decreased the frequency of PCP and other opportunistic infections. The incidence of TB in the United States, which was partly AIDS-related, started increasing in the mid-1980s, peaked in 1992, and has fallen steadily since then. The increasing use of one-at-a-time first-generation antiretroviral agents, such as zidovudine and didanosine, showed promise of lengthening life expectancy after a diagnosis of AIDS, but overall mortality rates remained extremely high.

Beginning in 1996, a sudden and dramatic epidemiologic reversal took place in high-income countries, due to the recent availability of potent combinations of antiretroviral therapy (ART) agents: nonnucleoside reverse transcriptase inhibitors (NNRTIs) and protease inhibitors (PIs), which were combined with nucleoside reverse transcriptase inhibitors. Properly selected ART regimens caused a remarkable decrease in both opportunistic and pathologic infections, some AIDS-related malignancies, the need for hospitalization, and AIDS mortality.

- The clinical benefits of ARTs are regularly accompanied by suppression of viral replication and reconstitution of CD4-T-cell counts; on the other hand, noncompliance with treatment, intolerable side effects, drug resistance, delayed AIDS diagnosis, and high drug costs compromise therapeutic efficacy.
- The collaborative results of 14 cohort studies of 43,355 patients infected with HIV who received effective ART drugs between 1996 and 2005 showed steadily decreasing mortality rates and improvements in life expectancy.[19] However, considerable variability was observed among risk groups; the life expectancy of women was higher and that of injection drug users was lower.
- In 2011, according to reports from the CDC in 2008, "1.2 million persons were living with HIV in the US, of whom 80 percent had been diagnosed."[20] The overall use of ART combinations depended on the age of recipients: 76% for persons aged 18 to 24 years versus 92% in those aged 55 years and older. In addition, the efficacy of viral suppression was 69% in persons aged 18 to 25 years versus 85% in those older than 55 years.
- Following the shift from single-agent antiretroviral drug treatment to combination therapy, there has been an impressive realignment of the prevailing types of HIV-associated pulmonary diseases. Bacterial pneumonias, especially pneumococcal, are now the most common cause of pulmonary disease in persons infected with HIV,[15] as discussed in subsequent sections.

Low-Income Countries, 1980–2000

Four cases of AIDS-related TB were reported in the 1984 NHLBI Workshop Summary[12] and other notifications from the United States soon followed.[17] But it took another 2 years to get the first glimpse of what proved to be the start of the still ongoing and far from finished AIDS-associated pandemic of TB that was about to ravage sub-Saharan Africa. In 1986, investigators from Project SIDA (the French translation of AIDS), a collaborative international Zairian, Belgian, and US-CDC research group, reported from Kinshasa on the first large cohort of HTLV-III/LAV (later known as HIV)-associated TB in a letter to the Journal of the American Medical Association.[21] Positive sputum smears for acid-fast bacilli (AFB) were found in 159 patients, of whom 96 (60%) were men and 63 (40%) were women; among these, 53 (33%) were repeatedly tested and found to be seropositive for HIV. Most clinical findings did not differ between HIV-positive and HIV-negative tuberculars, but those who were seropositive also had significant weight loss.

The enormity of the human catastrophe of HIV/AIDS in sub-Saharan Africa was slow to be recognized and even slower to be addressed. A few outposts of first-rate clinical and research activities, with Project SIDA at the vanguard, were formed in high-prevalence countries such as Uganda, Tanzania, Malawi, and Côte d'Ivoire. Moreover, the outcomes were not always beneficial. For example, Zaire was devastated in the mid-1990s and late-1990s by successive wars in the newly named Democratic Republic of Congo; progress in South Africa, the hardest hit country in the region, was stymied by President Mbeki's refusal to accept the viral origin of HIV infection. The challenges were enormous, but the achievements were important. Here are a few of the highlights.

- Within only 2 or 3 years of the emerging AIDS epidemic, it had become apparent that among its infectious and noninfectious complications, the HIV-seropositive rates in those with TB were high and increasing, and extrapulmonary disease was unusually common. It seemed clear that the already meager resources available for case-finding and treatment of TB were being overwhelmed.[22–24]
- In 1993, one of the earliest and by far the most extensive study of HIV/AIDS mortality and autopsy findings at the time was conducted in Abidjan, Côte d'Ivoire.[25] The results revealed that patients infected with HIV, were typically hospitalized for the first time and for advanced disease, and that mortality was high and swift. The most common cause of death in patients with HIV infection at autopsy was TB at 32%, nearly 3 times higher than the next most common cause (septicemia, 11%) (**Fig. 2**). Seropositive tuberculars were typically undiagnosed before death, and found to have disseminated multibacillary disease that was strongly correlated with diarrhea and wasting.
- Most reports from low-income countries include data that incorporate HIV-infected versus HIV-uninfected groups of selected patients with, for example, prevalences of either TB or KS or the effects of ARTs over a period of years. Only a few studies have attempted to catalog the broad spectrum of different pulmonary complications identified in sub-Saharan African countries. Two such reports (**Table 3**) were published in the mid-1990s from Burundi and Tanzania, neighboring countries that used fairly similar investigative techniques.[26,27]

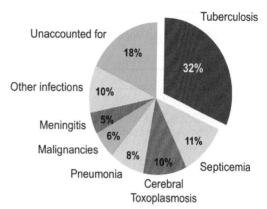

Fig. 2. Pie chart showing the prime causes of death among 230 HIV-positive patients who died of HIV-related disease confirmed by autopsy findings; study conducted in 1991 in Abidjan, Cote d'Ivoire. Nearly 3 times as many patients died of TB (32%) as septicemia (11%), the next most common cause. (*Data from* Lucas SB, Hounnos A, Peacock C, et al. The mortality and pathology of HIV infection in a West African City. AIDS 1993;7:1569–79.)

- TB is, by far, the most important cause of pulmonary and extrapulmonary disease in sub-Saharan Africa, followed by community-acquired pneumonia. As reported in 1993 and 1996, the prevailing HIV-infected seroprevalence rate was 4 to 6 times higher than in adults of similar age in the community.[26,27] (Currently, according to the WHO,[28] "[t]he risk of developing tuberculosis [TB] is estimated to be between 21–34 times greater in people living with HIV than among those without HIV infection.") The frequency of other HIV-associated infectious and noninfectious pulmonary disorders varies according to the geographic location and prevalence of indigenous disorders (eg, *Cryptococcus neoformans* and KS) and the availability of diagnostic resources (eg, blood cultures and bronchoscopy).
- In 1999, 2 breakthrough articles in the *Lancet* reported the beneficial results of separate randomized controlled trials in Abidjan, Côte d'Ivoire of cotrimoxazole (TMP-SMX) chemoprophylaxis for HIV-1 infection[29,30]; although not universal, benefits from other controlled studies supported the findings. (In 1986, studies in West Africa revealed a second HIV virus called HIV-2, which is far less common and less pathogenic than HIV-1; for the purposes of this discussion, only HIV-1, without the 1, is further considered.) In 2000, all low-income and middle-income infants exposed to PCP were advised to receive cotrimoxazole

Table 3
HIV/AIDS-related pulmonary complications in Burundi and Tanzania plus combined results

	Burundi, n (%)[a]	Tanzania, n (%)[b]	Combined, n (%)
Number of subjects	300 (100)	235 (100)	535 (100)
Prevalence of HIV	222 (74)	127 (54)	349 (65)
HIV-seropositive tuberculosis	109 (36)	95 (40)	204 (38)
HIV-seropositive community-acquired pneumonia	79 (26)	18 (8)	97 (18)
Pneumocystis pneumonia	11 (4)	1 (0.4)	12 (2)
Other	26 (9)	13 (6)	39 (7)

[a] *Data from* Kamanfu G, Mlika-Cabanne N, Girard PM, et al. Pulmonary complications of human immunodeficiency virus infection in Bujumbura, Burundi. Am Rev Respir Dis 1993;147:658–63.
[b] *Data from* Daley CL, Mugusi F, Chen LL, et al. Pulmonary complications of HIV infection in Dar es Salaam, Tanzania. Role of bronchoscopy and bronchoalveolar lavage. Am J Respir Crit Care Med 1996;154:1005–10.

prophylaxis until confirmatory HIV studies proved negative. Some doubters remained, but in 2005, a WHO Expert Consultation on Cotrimoxazole Prophylaxis in HIV Infection provided detailed guidelines that reinforced the standard of care. Compliance with this valuable recommendation, however, has remained a problem.[31]

Low-Income Countries, 2001–2012

Before 2000, access to HIV diagnosis and treatment was grossly inadequate, and world leaders began to address the colossal health inequalities between rich and poor countries. In this article, 2001 has been chosen as the watershed year for revamping international HIV/AIDS-related activities. The action started that year when the United Nations General Assembly Special Session of HIV/AIDS approved the Declaration of Commitment on HIV/AIDS. Special emphasis was targeted to ensure vastly improved access to ART agents, expanded use of antiretroviral agents to prevent mother-to-child transmission of HIV and, to mobilize available resources to prevent the development of HIV infection. Key events during the next 2 years included the inauguration of the Global Fund to Fight AIDS, Tuberculosis, and Malaria (2002), and 1 year later, the announcement of the United States President's Emergency Plan for AIDS Relief (PEPFAR); the largest single disease-related funding commitment in history. Both the Global Fund and PEPFAR have had their funding programs renewed for second 5-year cycles.

The political and financial commitments that were initiated in the early 2000s have created both a remarkable upsurge in the number of people receiving ART, and since 2005/2006, the number of people dying of AIDS-related causes has slowly begun to diminish.

- Patients with TB should know whether or not they have been tested for HIV and what the results are, particularly in high-prevalence countries. In 2010, 34% of the 2.1 million persons who had been tested were found to be HIV positive. Testing for HIV is especially important in the African region, home to 82% of the world's new cases of TB, and where 59% of cases with joint infections know their HIV status.[28]
- In 2010, according to WHO reports, there were an estimated 8.8 million incident cases of TB of which 1.1 million (13%) had both TB and HIV. Of the 1.1 million patients who died of TB, 350,000 (24%) were coinfected with HIV. Since 2004, the death rate from TB among people living with HIV infection has been gradually declining. Of the 1.8 million HIV-associated deaths, 350,000 (19%) were caused by TB, which remains the leading cause of AIDS-related mortality according to the CDC.[32]
- The benefits of isoniazid (INH) preventive therapy for tuberculosis infection for 6 to 12 months in non–HIV-infected persons have persisted for decades. But this has not proved to be the case in HIV-infected individuals with a positive tuberculin skin test. It seems that INH treatment in high-burden TB countries with high rates of HIV infection decreases the risk of developing active TB as long as chemoprophylaxis is provided. But after stopping INH in the face of ongoing exposure to *Mycobacterium tuberculosis* in HIV-coinfected persons, 36 months of prophylaxis may be insufficient, and even

longer courses of treatment may be needed.[33]

- The results of an international review of experts in 2011, which included a meta-analysis that specified 4 categories of CD4 counts at the start of ART (1, <200 cells/μL; 2, 200–350 cells/μL; 3, >350 cells/μL; and 4, any CD4 count) confirmed that the benefit of treating HIV-positive patients with ART combinations "is strongly associated with a reduction in the incidence of tuberculosis across all CD4 count strata."[34]

UNFINISHED BUSINESS

Early descriptions of the emerging and evolving HIV/AIDS pandemic were dominated by opportunistic pulmonary infections, particularly PCP. Chemoprophylaxis and aggressive antimicrobial treatment led to improvements in the outcomes of acute respiratory infections, but relentlessly worsening immunosuppression was an ever-threatening cause of morbidity and, ultimately, mortality, chiefly from respiratory diseases. But then a spectacular transformation occurred, starting in 1996, with the advent of powerful combinations of ART in high-income countries: HIV/AIDS switched within a few years from being mainly an acute routinely fatal disease to a chronic condition, with a projected life expectancy of 75 years, about the same longevity as in persons who smoke cigarettes.[35]

Prolonged survival requires first and foremost rigorous adherence to a widening range of potent antiretroviral agents and effective treatment regimens. That is the good news and formidable multidirectional progress to control the HIV pandemic is underway; witness the recent discoveries of effective oral and topical chemoprophylaxis.[36,37] But overdue advancements in new knowledge and upgrading clinical practices in both high-income and low-income countries for people living with HIV infection are urgently needed to solve existing problems concerning pathogenic and opportunistic pulmonary infectious diseases, and similar concerns pertain to the changing epidemiology of noninfectious pulmonary disorders.

Community-Acquired Bacterial Pneumonia

The inauguration and subsequent refinements of ART regimens have dramatically reshaped the pulmonary infectious disease landscape. Today, community-acquired bacterial pneumonia, particularly from *Streptococcus pneumoniae*, heads the list, but *Haemophilus influenzae* and *Staphylococcus aureus* are the second and third most common causative agents. Compared with the incidence before the availability of antiretroviral agents, *Pseudomonas aeruginosa* seems to have declined proportionately more than the other 3 leading bacterial species.

The incidence of invasive *S pneumoniae* infections in people with AIDS decreased by half, from 1094 cases/100,000 persons from July 1995 to June 1996 to 467 cases/100,000 persons from July 1999 to June 2000 due to the use of new ART combinations[38]; in 1999 to 2000, despite the impressive improvement in mortality, patients with AIDS remained at substantial increased risk of invasive pneumococcal disease. As increasingly powerful ART agents and regimens continue to improve, the risk of intercurrent pneumonias should diminish as protective CD4 counts increase.

Traditional risk factors for bacterial pneumonia such as older age, cigarette smoking, and use of intravenous drugs all amplify the clinical manifestations of HIV/AIDS. The incidence of bacterial pneumonia progressively increases during the course of untreated HIV infection as CD4 cell counts steadily decrease[39]; in addition, since 1992, the CDC has classified recurrent bacterial pneumonia as an AIDS-defining disorder.[40] Late diagnosis of advanced immunosuppression, the presence of respiratory failure, irregular administration or refusal to take ART, and adverse side effects of therapy all contribute to an unfavorable prognosis; early recognition and prompt ART are nearly always successful.

Legionella species, *Klebsiella pneumoniae*, *Mycoplasma pneumoniae*, and *Chlamydophila pneumoniae* seem to be infrequent and not well-characterized as HIV-related pulmonary infections. *Rhodococcus equi* and *Nocardia* species, which were occasionally encountered in extreme AIDS-related immunologic dysfunction, have mostly disappeared as a result of ART combinations.

The presiding jury at the time never returned a conclusive verdict regarding the value of pneumococcal vaccination for HIV-positive adults. Overall, several different pneumococcal vaccines seemed to provide favorable, but not necessarily definitive, results.[41] To further boost efficacy, the usual increases observed in CD4 cell counts resulting from ART should benefit future pneumococcal vaccination regimens.

Nosocomial Bacterial Pneumonia

Like virtually all HIV-related pulmonary diseases, hospital-acquired nosocomial bacterial pneumonias have decreased substantially since the advent of ART. According to Tumbarello and colleagues,[42] from 1994 to 1996, the incidence of nosocomial bacterial pneumonias caused by HIV infection more than halved from 13.9 per 10,000 patient-days to 5.9 per 10,000 patient-days after September 1996 after the introduction of ART in Italy. Nevertheless, these pulmonary infections remain an important cause of morbidity and mortality. A later study, also from Italy, revealed a noteworthy prevalence of *P aeruginosa* (33%), *S aureus* (25%), and *S pneumoniae* (21%); however, the sole predictor of increased mortality was methicillin-resistant staphylococci.[43]

Viral Infections

Several viral pulmonary infections (herpes simplex virus 1 and 2, human CMV, Epstein-Barr virus, and varicella zoster virus) may be either newly triggered or exacerbated from a latent state by severe immunosuppression, including by HIV infection. In theory at least, immune reconstitution by potent ART should prevent or attenuate such previously recognized viral breakthroughs.

Coinfections with PCP and CMV during the era before antiretroviral agents were common, and it was soon learned that anti-*Pneumocystis* treatment alone led to clinical improvement; CMV became regarded more as a passenger than a pathogen. Marked AIDS-related immunosuppression was indeed a recognized cause of severe CMV disease, but far more frequently of systemic than of pulmonary origin.[44] Effective ART should minimize or even eradicate such occurrences.

According to the CDC, "([p])eople with HIV/AIDS are considered at increased risk from serious influenza-related complications."[45] Most people with HIV infections should receive inactivated influenza vaccine during the flu season; other high-risk individuals with severe HIV-induced immune depression may need antiinfluenza medications to prevent flu during the entire season if they are likely to be exposed to infectious contacts. Health care workers who are involved in direct care of patients infected with HIV should be vaccinated or receive the nasal-spray flu vaccine.

Pneumocystis Pneumonia

Pneumocystis jirovecii is a ubiquitous, resilient microorganism, which keeps finding ways to cause disease. By the age of 2 to 4 years, more than 80% of children in the United States and many other countries have developed species-specific antibodies.[16] Originally, PCP was believed to be caused chiefly by reactivation of latent *Pneumocystis* organisms due to severe AIDS-related immunosuppression, but acquisition of recent transmission and spread by airborne infection

provide additional routes for new disease. In the early days, 70% to 80% of patients with AIDS developed PCP, of whom 20% to 40% died. Chemoprophylaxis and ART have markedly reduced the incidence of PCP in the United States and western Europe to about 2 to 3 cases per 100 person-years.[16] Currently, most patients with PCP in rich countries are either unaware of their HIV status or have advanced immunosuppression; in either case, such patients are likely to have CD4 counts less than 100 cells/μL when the diagnosis is made and the prognosis is guarded.

Chest radiographs often show typical bilateral infiltrations radiating from both hilae, but many different radiographic findings may occur; no pattern is pathognomonic for PCP, so specific microscopic diagnosis is mandatory. Diagnosis may be complicated by a 13% to 18% incidence of coexisting pulmonary infection or other competing condition. The diagnosis of PCP is usually made fairly easily by fiber-optic bronchoscopy with BAL; several tinctorial stains and immunofluorescence generally have high yields in experienced laboratories. Extrapulmonary *P jirovecii* may involve any organ, but is uncommon.

Within the foreseeable future, most of the rich countries of the world should be liberated from using cotrimoxazole, except, of course, for occasional diehards, such as people who refuse to make an early diagnosis of HIV infection or who are ignorant of their CD4 counts. As long as ART alone keeps CD4 counts consistently above the threshold of 200 cells/μL, cotrimoxazole is unnecessary. On those occasions when chemoprophylaxis might be warranted, CD4 counts should be monitored as long as needed, but when counts are greater then 200 cells/μL for more than 3 to 6 months, prophylaxis can be discontinued.

GAINING GROUND ON TB

Experts from the United States during the first few years of the HIV/AIDS pandemic took note of the 1986 brief communication from Kinshasa, Zaire (now the Democratic Republic of Congo), which reported a 33% HIV seroprevalence rate among 159 patients with TB, all of whom had positive smears for AFB. Reports from other major cities confirmed that TB was "clearly the sovereign HIV-associated lung disease throughout sub-Saharan Africa,"[26] with an already alarming and steadily increasing number of cases. From 1985 to 1999, for example, data from Tanzania (**Fig. 3**) reveal a progressive increase in smear-positive, smear-negative, and extrapulmonary forms of TB, most of which were related to increasing rates of coexisting HIV and TB.[46] In many sub-Saharan

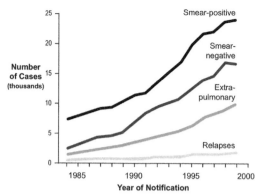

Fig. 3. Notifications of tuberculosis by type of disease (smear-positive, smear-negative, extrapulmonary, and relapses) in Tanzania from 1984 to 1999. (*Data from* Tanzania NTLP/IUATLD. Progress report 1996, No.36. Tanzania NTLP/KNCV. Report 2000, No. 7; and *Courtesy of* Dr Hans Rieder, with permission.)

African countries, the TB-HIV partnership increased from 60% to 80%.

Trends in the Epidemiology of Tuberculosis

In the mid-1980s to early 1990s, the United States had its own recrudescence of TB, which was in part related to HIV, but which was also exacerbated by an influx of high-risk immigrants, closure of mental health institutions, and reductions in federal funding of TB services. Reason and funds were restored in 1993, resulting in a fairly orderly subsequent decline to 10,521 new TB cases in 2011, an incidence of 3.4 cases/100,000 population, the lowest rate ever recorded since national reporting began 58 years ago.[47] Moreover, of the 10,521 cases of TB throughout the United States, only 831 (9.7%) had both TB and HIV infection. The fact that 81% of all persons with TB were tested for HIV in 2011 is an important advance; the previous figure was 66.3% in 2010. The goal, however, should be even higher; the American Thoracic Society (ATS) and the IDSA recommend that 100%, of patients with TB should be tested for HIV.

Early in the unfolding HIV/AIDS pandemic, 2 strikingly different clinical, radiographic, and laboratory disease patterns of HIV-associated TB were described: one was characterized as chronic and the other as aggressive. The chronic presentation encompasses an indolent clinical course similar to patients with ordinary HIV-seronegative TB, which includes predominant upper lung zone infiltrations, frequently with cavitation, positive AFB smears, a low prevalence of extrapulmonary disease, plus several hundred CD4 T cells/μL; by contrast, the aggressive group of HIV-infected

tuberculars have an acute or subacute progression of disease, often with lower lung zone miliary infiltrations, multiple sites of extrapulmonary involvement, negative AFB smears, and low values (<200 cell/μL) of CD4 T cells. In 2010, Chamie and colleagues[48] greatly extended these findings in Ugandan patients with pulmonary TB according to their HIV status and across 11 CD4 cell count strata, and reported trends in both radiographic findings and AFB smears; the continuous trends in variations in chest radiographic findings and in acid-fast counts correlated significantly with decreases in CD4 cell counts.

One measure of the transmissibility of TB is the duration of infectivity of M tuberculosis, usually taken as the presence of AFB in direct sputum smears. Some HIV-infected persons progress much more rapidly than their non–HIV-infected counterparts, many of whom have extensive extrapulmonary TB, which may be widely disseminated but negative on an AFB smear. The duration of clinically active TB from beginning to end in patients infected with HIV was only 18 weeks compared with 83 weeks for patients without HIV infection in Harare, Zimbabwe.[49] These findings raise the possibility that the chief transmitter of M tuberculosis is close contacts with chronic HIV-negative, smear-positive TB, but the experience of Chamie and colleagues[48] suggests that transmission of M tuberculosis takes place at all clinical strata of HIV infections, both positive and negative, and with declining frequency as CD4 counts decrease.

When to Start ART for HIV-associated TB

Studies soon made it clear that starting ART usually improved the clinical outcome in persons with TB, but it took time to optimize the routine. Favoring early administration of ART was the obvious and critical need to prevent premature deaths from TB and other complications in profoundly immunosuppressed patients. Favoring a later start of ART avoided some of the adverse consequences of the immune reconstitution inflammatory syndrome (IRIS); it also reduced drug toxicity and it spared users the complexities of a high pill burden.

In October 2011, clinicians profited from 3 valuable research studies published in the *New England Journal of Medicine* dealing with the optimal time to start ART in HIV-associated TB, plus a companion editorial that summarized the results.[50–53] With one important exception, the evidence supports starting ART in nearly all patients with HIV-associated TB at around 8 weeks (ie, toward the end of the 2-month intensive phase of anti-TB treatment or beginning of the continuation phase). The exception is patients infected with HIV with advanced immunosuppression (CD4 T-cell counts <50 cells/μL), who require early initiation (no later than 2 weeks of ART); this deliberate switch in timing creates a trade-off between reducing early deaths from severe coexisting TB disease and the competing adverse clinical effects of early-onset IRIS, which can be severe but is usually manageable. Another caveat arose in the knowledge that early ART had unfavorable consequences and may prove fatal in patients with tuberculous meningitis, so an approximately 8-week delay in starting ART seems indicated in that setting.[54]

The most recent (2012) HIV/TB WHO guidelines differ in one important consideration from those summarized earlier[50–53]: recommendation C.5 in the WHO document states that ART should start "within 8 weeks," which means treatment is limited to only the intensive phase of TB treatment, rather than a somewhat longer delay of around 8 weeks.[55] Both the WHO and New England Journal of Medicine recommend ART "immediately within the first 2 weeks of initiating TB treatment" for patients with profound immunosuppression (ie, CD4 T-cell counts <50 cells/μL).

Immune Reconstitution Inflammatory Syndrome

Most, but by no means all, cases of IRIS are caused by HIV-associated TB in low-income countries. Three clinical scenarios may accompany the onset of IRIS. Basically any HIV-related pathogen in the face of (usually) severe immunosuppression can trigger IRIS when "pathogen-specific immune responses recover" during ART[56]; typically, the time course incorporates clinical features of both resolving TB and new-onset IRIS. Second, subclinical HIV-associated opportunistic infections may be invigorated by the clinical manifestations of immune recovery that follow ART; and third, another variation on the IRIS theme causes a second wave of inflammation that comes on a few months after the initial pathogenic response subsides, sometimes called a paradoxic relapse, which may be clinically more severe than the initial reaction.

Reports of TB-activated IRIS in low-income countries show an incidence of 8% to 43%; in addition, according to French,[56] IRIS-linked M tuberculosis causes substantial morbidity and C neoformans substantial mortality in resource-poor countries, exacerbating an already excessive clinical burden. As discussed, it looks as though most cases of IRIS can be successfully treated

by waiting 8 weeks, plus or minus a week or two, to start ART; by comparison, in patients with advanced immunosuppression signaled by extremely reduced CD4 T-cell counts (<50 cells/μL), starting ART within 2 weeks seems to be indicated. However, the SAPiT Trial, which also sought to establish the best time to initiate ART in patients with TB, as discussed in the previously referenced series of articles, early (within 4 weeks of TB treatment) led to high rates of IRIS, longer time to resolution, and particularly severe disease, especially in patients with counts less than 50 cells/μL[57]; further experience and studies are needed to determine the outcome of the trade-off between reducing early deaths from near lethal TB versus serious IRIS. Most patients respond to nonsteroidal antiinflammatory agents (NSAIDS), although corticosteroids may be required to control life-threatening IRIS.

Multidrug-Resistant and Extensively Drug-Resistant TB with HIV Infection

Short-course anti-TB chemotherapy with INH, rifampin (rifampicin or RIF), pyrazinamide, and ethambutol, with authorized variations in alternative agents and in dosing schedules, strengthened the potency and shortened the duration of standard treatment. In theory, at least, these regimens should streamline anti-TB therapy by making it more efficacious than previous regimens. Unfortunately, just the opposite outcome has come to light, and both multidrug-resistant (MDR) and extensively drug-resistant (XDR) TB pose significant clinical burdens that require second-line treatment regimens, which necessitate longer courses of treatment, use of drugs with considerable toxicity, and greatly amplified costs and mortality rates. MDR TB means that patients no longer respond to at least 2 of the most effective anti-TB drugs in current use: INH and RIF. A relatively new designation (since 2006) includes patients with XDR TB who not only fail to respond to INH and RIF, but who also do not respond to 2 or more second-line agents, including any fluoroquinolone, and at least 1 of 3 injectable drugs: capreomycin, kanamycin, and amikacin.

In 2010, estimates by the WHO suggested that there were about 650,000 cases of MDR TB; of these, 9%, or around 60,000 cases were XDR TB. But these estimates must be fairly rough, because the WHO admits that "[l]ess than 5 percent of new and previously treated TB patients were tested for MDR TB in most countries in 2010."[58] Epidemiologists have known since the breakup of the former Soviet Union that the prevalence of MDR TB in many affected countries was in the 20% to 30% range, but detailed information is lacking from large regions of eastern Europe and central Asia. The problem is compounded by the virtual absence of drug susceptibility data from all but the southern part of sub-Saharan Africa. The accessibility of molecular technologies, such as GeneXpert MTB/RIF, which can detect RIF resistance in less than 2 hours, should substantially advance the surveillance of drug-resistant TB in countries that are able to utilize new diagnostic resources. Combining knowledge about HIV serologic status and TB drug susceptibility studies is a must.

Recently, a national survey of MDR TB was carried out in China among 3037 patients with newly diagnosed TB and 892 with previously treated TB; of these, 5.7% and 25.6%, respectively, had MDR TB[59]; moreover, among all patients with MDR TB, approximately 8% had XDR TB. Primary transmission of *M tuberculosis* is responsible for most cases of MDR disease; unfortunately, the prevalence of HIV infection was not studied.

Several studies in the last few years, the original of which created the term extensively drug-resistant TB, documented increasing numbers of cases of MDR and XDR TB from South Africa and neighboring countries with increased prevalences of HIV infection and with exceptionally high mortality rates. The first report came to light in a rural area of South Africa in which 221 patients with MDR TB were detected, of whom 53 had XDR TB, all of whom were HIV seropositive. Of particular note, 52 of 53 patients (98%) with XDR TB died after a median survival time of 16 days from the date of diagnosis.[60] Recent reports confirm the high rates of death from both HIV-associated MDR TB (n = 123, mortality 63%) and, especially, XDR TB (n = 139, mortality 80%) in southern Africa[61]; new models of treatment of HIV-positive MDR TB show promise, but more time and operational details are required.[62] Information about these important countrywide events is difficult to generalize, however, and additional data are urgently needed.

NONINFECTIOUS HIV-ASSOCIATED PULMONARY COMPLICATIONS

KS and non-Hodgkin lymphoma (NHL), both of which may involve the lungs and respiratory organs, and cervical cancer are AIDS-defining malignancies; in addition, lymphocytic interstitial pneumonitis is also an AIDS-defining condition in children aged 13 years and younger. Furthermore, it now seems clear that a few other lung diseases show meaningful statistical relationships with HIV

infection. This discussion briefly reviews the epidemiologic features of AIDS-defining KS and NHL, as well as the clinically apparent HIV connections with cancer of the lung, chronic obstructive pulmonary disease (COPD), and pulmonary hypertension. The individual members of this group of players are all influenced in one way or another by the effects of ART, so are predominantly in the high-income category of lung diseases.

KS

KS has been the most common AIDS-associated malignancy since the early 1980s, but its prevalence has decreased largely as a result of the use of ART in high-income countries. Human herpes virus 8, also known as KS-associated herpes virus, has a key role in pathogenesis, and men who have sex with men have a significantly higher incidence of KS than other risk groups. About one-third of patients with KS have clinical pulmonary manifestations and an even higher percentage, roughly one-half, have lung involvement on pathologic examination.

In 2008, the findings from 114 patients with KS showed that both chemotherapy and ART led to improvement, but only ART produced tumor resolution[63]; residual KS caused clinical problems and only half the treated patients achieved complete resolution of their disease. In an analysis of 305 patients with KS treated with ART, 25 with pulmonary KS and 280 without pulmonary involvement, those with pulmonary KS had lower CD4 cell counts at the time of diagnosis than those of African descent[64]; 5-year survival was 49% in patients with pulmonary KS compared with 82% in those without pulmonary features, highlighting the poorer prognosis of the presence of lung disease.

NHL

After KS, NHL is the second most common AIDS-defining malignancy; NHL has varying kinds of clinical pulmonary complications in up to 30% of patients, and an even higher percentage of pulmonary disease is found at autopsy. In the early days of using ART, there was some uncertainty about the timing of chemotherapy and when to start ART, but standard treatment now regularly includes combined chemotherapy and ART, which has greatly improved survival. Compared with pre-ART outcomes, survival of patients with NHL has substantially increased from 8.3 to 43.2 months,[65] with a goal of combined treatment of complete remission rather than merely palliation.[66]

Cancer of the Lung

Among patients infected with HIV, lung cancer has become the most common cause of non–AIDS-defining malignancies. The results of several epidemiologic studies have now conclusively shown that HIV-associated lung cancer is becoming an increasing clinical problem, possibly because patients with HIV/AIDS are living longer than before, thanks to ART. Patients with HIV infection and lung cancer tend to be young (average age around 50 years) and nearly all are smokers, but otherwise tend to have similar clinical findings patients with lung cancer without HIV infection[67]; 1 study revealed that women infected with HIV with lung cancer, in contrast to men, seemed to have accelerated development of their cancers. Administration of ART increases CD4 cell counts and may retard clinical progression of disease, but HIV-linked lung cancer continues to have a poor prognosis.[68]

COPD

An association between COPD and HIV infection was first reported during the pre-ART period of HIV/AIDS as a result of findings that suggested the presence of disease at a lower age of onset than usual, and with a predominance of bullous disease demonstrated by computed tomography scanning; pulmonary function studies confirmed the presence of reduced carbon monoxide diffusing capacity. Smoking, previous lung infections, and drug abuse were certainly implicated, but so were latent chronic pulmonary infections and cytotoxic lymphocytes in BAL liquid, which might be playing a pathogenic role.[69] Additional studies further strengthened the finding that HIV infection hastens and worsens the susceptibility to COPD, particularly with bullous radiographic abnormalities, and independent of cigarette smoking status.[70] Not surprisingly, other findings include increased frequency of symptoms such as shortness of breath.

But the new and interesting aspect of the HIV-COPD story is that ART may actually worsen the outcome of the interaction between the 2 conditions. There is not much information to go on, and one obvious factor is that the effect of aging per se on the HIV population, with or without smoking, leads to emphysema. Morris and colleagues[71] recently reviewed 3 prospective studies on the respiratory complications of several hundred persons infected with HIV[72–74]; 2 of the 3 studies showed an independent relationship between the use of ART and the presence of airway obstruction. No one knows why ART might increase the prevalence of COPD and its various airway derivatives. Several risk factors alone or in combination may be responsible, such as ART itself, previous or occult pulmonary infections, increased oxidative stress, and heightened apoptosis. Smoking and drug use typically exacerbate COPD and other airway consequences of HIV infection, but they also occur in the absence of these insults. The paradox, of course, is that ART characteristically attenuates a host of HIV-induced inflammatory responses, whereas COPD and airway abnormalities seem to generate exactly the opposite effects. Future results of ongoing studies are eagerly awaited.

Pulmonary Hypertension

Among all AIDS-defining and non–AIDS-defining pulmonary complications, HIV-associated pulmonary arterial hypertension (PAH) has got to be the most vexing, because of its numerous prevailing inconsistencies. Now, there is a good reason for that. At first it was believed that the incidence of HIV-related PAH, calculated by Doppler echocardiographic findings, showed that median pulmonary artery systolic pressure (PASP) was 27.5 mm Hg and that 35.2% of patients had PASP greater than 30 mm Hg.[75] Alas, comparisons of 160 patients with simultaneous echocardiographic and right heart catheterization measurements have shown that PASP is undependable and cannot be relied on to make the diagnosis of HIV-associated PAH or monitor the outcome of ART.[76]

Basically, it looks like all bets are currently off, at least most of them. For example, the role of ART in patients infected with HIV who have PAH assessed by echocardiography, not surprisingly, is controversial. Some reports indicate improvement, others no change, and still others worsening. Catheter techniques to measure PAH in patients who do not have HIV infection have a long history and well-defined pathophysiology; but in the presence of HIV infection, the time course and response to therapy may be different. Obviously, improved techniques for measuring HIV-linked PAH and deciphering its mechanisms, which underlie excessive endothelial cell and vascular smooth muscle cell proliferation, are badly needed to allow for accurate characterization of this mysterious syndrome.

SUMMARY

The epidemiology of HIV/AIDS has changed totally and remarkably since the early 1980s, due largely to potent antiretroviral agents used in combination. Instead of progressive immunologic suppression with inevitable clinical deterioration leading to

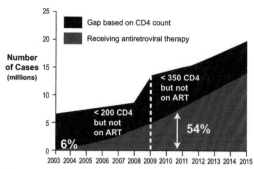

Fig. 4. Number of HIV-infected persons from 2003 to 2015 receiving ART (*in red*) and the gap in the numbers with CD4 cell counts <200 cells/μL (before 2008) and <350 cells/μL (after 2009) (*in blue*). (*From* Harries AD. The strategic use of antiretrovirals to help end the HIV epidemic. Geneva, Switzerland: WHO Press, World Health Organization; 2012; with permission.)

death, the lucky ones, people living with HIV and others within reach of ART, can now survive for decades. That nirvana is only about halfway finished. As **Fig. 4** shows, there is a long way to go to complete the job of ensuring that everyone with HIV infection is restored to health and kept there with proper surveillance, medications, and management. New means of preventing HIV infection also show great promise.

REFERENCES

1. CDC. Pneumocystis pneumonia—Los Angeles. MMWR Morb Mortal Wkly Rep 1981;30:250–2.

2. CDC. Kaposi's sarcoma and Pneumocystis pneumonia among homosexual men—New York City and California. MMWR Morb Mortal Wkly Rep 1981;30:306–8.

3. Hymes KB, Greene JB, Marcus A. Kaposi's sarcoma in homosexual men: a report of 8 cases. Lancet 1981;2:598–600.

4. Gottlieb MS, Schnoff R, Schanker HM, et al. *Pneumocystis carinii* pneumonia and mucosal candidiasis in previously healthy homosexual men—evidence of a new acquired cellular immunodeficiency. N Engl J Med 1981;305:1425–31.

5. Masur H, Michelis MA, Greene JB, et al. An outbreak of community-acquired *Pneumocystis carinii* pneumonia—initial manifestation of cellular immune dysfunction. N Engl J Med 1981;305:1431–8.

6. Siegal FP, Lopez C, Hammer GS, et al. Severe immune deficiency in male homosexuals, manifested by chronic perianal ulcerative Herpes simplex lesions. N Engl J Med 1981;305:1439–44.

7. Durack DT. Opportunistic infections and Kaposi's sarcoma in homosexual men. N Engl J Med 1981; 305:1465–7.

8. Barre-Sinoussi F, Chermann J-C, Ray F, et al. Lymphotropic retrovirus from a patient at risk for acquired immune deficiency syndrome (AIDS). Science 1983;220(4599):868–71.

9. Popovic M, Sangadharan MG, Read E, et al. Detection, isolation, and continuous production of cytopathic retroviruses (HTLV-III) from patients with AIDS and pre-AIDS. Science 1984;224(4648):497–500.

10. Bureau of Hygiene & Tropical Diseases. AIDS Newsletter 1986;2(2).

11. Mann JM. A worldwide pandemic. In: Gottlieb MS, Jeffries DJ, Mildvan D, et al, editors. Current topics in AIDS, vol. 2. Chichester (United Kingdom): John Wiley; 1989.

12. Murray JF, Felton CP, Garay SM, et al. Pulmonary complications of the acquired immunodeficiency syndrome. Report of a National Heart, Lung, and Blood Institute Workshop. N Engl J Med 1984;310: 1682–8.

13. Murray JF, Garay SM, Hopewell PC, et al. NHLBI workshop summary. Pulmonary complications of the acquired immunodeficiency syndrome: an update. Report of the 2nd NHLBI workshop. Am Rev Respir Dis 1987;135:504–9.

14. CDC. Epidemiology of HIV/AIDS—United States, 1981–2005. MMWR Morb Mortal Wkly Rep 2006; 55:589–92.

15. Benitio N, Moreno A, Miro JM, et al. Pulmonary infections in HIV-infected patients: an update in the 21st century. Eur Respir J 2012;39:730–45.

16. Kaplan JE, Benson C, Holmes KK, et al. Guidelines for prevention and treatment of opportunistic infections in HIV-infected adults and adolescents. Recommendations from CDC, the National Institutes of Health, and the HIV Medicine Association of the Infectious Diseases Society of America. MMWR Recomm Rep 2009;58:1–207.

17. Pitchenik AE, Cole C, Russell RW, et al. Tuberculosis, atypical myobacteriosis, and the acquired immunodeficiency syndrome among Haitian and non-Haitian patients in south Florida. Ann Intern Med 1984;101:641–5.

18. The National Institutes of Health—University of California Expert Panel for Corticosteroids as Adjunctive Therapy for Pneumocystis Pneumonia. Consensus statement on the use of corticosteroids as adjunctive therapy for Pneumocystis pneumonia in the acquired immunodeficiency syndrome. N Engl J Med 1990;323:1500–4.

19. The Antiretroviral Therapy/Cohort Collaboration. Life expectancy of individuals on combination antiretroviral therapy in high-income countries: a collaborative analysis of 14 cohort studies. Lancet 2008; 372:293–9.

20. CDC. Vital signs: HIV prevention through care and treatment – United States. MMWR Morb Mortal Wkly Rep 2011;60:1618–23.

21. Mann J, Snider DF, Francis H, et al. Association between HTLV-III/LAV infection and tuberculosis in Zaire. JAMA 1986;256:346.

22. Colebunders RL, Ryder RW, Nzliambi N, et al. HIV infection in patients with tuberculosis in Kinshasa, Zaire. Am Rev Respir Dis 1989;139:1082–5.

23. Harries AD. Tuberculosis and human immunodeficiency virus infection in developing countries. Lancet 1990;335(8686):387–90.

24. Murray JF. Tuberculosis and human immunodeficiency virus infection during the 1990s. Bull Int Union Tuberc Lung Dis 1991;86:21–5.

25. Lucas SB, Hounnou A, Peacock C, et al. The mortality and pathology of HIV infection in a West African city. AIDS 1993;7:1569–79.

26. Kamanfu G, Mlika-Cabanne N, Girard PM, et al. Pulmonary complications of human immunodeficiency virus infection in Bujumbura, Burundi. Am Rev Respir Dis 1993;147:658–63.

27. Daley CL, Mugusi F, Chen LL, et al. Pulmonary complications of HIV infection in Dar Es Salaam, Tanzania. Role of bronchoscopy and bronchoalveolar lavage. Am J Respir Crit Care Med 1996;154:105–10.

28. WHO. Global tuberculosis control report. Chapter 6. World Health Organization; 2011. Available at:. http://www.who.int/tb/publications/global_report/en/. Accessed October 1, 2012.

29. Anglaret X, Chene G, Attia A, et al. Early chemoprophylaxis with trimethoprim-sulfamethoxazole for HIV-1 infected adults in Abidjan, Cote d'Ivoire: a randomized trial. Cotrimo-CI Study Group. Lancet 1999;353(9163):1463–8.

30. Wiktor SZ, Sassan-Morokro M, Grant AD, et al. Efficacy of trimethoprim-sulfamethoxazole prophylaxis to decrease morbidity and mortality in HIV-1-infected patients with tuberculosis in Abidjan, Cote d'Ivoire: a randomized controlled trial. Lancet 1999;353(9163):1469–75.

31. WHO Expert Consultation of Cotrimoxazole Prophylaxis in HIV Infection: report of a WHO expert consultation, Geneva, 10–12 May 2005. Geneva (Switzerland): World Health Organization; 2006. Available at: http://www.int/hiv/pub/meetingreports/ctxprophylaxismeeting.pdf. Accessed August 12, 2012.

32. CDC. Reported tuberculosis in the United States, 2010. Atlanta (GA): US Department of Health and Human Services, CDC; 2011. Available at: http://www.cdc.gov/tb/statistics/reports/2010/default.htm. Accessed August 12, 2012.

33. Samandari T, Agizew TB, Nyirenda S, et al. 6-month versus 36-month isoniazid preventive treatment for tuberculosis in adults with HIV infection in Botswana: a randomized, double-blind, placebo-controlled trial. Lancet 2011;377(9777):1588–98.

34. Suthar AB, Lawn SD, del Amo J, et al. Antiretroviral therapy for prevention of tuberculosis in adults with HIV: a systematic review and meta-analysis. PLoS Med 2012;9(7):e1001270. http://dx.doi.org/10.1371/journal.pmed.1001270.

35. Nakagawa F, Lodwick RK, Smith CJ, et al. Projected life expectancy of people with HIV according to timing of diagnosis. AIDS 2012;26:335–43.

36. Grant RM, Larra JR, Anderson PL, et al. Preexposure chemoprophylaxis for HIV prevention in men who have sex with men. N Engl J Med 2010;363:2587–90.

37. Abdool Karim Q, Abdool Karim SS, Frolich JA, et al. Effectiveness and safety of tenofovir gel, an antiretroviral microbicide for the prevention of HIV infection in women. Science 2010;329:1168–74.

38. Heffernan RT, Garrett NL, Gallagher KM, et al. Declining incidence of invasive *Streptococcus pneumoniae* infections among persons with AIDS in an era of highly active antiretroviral therapy, 1995-2000. J Infect Dis 2005;191:2038–45.

39. Hirshtick RE, Glassroth J, Jordan MC, et al. Bacterial pneumonia in persons infected with the human immunodeficiency virus. N Engl J Med 1995;333:845–51.

40. Castro KG, Ward JW, Aluraker L, et al. 1993 revised classification system for HIV infection and expanded surveillance case definition for AIDS among adolescents and adults. MMWR Recomm Rep 1992;41(RR-17):1–19.

41. Hull MW, Phillips P, Montaner JSG. Changing global epidemiology of pulmonary manifestations of HIV.AIDS. Chest 2008;134:1287–98.

42. Tumbarello M, Tacconelli E, de Gaetano Donati K, et al. Nosocomial bacterial pneumonia in human immunodeficiency virus infected subjects: incidence, risk factors and outcome. Eur Respir J 2001;17:636–40.

43. Franzetti F, Grassini A, Piazza M, et al. Nosocomial bacterial pneumonia in HIV-infected patients: risk factors for adverse outcome and implications for rational empiric antibiotic therapy. Infection 2006;34:9–16.

44. Bozzette SA, Arcia J, Bartok AE, et al. Impact of *Pneumocystis carinii* and cytomegalovirus on the course and outcome of atypical pneumonia in advanced human immunodeficiency virus disease. J Infect Dis 1992;165:93–8.

45. CDC. Seasonal influenza (Flu) – HIV/AIDS and the flu. Available at: http://www.cdc.gov/flu/protect/hiv-flu.htm. Accessed August 15, 2012.

46. Notifications of tuberculosis by type of disease, Tanzania, 1984-1999. Tanzania NTLP/IUATLD. Progress report 1996, No. 36; Tanzania NTLP/KNCV. Report 2000; No.7.

47. CDC. HIV and TB. Available at: www.cdc.gov/hiv/resources/factsheet/hivtb.htm. Accessed August 25, 2012.

48. Chamie G, Luetkemeyer A, Walusimbi-Nanteza M, et al. Significant variation in presentation of pulmonary tuberculosis across a high resolution of CD4 strata. Int J Tuberc Lung Dis 2010;14:1295–302.

49. Corbett EL, Charalambous T, Cheung YB, et al. Epidemiology of tuberculosis in a high HIV prevalence population provided with enhanced diagnosis of symptomatic disease. PLoS Med 2007; 4:e22.

50. Blanc FX, Sok T, Laureillard D, et al. Earlier versus later start of antiretroviral therapy in HIV-infected adults with tuberculosis. N Engl J Med 2011;365: 1471–81.

51. Havlir DV, Kendall MA, Ive P, et al. Timing of antiretroviral therapy for HIV-1 infection and tuberculosis. N Engl J Med 2011;365:1482–91.

52. Abdool Karim SS, Naidoo K, Grobler A, et al. Integration of antiretroviral therapy with tuberculosis treatment. N Engl J Med 2011;365:1492–501.

53. Torok ME, Farrar JJ. When to start antiretroviral therapy in HIV-associated tuberculosis. N Engl J Med 2011;365:1538–40.

54. Torok ME, Yee NT, Chau TT, et al. Timing of initiation of antiretroviral therapy in human immunodeficiency virus (HIV)-associated tuberculosis meningitis. Clin Infect Dis 2011;52:1374–83.

55. WHO. WHO policy on collaborative TB/HIV activities. Guidelines for national programmes and other stakeholders. Geneva (Switzerland): WHO; 2012. WHO/HIV/2012.1.

56. French MA. Immune reconstitution inflammatory syndrome: a reappraisal. Clin Infect Dis 2009;48: 101–7.

57. Naidoo K, Yende-Zumz N, Padayatchi N, et al. The immune reconstitution inflammatory syndrome after antiretroviral therapy initiation in patients with tuberculosis: findings from the SAPiT Trial. Ann Intern Med 2012;157:313–24.

58. WHO. Tuberculosis control report. Executive Summary. World Health Organization; 2011. Available at: www.who.int/tb/publications/global_report/en/. Accessed October 1, 2012.

59. Zhao Y, Xu S, Wang L, et al. National survey of drug-resistant tuberculosis in China. N Engl J Med 2012; 366:2161–70.

60. Gandhi NR, Moll A, Sturm AW, et al. Extensively drug-resistant tuberculosis as a cause of death in patients co-infected with tuberculosis and HIV in a rural area of South Africa. Lancet 2006;368: 1575–80.

61. Gandhi NR, Andrews JR, Brust JC, et al. Risk factors for mortality among MDR- and XDR-TB in a high HIV prevalence setting. Int J Tuberc Lung Dis 2012;16: 90–7.

62. Brust JC, Shah NS, Scott M, et al. Integrated, home-based treatment for MDR-TB and HIV in rural South Africa: an alternate model of care. Int J Tuberc Lung Dis 2012;16:998–1004.

63. Nguyen HQ, Magaret AS, Kitahata MM, et al. Persistent Kaposi sarcoma in the era of highly active anti-retroviral therapy: characterizing the predictors of clinical response. AIDS 2008;11:937–45.

64. Palmieri C, Dhillon T, Thirlwell C, et al. Pulmonary Kaposi sarcoma in the era of highly active antiretroviral therapy. HIV Med 2006;7:291–3.

65. Lim ST, Karim R, Tulpule A, et al. Prognostic factors in HIV-related large-cell lymphoma before versus after highly active antiretroviral therapy. J Clin Oncol 2005;23:8477–82.

66. Palmieri C, Triebel T, Large O, et al. AIDS-related non-Hodgkin's lymphoma in the first decade of highly active antiretroviral therapy. QJM 2006;99:811–26.

67. Pakkala S, Chen Z, Rimland D, et al. Human immunodeficiency virus-associated lung cancer in the era of highly active antiretroviral therapy. Cancer 2012;118:164–72.

68. D'Jaen GA, Pantanowiitz L, Bower M, et al. Human immunodeficiency virus-associated primary lung cancer in the era of highly active antiretroviral therapy: a multi-institutional collaboration. Clin Lung Cancer 2010;11:396–404.

69. Diaz PT, King MA, Pacht ER, et al. Increased susceptibility to pulmonary emphysema among HIV-seropositive smokers. Ann Intern Med 2000; 132:369–72.

70. Petrache I, Diab K, Knox KS, et al. HIV associated pulmonary emphysema: a review of the literature and inquiry into its mechanism. Thorax 2008;63: 463–9.

71. Morris A, George MP, Crothers K, et al. HIV and chronic obstructive pulmonary disease. Is it worse and why? Proc Am Thorac Soc 2011;8:320–5.

72. George MP, Kannass M, Huang L, et al. Respiratory symptoms and airway obstruction in HIV-infected subjects in the HAART era. PLoS One 2009;4:e6328.

73. Cui O, Carruthers S, McIvor A, et al. Effect of smoking on lung function, respiratory symptoms and respiratory diseases amongst HIV-positive subjects: a cross-sectional study. AIDS Res Ther 2009;7:6.

74. Gingo ER, George MP, Kessinger C, et al. Pulmonary function abnormalities in HIV-infected patients during the current antiretroviral therapy era. Am J Respir Crit Care Med 2010;182:790–6.

75. Hsue PY, Deeks SG, Farah HH, et al. Role of HIV and human herpesvirus-8 infection in pulmonary arterial hypertension. AIDS 2008;23:825–33.

76. Rich JD, Shah SJ, Swamy RS, et al. Inaccuracy of Doppler echocardiographic estimates of pulmonary artery pressures in patients with pulmonary hypertension: implications for clinical practice. Chest 2011;139:988–93.

Tobacco Use and Cessation in HIV-Infected Individuals

Kristine K. Browning, PhD[a],*,
Mary Ellen Wewers, PhD, MPH[b], Amy K. Ferketich, PhD[c],
Philip Diaz, MD[d]

KEYWORDS

- HIV • Tobacco dependence treatment • Smoking cessation • Tobacco dependence treatment trials

KEY POINTS

- Smoking prevalence among human immunodeficiency virus (HIV)-infected individuals remains much higher than the US adult smoking prevalence.
- HIV-infected smokers have an increased risk for developing numerous health-related complications such as bacterial pneumonia, pneumocystis pneumonia (PCP), tuberculosis (TB), lung cancer, chronic obstructive pulmonary disease (COPD), and cardiovascular (CV) disease.
- To date, a small number of tobacco dependence treatment trials among HIV-infected smokers have been conducted; most have used nicotine replacement therapy (NRT) with cognitive behavioral therapy. The abstinence rates were low.
- A recent preliminary study found the use of varenicline to be well tolerated, and it may increase abstinence rates with HIV-infected individuals.
- Clinicians should be aggressive in using available resources (ie, United States Public Health Service [USPHS] *Treating Tobacco Use and Dependence Guideline*), including pharmacologic management and counseling to address tobacco dependence in this population.
- Recommendations for future research include examining underlying factors that contribute to persistent smoking and barriers to abstinence, identifying ways to increase motivation for quit attempts, and increasing the number of multicentered 2-arm tobacco dependence treatment trials.

The prevalence of current smoking among HIV-infected individuals ranges between 40% and 84% in various studies.[1–6] These estimates for the HIV-infected population are several-fold higher than the current 20% overall adult prevalence in the United States.[7] With the aging of the HIV-infected population, such a high smoking prevalence has profound health implications for this group of individuals. This review (1) identifies clinical and sociodemographic characteristics associated with tobacco use in this population; (2) discusses the health risks and consequences (pulmonary and nonpulmonary) of tobacco use that are associated with HIV infection; (3) summarizes results of

Support: This work was supported by the National Institutes of Health, R01HL090313-01, "Smoking Cessation and the Natural History of HIV-Associated Emphysema" and award number UL1RR025755 from the National Center for Advancing Translational Sciences.

Financial disclosure: The authors did not engage in any relationships with commercial companies that had a direct financial interest in the subject matter or material discussed in this Article.

[a] The Ohio State University College of Nursing and Comprehensive Cancer Center-James Cancer Hospital, 370 Newton Hall, 1585 Neil Avenue, Columbus, OH 43210, USA; [b] Division of Health Behavior and Health Promotion, The Ohio State University College of Public Health, 349 Cunz Hall, 1841 Neil Avenue, Columbus, OH 43210, USA; [c] Division of Epidemiology, The Ohio State University College of Public Health, 310 Cunz Hall, 1841 Neil Avenue, Columbus, OH 43210, USA; [d] Division of Pulmonary, Allergy, Critical Care, and Sleep Medicine, The Ohio State University College of Medicine, 201 DHLRI, 273 West 12th Avenue, Columbus, OH 43210, USA
* Corresponding author.
E-mail address: browning.99@osu.edu

Clin Chest Med 34 (2013) 181–190
http://dx.doi.org/10.1016/j.ccm.2013.01.005
0272-5231/13/$ – see front matter © 2013 Elsevier Inc. All rights reserved.

chestmed.theclinics.com

tobacco dependence treatment studies among HIV-infected smokers; (4) discusses strategies for smoking cessation, highlighting key components of the USPHS *Treating Tobacco Use and Dependence Guideline*; and (5) provides recommendations for future directions of research.

CHARACTERISTICS OF HIV-INFECTED SMOKERS

Several studies have examined the characteristics of HIV-infected smokers in the United States. Gritz and colleagues[2] examined 348 low-income HIV-infected individuals who received care at an HIV/AIDS care facility where the smoking prevalence was 47%. In a multivariable model they found that age, white race (vs Hispanic ethnicity), and heavy alcohol drinking were positively associated with current smoking. In another low-income sample of HIV-infected individuals receiving Medicaid benefits, the current smoking prevalence was 66% and smoking was positively related to age, low level of education, heavy drinking, and illicit substance use.[3] Shuter and colleagues[8] found that almost 50% of HIV-infected smokers reported both current cocaine and marijuana use, 33% reported current heroin use, and almost 40% had depressive symptoms and symptoms of anxiety.

Webb and colleagues[4] examined predictors of various levels of smoking (light smoking, 1–10 cigarettes per day [CPD]; moderate smoking, 11–19 CPD; and heavy smoking, 20 or more CPD) in a sample of 221 HIV-infected individuals recruited from an infectious disease clinic. The prevalence estimates of light, moderate, and heavy smoking were 25%, 22%, and 27%, respectively. Heavy drinking was the only consistent variable related to smoking status; however, age, education, income, race, marijuana use, and social support were significantly related to smoking in one or more of the models. In a large ($n = 1094$) representative sample of HIV-infected individuals in New York state, Tesoriero and colleagues[1] reported a smoking prevalence of 59%. Similar to other studies, smoking was positively associated with younger age and a low level of education. In addition, those who self-reported as being of "other" race/ethnicity, which did not include African American, or Hispanic, were significantly less likely than whites to be current smokers.

At least 4 studies have examined characteristics related to smoking cessation. Burkhalter and colleagues[3] found that about one-third of smokers had not made a quit attempt since diagnosis and that only 82% of smokers were in either the precontemplation (not interested in trying to quit in

the next 6 months) or contemplation (interested in quitting in the next 6 months but not the next 30 days) stage of quitting. Furthermore, only 38% of smokers reported trying any cessation treatment and less than half reported interest in using a cessation program if available. However, Shuter and colleagues[8] report that 66% of participants were in the preparation (ready to quit in the next 30 days) or action stages of quitting.

Tesoriero and colleagues[1] reported that nearly half of the smokers in their sample did not change their level of smoking after receiving their HIV diagnosis, whereas a similar percentage reported smoking more (23%) or smoking less (29%) after diagnosis. Almost two-thirds (64%) reported a serious quit attempt, defined as not smoking for 24 hours or more in the past year and 75% indicated that they wanted to quit smoking.[1] In another study, 40% of HIV-infected smokers were motivated to quit smoking and 70% reported at least one serious quit attempt in the past.[9]

In summary, studies reporting the interest or motivation to quit among HIV-infected smokers are mixed. Furthermore, it is likely that characteristics associated with increased smoking prevalence in the general population play a role in the high smoking rates among HIV-infected individuals.[10] These characteristics may represent important barriers to smoking cessation for HIV-infected smokers and include lower level of education and socioeconomic status,[10] alcohol and drug abuse,[2,3,8,11] and psychiatric comorbidities.[11]

CIGARETTE SMOKING AND HEALTH IMPLICATIONS FOR THE HIV-INFECTED POPULATION
Smoking and Pulmonary Complications

Because details of pulmonary complications and their relationship to cigarette smoking are elucidated in articles reviewing specific complications, only a brief summarization of the pulmonary effects of smoking in the HIV-infected population are provided. In the current antiretroviral therapy (ART) era, bacterial pneumonia has become the most important pulmonary infectious complication in the HIV-infected population.[12] Bacterial pneumonia is closely linked to cigarette smoking, and studies in both the pre-ART and ART eras have demonstrated a greatly increased risk of bacterial pneumonia in HIV-infected smokers.[6,13–15] Furthermore, evidence now exists that cigarette smoking has become the single most important clinical risk factor for bacterial pneumonia in the HIV-infected population.[14,15] Smoking effects on lung host defense, including adverse effects on alveolar macrophage function and chemotactic properties, may be an important contributing mechanism.[16–18] Importantly, evidence exists that the risk of bacterial pneumonia in the HIV-infected population is much greater in current than former smokers, underscoring the importance of smoking cessation in this population.[19]

Cigarette smoking may also be an important risk factor for other lower respiratory tract infections in the HIV-infected population. For example, Miguez-Burbano and colleagues[20] have demonstrated that smoking may be an important risk factor for PCP among hospitalized individuals with HIV. Furthermore, in a murine model of PCP, cigarette smoke greatly increases the organism load in the lung.[21] In addition, smoking increases the risk for developing TB,[22–24] and it has been suggested that HIV combined with high smoking rates will be critical determinants of the global burden of TB in the coming years.[25]

Numerous studies have demonstrated that HIV-infected individuals are at increased risk for lung cancer.[26–29] Given the high prevalence of cigarette smoking in this population, it has been difficult to determine whether this risk is primarily related to a higher smoking prevalence.[28] However, recent data suggest that HIV infection may represent an independent risk factor for lung cancer development.[26,29] Similarly, data from the pre-ART and ART eras are consistent in demonstrating that HIV is an independent risk factor for COPD,[30,31] which may involve an interaction of HIV with smoking to increase the susceptibility of COPD in this population.[30]

In summary, evidence indicates that the lungs of persons infected with HIV are unusually susceptible to the adverse effects of cigarette smoking. These adverse effects include a heightened risk for lower respiratory tract infections, lung cancer, and COPD. As such, it can be argued that the single most important issue relevant to the natural history of HIV-related pulmonary complications today is the exceedingly high prevalence of cigarette smoking in this population.

Smoking and Nonpulmonary Complications

Numerous other complications in the HIV-infected population have been linked to cigarette smoking. These complications include an increase in perinatal mortality among infants born to HIV-infected women,[32] periodontal disease,[33] accelerated bone loss,[34] and a significantly poorer health-related quality of life.[35] Crothers and colleagues[36] in the Veterans Aging Cohort Study compared HIV-infected and noninfected veterans and found that smoking was associated with increased comorbid conditions and mortality in the HIV-infected group.

Lifson and colleagues[6] using data from the Strategies for Management of Antiretroviral Therapy (SMART) study demonstrated that compared with nonsmokers, smokers had a significantly greater risk of all-cause mortality and an increased adjusted hazard ratio for bacterial pneumonia, non-AIDS malignancies, and major CV disease.

Comorbid conditions of increasing relevance to the HIV-infected population include the increased risk of atherosclerosis and coronary artery disease.[37–43] Numerous reports have documented that the HIV-infected population has an increased disease burden of atherosclerotic vascular disease including increase in coronary calcium scores,[37] progression of carotid and coronary artery disease documented by imaging studies,[38] and an increased risk of CV complications, including acute myocardial infarction,[39–41] hospitalization for cardiac ischemia,[42] and sudden cardiac death.[43]

Notably, studies have demonstrated that even when accounting for demographics and traditional risk factors, HIV-infected individuals have a significantly greater risk for the development of CV disease, suggesting that several HIV-specific factors may be involved in the pathogenesis, including adverse effects of certain antiretroviral medications, heightened inflammation, and immune dysfunction.[44–50]

Given that HIV infection may independently raise CV risk, it is imperative that adequate attention to traditional risk factor modification be given.[51,52] Indeed, cigarette smoking has been shown to be a far greater risk factor for CV morbidity than ART[53] and smoking has been shown to be the most common traditional CV risk factor in a cohort of HIV-infected individuals.[54] Furthermore, smoking cessation has been shown to decrease the risk of acute myocardial infarction rates in an HIV-infected population.[54] In fact, Triant[55] has suggested that smoking cessation is the most important specific management principle in modifying CV risk in the HIV-infected population.

TOBACCO DEPENDENCE TREATMENT STUDIES

In the decade after the HIV epidemic emerged in the United States, *JAMA* published a commentary in 1994 noting that stopping smoking may provide short-term health benefits to patients with HIV infection who continue to smoke.[56] Furthermore, the article emphasized to clinicians that tobacco dependence treatment was warranted to reduce the incidence of complications related to smoking in HIV-infected smokers. Shortly afterward, investigators started to design and test tobacco dependence treatment approaches for HIV-infected

Table 1
Published controlled studies of tobacco dependence treatment trials in HIV-infected smokers

Study	Sample	Intervention	Abstinence Outcomes	Comments
Wewers et al,[57] 2000	AIDS clinical trials unit patients Intervention n = 8 100% male Mean age = 42 y CPD = 27 Control n = 7 100% male Mean age = 37 y CPD = 28	Intervention: 8 wk of weekly peer support telephone counseling + NRT Control: written self-help materials	Intervention: 62.5% at 8 wk 50% at 8 mo Control: 0% at 8 wk 0% at 8 mo	Intent-to-treat analysis with randomization; biochemical confirmation of abstinence; small sample size
Elzi et al,[61] 2006	Swiss HIV cohort study Intervention n = 34 82% male Median age = 43 y CPD = 28 Control n = 383 67% male Median age = 40 y CPD = 21	Intervention: 12 mo of counseling + NRT Control: no treatment	Intervention: 38% at 12 mo Control: 7% at 12 mo	Intent-to-treat analysis without randomization; self-reported abstinence; pilot study
Lloyd-Richardson et al,[58] 2009	Immunology clinic patients Intervention n = 232 67.7% male Mean age = 41.2 y CPD = 18.3 Control n = 212 58.5% male Mean age = 42.9 y CPD = 18.2	Intervention: 4 sessions of tailored motivational counseling + quit day counseling call + NRT for those willing to quit Control: 2 counseling sessions with health educator + NRT for those willing to quit	Intervention: 12% at 2 mo 9% at 4 mo 9% at 6 mo Control: 13% at 2 mo 10% at 4 mo 10% at 6 mo	Intent-to-treat analysis with randomization; biochemical confirmation of abstinence; only those ready to quit were offered NRT
Ingersoll et al,[62] 2009	Infectious disease clinic patients Whole sample n = 40 55% male Mean age = 42 y CPD = 17.3	Intervention: single motivational interviewing session + NRT (n = 22) Control: Written materials + NRT (n = 18)	No differences between groups; 22.5% of whole sample abstinent at 3 mo	Intent-to-treat analysis with randomization; biochemical confirmation of abstinence; small sample size

Study	Setting/Participants	Intervention/Control	Results	Comments
Vidrine et al,[59] 2012	Primary care/HIV care clinic Intervention n = 236 71.9% male Mean age = 43.9 y CPD = 18.6 Control n = 238 68.9% male Mean age = 45.7 y CPD = 19.7	Intervention: Physician advice to quit + setting a quit date+ NRT + personalized quit plan and written materials + 2 mo proactive cell phone counseling + hotline access Control: Physician advice to quit + setting a quit date + personalized quit plan and written materials + NRT	Intervention: 11.9% 7-d point prevalence at 3 mo 8.9% continuous at 3 mo Control: 3.4% 7-d point prevalence at 3 mo 2.1% continuous at 3 mo	Intent-to-treat analysis with randomization; biochemical confirmation of abstinence; continuation of Vidrine et al,[59] 2006 pilot study with updated results at 3 mo postintervention
Moadel et al,[64] 2012	Infectious disease clinic Intervention n = 73 49.3% male Mean age = 49.2 y CPD = 12.8 Control n = 72 48.6% male Mean age = 47.9 y CPD = 11.1	Intervention: 8-session group intervention; offer of 3 mo supply of NRT Control: physician advice to quit; written materials; offer of 3 mo supply of NRT	Intervention: 19.2% at 3 mo Control: 9.7% at 3 mo	Intent-to-treat analysis with randomization; biochemical confirmation of abstinence; small sample size
Ferketich et al,[60] 2013	Infectious Disease Clinic Intervention n = 228 85.1% male Mean age = 42.7 y CPD = 19.8	Intervention: 12 wk of nurse counseling + varenicline or NRT	Varenicline: 25.6% at 3 mo NRT: 11.8% at 3 mo	Intent-to-treat analysis without randomization; biochemical confirmation of abstinence

smokers. To date, only a small number of tobacco dependence treatment trials have been conducted. The first feasibility trial was conducted in 2000[57]; more recently, findings from larger trials have been published.[58–60] **Table 1** provides a chronologic listing and summary of published studies, which includes a 2-group design to examine the feasibility and efficacy of treatment approaches.[57–64]

All studies summarized in **Table 1** included treatment that consisted of behavioral counseling and pharmacotherapy; all investigations were grounded in evidence-based treatment strategies recommended by the USPHS *Treating Tobacco Use and Dependence Clinical Practice Guideline*.[65,66] With the exception of the Swiss HIV Cohort investigation,[61] all studies included cognitive behavioral strategies tailored for smokers with HIV infection.

The pharmacotherapeutic agent of choice in all but one of the above-mentioned studies was nicotine replacement. Concern about drug interactions for HIV-infected smokers receiving ART may have contributed to the paucity of studies examining the efficacy of other agents. However, Pedrol-Clotet and colleagues[67] conducted a single-arm trial testing the use of bupropion with 21 HIV-positive patients and reported a 38% success rate for more than 1 year posttreatment. In this trial, no clinically significant drug interactions were noted.

Ferketich and colleagues[60] have recently reported the largest experience of varenicline in HIV-infected smokers, comparing the success rate of NRT and varenicline among 228 HIV-infected smokers involved in a smoking cessation study. Both groups also received a weekly telephone smoking cessation counseling from a nurse specialist. The rates of biochemically confirmed abstinence at 3 months were higher in the varenicline group compared with the NRT group (25.6% vs 11.8%). Although the design was nonrandomized, inverse probability of treatment-weighted logistic regression modeling was used to compare the 2 groups and the odds ratio of successful abstinence was significantly greater with varenicline (adjusted odds ratio, 2.72; 95% confidence interval, 1.50–4.94).

Importantly, varenicline was reasonably well tolerated in the HIV population with the most common side effects being nausea (32.2%), abnormal dreams (22.9%), and difficulty sleeping (17.8%). About 14% had to discontinue therapy because of adverse effects. Of note, no coronary events were observed. One patient reported suicidal ideation, but the symptoms resolved after stopping the use of varenicline. There were no differences in the side effect profile between those on ART and those not on ART.[60]

RECOMMENDATIONS FOR SMOKING CESSATION FOR THE HIV-INFECTED SMOKER

In general, the approach for smoking cessation with an HIV-infected population should follow the USPHS *Treating Tobacco Use and Dependence* Guideline. The guideline, now in its third update, is composed of a systematic review of approximately 8700 research articles that address the assessment and treatment recommendations for tobacco dependence. Clinicians can make a difference when providing tobacco dependence treatment even when it is minimal (eg, <3 minutes). When patients are not willing to make a quit attempt, clinician-delivered brief interventions can increase motivation and the likelihood of future quit attempts. Furthermore, there is evidence that smokers who receive advice and assistance on quitting from their clinician have greater satisfaction with their health care.[68–70] The guideline also provides key strategies and recommendations that are designed to assist the clinician in delivering evidence-based tobacco dependence treatment. **Table 2** summarizes the key recommendations.

The USPHS guideline recommendations are based on research that included a wide-range of populations. Clearly, the HIV-infected population is a special population with substantial barriers to smoking abstinence. Nevertheless, the potential benefits to smoking cessation are considerable given the increased risk of numerous complications, including bacterial pneumonia, PCP, TB, COPD, lung cancer, and coronary artery disease. Clinicians should be aggressive in using available resources, including pharmacologic management and counseling to address tobacco dependence in this population. As noted above, preliminary evidence suggests that varenicline has an acceptable safety profile and may be more effective than NRT for this population.

RECOMMENDATIONS FOR FUTURE DIRECTIONS OF RESEARCH

Smoking prevalence remains high among HIV-infected individuals, despite important disease-related consequences of continued smoking. The success of ART has resulted in increased survival for individuals living with HIV.[71] Thus, careful examination and efficacy testing of successful tobacco dependence treatment strategies in the general population are important in this special population of smokers. Recommendations for

Table 2
USPHS recommendations for treating tobacco use and dependence

USPHS Components	Recommendation
Tobacco dependence is a chronic disease	• Requires repeated intervention • Often multiple quit attempts

The 5 A's model (ask, advise, assess, assist, arrange)	• Clinicians should offer 5 A's to *every* patient at *each* visit
	• Systematically, *ask* tobacco use status:
	  ○ Identify all users at each visit
	  ○ Document on each user at each visit
	  ○ Encourage every willing patient to quit
	• In a clear, strong personalized message, *advise* all tobacco users to quit
	• For current tobacco users, *assess* willingness to make a quit attempt
	  ○ For patients *willing* to make a quit attempt, *assist* with a quit plan
	  ○ For patients *unwilling* to quit, provide interventions to increase quit attempts in the future
	  ○ For recent quitters, provide relapse prevention
	• All patients receiving previous A's, *arrange* for follow-up

Individual, group, and telephone counseling are effective	• Effectiveness increases with treatment intensity
	• Most effective components
	  ○ Problem solving and skills training
	  ○ Social support

7 first-line medications that increase long-term smoking abstinence rates	• Bupropion (Zyban) • Nicotine gum • Nicotine inhaler • Nicotine lozenge • Nicotine nasal spray • Nicotine patch • Varenicline (Chantix)
Counseling and medication	• Effective when used alone, *more effective* when used together • Clinically and highly cost effective
Telephone quitline counseling	• Effective, particularly with diverse populations

Adapted from Fiore MC, Jaén CR, BT, et al. Treating tobacco use and dependence: 2008 Update. Clinical practice guideline. Rockville (MD): U.S. Department of Health and Human Services. Public Health Service; 2008; with permission.

future research among HIV-infected smokers include (1) examining the underlying factors that contribute to persistent smoking as well as barriers to abstinence, (2) identifying ways to increase motivation for quit attempts, (3) increasing the number of multicentered 2-arm tobacco dependence treatment trials, and (4) using highly efficacious first-line pharmacotherapy in tobacco dependence treatment intervention studies. Although continued implementation of clinician and system-level tobacco dependence treatment interventions for HIV-infected individuals is warranted, addressing the above-mentioned research gaps could help to substantially reduce smoking-related comorbidities in the future.

REFERENCES

1. Tesoriero JM, Gieryic SM, Carrascal A, et al. Smoking among HIV positive New Yorkers: prevalence, frequency, and opportunities for cessation. AIDS Behav 2010;14(4):824–35.

2. Gritz ER, Vidrine DJ, Lazev AB, et al. Smoking behavior in a low-income multiethnic HIV/AIDS population. Nicotine Tob Res 2004;6(1):71–7.

3. Burkhalter JE, Springer CM, Chhabra R, et al. Tobacco use and readiness to quit smoking in low-income HIV-infected persons. Nicotine Tob Res 2005;7(4):511–22.

4. Webb MS, Vanable PA, Carey MP, et al. Cigarette smoking among HIV+ men and women: examining health, substance use, and psychosocial correlates across the smoking spectrum. J Behav Med 2007;30(5):371–83.

5. Marshall MM, Kirk GD, Caporaso NE, et al. Tobacco use and nicotine dependence among HIV-infected and uninfected injection drug users. Addict Behav 2011;36(1–2):61–7.

6. Lifson AR, Neuhaus J, Arribas JR, et al. Smoking-related health risks among persons with HIV in the Strategies for Management of Antiretroviral Therapy clinical trial. Am J Public Health 2010;100(10):1896–903.

7. Barnes PM, Ward BW, Freeman G, et al. Early release of selected estimates based on data from the January-September 2010 National Health Interview Survey. Government Report. March 2011; 2012(August 23).

8. Shuter J, Bernstein SL, Moadel AB. Cigarette smoking behaviors and beliefs in persons living with HIV/AIDS. Am J Health Behav 2012;36(1): 75–85.

9. Benard A, Bonnet F, Tessier JF, et al. Tobacco addiction and HIV infection: toward the implementation of cessation programs. ANRS CO3 Aquitaine Cohort. AIDS Patient Care STDS 2007;21(7):458–68.

10. Centers for Disease Control and Prevention. Vital signs: current cigarette smoking among adults aged ≥18 years—United States, 2009. MMWR Morb Mortal Wkly Rep 2010;59(35):1135–40.

11. Bing EG, Burnam MA, Longshore D, et al. Psychiatric disorders and drug use among human immunodeficiency virus-infected adults in the United States. Arch Gen Psychiatry 2001;58(8):721–8.

12. Crothers K, Huang L, Goulet JL, et al. HIV infection and risk for incident pulmonary diseases in the combination antiretroviral therapy era. Am J Respir Crit Care Med 2011;183(3):388–95.

13. Hirschtick RE, Glassroth J, Jordan MC, et al. Bacterial pneumonia in persons infected with the human immunodeficiency virus. Pulmonary Complications of HIV Infection Study Group. N Engl J Med 1995; 333(13):845–51.

14. Gordin FM, Roediger MP, Girard PM, et al. Pneumonia in HIV-infected persons: increased risk with cigarette smoking and treatment interruption. Am J Respir Crit Care Med 2008;178(6):630–6.

15. Kohli R, Lo Y, Homel P, et al. Bacterial pneumonia, HIV therapy, and disease progression among HIV-infected women in the HIV epidemiologic research (HER) study. Clin Infect Dis 2006;43(1):90–8.

16. Elssner A, Carter JE, Yunger TM, et al. HIV-1 infection does not impair human alveolar macrophage phagocytic function unless combined with cigarette smoking. Chest 2004;125(3):1071–6.

17. Wewers MD, Diaz PT, Wewers ME, et al. Cigarette smoking in HIV infection induces a suppressive inflammatory environment in the lung. Am J Respir Crit Care Med 1998;158(5 Pt 1):1543–9.

18. Twigg HL 3rd, Soliman DM, Spain BA. Impaired alveolar macrophage accessory cell function and reduced incidence of lymphocytic alveolitis in HIV-infected patients who smoke. AIDS 1994;8(5): 611–8.

19. Benard A, Mercie P, Alioum A, et al. Bacterial pneumonia among HIV-infected patients: decreased risk after tobacco smoking cessation. ANRS CO3 Aquitaine Cohort, 2000-2007. PLoS One 2010;5(1):e8896.

20. Miguez-Burbano MJ, Ashkin D, Rodriguez A, et al. Increased risk of Pneumocystis carinii and community-acquired pneumonia with tobacco use in HIV disease. Int J Infect Dis 2005;9(4): 208–17.

21. Christensen PJ, Preston AM, Ling T, et al. Pneumocystis murina infection and cigarette smoke exposure interact to cause increased organism burden, development of airspace enlargement, and pulmonary inflammation in mice. Infect Immun 2008; 76(8):3481–90.

22. Slama K, Chiang CY, Enarson DA, et al. Tobacco and tuberculosis: a qualitative systematic review and meta-analysis. Int J Tuberc Lung Dis 2007; 11(10):1049–61.

23. Lin HH, Ezzati M, Murray M. Tobacco smoke, indoor air pollution and tuberculosis: a systematic review and meta-analysis. PLoS Med 2007;4(1):e20.

24. Bates MN, Khalakdina A, Pai M, et al. Risk of tuberculosis from exposure to tobacco smoke: a systematic review and meta-analysis. Arch Intern Med 2007;167(4):335–42.

25. van Zyl Smit RN, Pai M, Yew WW, et al. Global lung health: the colliding epidemics of tuberculosis, tobacco smoking, HIV and COPD. Eur Respir J 2010;35(1):27–33.

26. Kirk GD, Merlo C, O'Driscoll P, et al. HIV infection is associated with an increased risk for lung cancer, independent of smoking. Clin Infect Dis 2007; 45(1):103–10.

27. Guiguet M, Boue F, Cadranel J, et al. Effect of immunodeficiency, HIV viral load, and antiretroviral therapy on the risk of individual malignancies (FHDH-ANRS CO4): a prospective cohort study. Lancet Oncol 2009;10(12):1152–9.

28. Clifford GM, Lise M, Franceschi S, et al. Lung cancer in the Swiss HIV Cohort Study: role of smoking, immunodeficiency and pulmonary infection. Br J Cancer 2012;106(3):447–52.

29. Sigel K, Wisnivesky J, Gordon K, et al. HIV as an independent risk factor for incident lung cancer. AIDS 2012;26(8):1017–25.

30. Diaz PT, King MA, Pacht ER, et al. Increased susceptibility to pulmonary emphysema among HIV-seropositive smokers. Ann Intern Med 2000; 132:369–72.

31. Crothers K, Butt AA, Gibert CL, et al. Increased COPD among HIV-positive compared to HIV-negative veterans. Chest 2006;130(5):1326–33.

32. Aliyu MH, Weldeselasse H, August EM, et al. Cigarette smoking and fetal morbidity outcomes in a large cohort of HIV-infected mothers. Nicotine Tob Res 2013;15(1):177–84.

33. Jeganathan S, Batterham M, Begley K, et al. Predictors of oral health quality of life in HIV-1 infected patients attending routine care in Australia. J Public Health Dent 2011;71:248–51.

34. Walker Harris V, Brown TT. Bone loss in the HIV-infected patient: evidence, clinical implications,

and treatment strategies. J Infect Dis 2012; 205(Suppl 3):S391–8.

35. Crothers K, Griffith TA, McGinnis KA, et al. The impact of cigarette smoking on mortality, quality of life, and comorbid illness among HIV-positive veterans. J Gen Intern Med 2005;20(12):1142–5.

36. Crothers K, Goulet JL, Rodriguez-Barradas MC, et al. Impact of cigarette smoking on mortality in HIV-positive and HIV-negative veterans. AIDS Educ Prev 2009;21(Suppl 3):40–53.

37. Fitch KV, Lo J, Abbara S, et al. Increased coronary artery calcium score and noncalcified plaque among HIV-infected men: relationship to metabolic syndrome and cardiac risk parameters. J Acquir Immune Defic Syndr 2010;55(4):495–9.

38. Mangili A, Polak JF, Skinner SC, et al. HIV infection and progression of carotid and coronary atherosclerosis: the CARE study. J Acquir Immune Defic Syndr 2011;58(2):148–53.

39. Triant VA, Lee H, Hadigan C, et al. Increased acute myocardial infarction rates and cardiovascular risk factors among patients with human immunodeficiency virus disease. J Clin Endocrinol Metab 2007;92(7):2506–12.

40. Lang S, Mary-Krause M, Cotte L, et al. Increased risk of myocardial infarction in HIV-infected patients in France, relative to the general population. AIDS 2010;24(8):1228–30.

41. Durand M, Sheehy O, Baril JG, et al. Association between HIV infection, antiretroviral therapy, and risk of acute myocardial infarction: a cohort and nested case-control study using Quebec's public health insurance database. J Acquir Immune Defic Syndr 2011;57(3):245–53.

42. Obel N, Thomsen HF, Kronborg G, et al. Ischemic heart disease in HIV-infected and HIV-uninfected individuals: a population-based cohort study. Clin Infect Dis 2007;44(12):1625–31.

43. Tseng ZH, Secemsky EA, Dowdy D, et al. Sudden cardiac death in patients with human immunodeficiency virus infection. J Am Coll Cardiol 2012; 59(21):1891–6.

44. Padilla S, Masia M, Garcia N, et al. Early changes in inflammatory and pro-thrombotic biomarkers in patients initiating antiretroviral therapy with abacavir or tenofovir. BMC Infect Dis 2011;11:40.

45. Kuller LH, Tracy R, Belloso W, et al. Inflammatory and coagulation biomarkers and mortality in patients with HIV infection. PLoS Med 2008;5(10):e203.

46. Neuhaus J, Jacobs DR Jr, Baker JV, et al. Markers of inflammation, coagulation, and renal function are elevated in adults with HIV infection. J Infect Dis 2010;201(12):1788–95.

47. Calmy A, Gayet-Ageron A, Montecucco F, et al. HIV increases markers of cardiovascular risk: results from a randomized, treatment interruption trial. AIDS 2009;23(8):929–39.

48. Triant VA, Regan S, Lee H, et al. Association of immunologic and virologic factors with myocardial infarction rates in a US healthcare system. J Acquir Immune Defic Syndr 2010;55(5):615–9.

49. Lichtenstein KA, Armon C, Buchacz K, et al. Low CD4+ T cell count is a risk factor for cardiovascular disease events in the HIV outpatient study. Clin Infect Dis 2010;51(4):435–47.

50. Ferry T, Raffi F, Collin-Filleul F, et al. Uncontrolled viral replication as a risk factor for non-AIDS severe clinical events in HIV-infected patients on long-term antiretroviral therapy: APROCO/COPILOTE (ANRS CO8) cohort study. J Acquir Immune Defic Syndr 2009;51(4):407–15.

51. Ford ES, Greenwald JH, Richterman AG, et al. Traditional risk factors and D-dimer predict incident cardiovascular disease events in chronic HIV infection. AIDS 2010;24(10):1509–17.

52. Reinsch N, Neuhaus K, Esser S, et al. Are HIV patients undertreated? Cardiovascular risk factors in HIV: results of the HIV-HEART study. Eur J Prev Cardiol 2012;19(2):267–74.

53. DAD Study Group, Friis-Moller N, Reiss P, et al. Class of antiretroviral drugs and the risk of myocardial infarction. N Engl J Med 2007;356(17): 1723–35.

54. Petoumenos K, Worm S, Reiss P, et al. Rates of cardiovascular disease following smoking cessation in patients with HIV infection: results from the D: a:D study(*). HIV Med 2011;12(7):412–21.

55. Triant VA. HIV infection and coronary heart disease: an intersection of epidemics. J Infect Dis 2012; 205(Suppl 3):S355–61.

56. Chaisson RE. Smoking cessation in patients with HIV. JAMA 1994;272(7):564.

57. Wewers ME, Neidig JL, Kihm KE. The feasibility of a nurse-managed, peer-led tobacco cessation intervention among HIV-positive smokers. J Assoc Nurses AIDS Care 2000;11(6):37–44.

58. Lloyd-Richardson EE, Stanton CA, Papandonatos GD, et al. Motivation and patch treatment for HIV+ smokers: a randomized controlled trial. Addiction 2009;104(11):1891–900.

59. Vidrine DJ, Marks RM, Arduino RC, et al. Efficacy of cell phone-delivered smoking cessation counseling for persons living with HIV/AIDS: 3-month outcomes. Nicotine Tob Res 2012;14(1):106–10.

60. Ferketich AK, Diaz P, Browning KK, et al. Safety of varenicline among smokers enrolled in the lung HIV study. Nicotine Tob Res 2013;15(1):247–54.

61. Elzi L, Spoerl D, Voggensperger J, et al. A smoking cessation programme in HIV-infected individuals: a pilot study. Antivir Ther 2006;11(6):787–95.

62. Ingersoll KS, Cropsey KL, Heckman CJ. A test of motivational plus nicotine replacement interventions for HIV positive smokers. AIDS Behav 2009;13(3): 545–54.

63. Vidrine DJ, Arduino RC, Gritz ER. Impact of a cell phone intervention on mediating mechanisms of smoking cessation in individuals living with HIV/AIDS. Nicotine Tob Res 2006;8(Suppl 1):S103–8.

64. Moadel AB, Bernstein SL, Mermelstein RJ, et al. A randomized controlled trial of a tailored group smoking cessation intervention for HIV-infected smokers. J Acquir Immune Defic Syndr 2012;61(2):208–15.

65. Fiore MC, Jaén CR, Baker TB, et al. Treating tobacco use and dependence: 2008 Update. Clinical practice guideline. Rockville (MD): U.S. Department of Health and Human Services. Public Health Service; 2008.

66. Fiore M, Bailey W, Cohen S, et al. Treating tobacco use and dependence: clinical practice guideline. Goverment Report. 2000.

67. Pedrol-Clotet E, Deig-Comerma E, Ribell-Bachs M, et al. Bupropion use for smoking cessation in HIV-infected patients receiving antiretroviral therapy. Enferm Infecc Microbiol Clin 2006;24(8):509–11.

68. Solberg LI, Boyle RG, Davidson G, et al. Patient satisfaction and discussion of smoking cessation during clinical visits. Mayo Clin Proc 2001;76(2):138–43.

69. Barzilai DA, Goodwin MA, Zyzanski SJ, et al. Does health habit counseling affect patient satisfaction? Prev Med 2001;33(6):595–9.

70. Quinn V, Stevens V, Hollis J, et al. Tobacco-cessation services and patient satisfaction in nine nonprofit HMOs. Am J Prev Med 2005;29(2):77–84.

71. Patel N, Talwar A, Reichert VC, et al. Tobacco and HIV. Clin Occup Environ Med 2006;5(1):193–207.

Evaluation of Respiratory Disease

Sofya Tokman, MD*, Laurence Huang, MD

KEYWORDS

• HIV • AIDS • Lung diseases • CD4 count • Chest radiograph • Diagnosis

KEY POINTS

- The spectrum of HIV-associated pulmonary diseases is broad.
- Opportunistic infections and neoplasms remain important considerations in persons infected with HIV even in the current combination antiretroviral therapy (ART) era.
- Lung diseases such as chronic obstructive pulmonary disease (COPD) and lung cancer are prevalent in persons infected with HIV.
- Clinicians caring for persons infected with HIV must have a systematic approach. The approach begins with a thorough history and physical examination and often involves selected laboratory tests and a chest radiograph.
- The goal of the diagnostic evaluation is to arrive at a specific diagnosis or, at most, a few diagnoses, which then prompts specific diagnostic testing and treatment.

INTRODUCTION

The spectrum of HIV-associated pulmonary diseases is broad and the lungs continue to be one of the most frequently affected organ systems in persons infected with HIV. Opportunistic infections and neoplasms are common even in the current combination antiretroviral therapy (ART) era. The extent of immunosuppression, use of ART and antimicrobial prophylaxis, prior history of illness, geographic setting, and life style choices influence the cause and relative frequency of observed respiratory disease. In addition to pulmonary infections classically associated with advanced immunosuppression, such as *Pneumocystis* pneumonia (PCP), persons infected with HIV are also susceptible to community-acquired pathogens, such as *Streptococcus pneumoniae*, and to hospital-acquired pathogens, such as methicillin-resistant *Staphylococcus aureus*. Worldwide, *Mycobacterium tuberculosis* is a dominant cause of pneumonia in persons infected with HIV. Furthermore, lung diseases commonly seen in individuals without HIV, including chronic obstructive pulmonary disease (COPD) and lung cancer, are prevalent in those with HIV and there is growing evidence that HIV infection predisposes patients to develop COPD and lung cancer and to present with these diseases at a younger age. Risk factors for HIV infection, such as injection drug use, also make patients susceptible to a wide variety of pulmonary complications, such as aspiration pneumonia, septic emboli from right-sided endocarditis, and talc granulomatosis. Given the breadth of pulmonary illnesses faced by people living with HIV, clinicians must have a systematic approach to evaluate this patient population. This article presents an overview of the evaluation of respiratory disease in persons with HIV/AIDS.

Dr Tokman is supported by NIH T32 HL007185.
Dr Huang is supported by NIH K24 HL087713, R01 HL090335, and U01 HL098964.
HIV/AIDS Division, Division of Pulmonary and Critical Care Medicine, Department of Medicine, San Francisco General Hospital, UCSF, 995 Potrero Avenue, Ward 84, Box 0874, San Francisco, CA 94110, USA
* Corresponding author.
E-mail address: sofya.tokman@ucsf.edu

Clin Chest Med 34 (2013) 191–204
http://dx.doi.org/10.1016/j.ccm.2013.02.005
0272-5231/13/$ – see front matter © 2013 Elsevier Inc. All rights reserved.

chestmed.theclinics.com

EVALUATION OF RESPIRATORY DISEASE

The evaluation of respiratory disease in persons infected with HIV begins with a thorough history and physical examination. The information from the history and physical examination can then be used to determine whether additional testing (eg, laboratory tests, chest radiograph) is indicated. Frequently, the clinical, laboratory, and chest radiographic presentation suggests a specific diagnosis or, at most, a few diagnoses, which then prompts specific diagnostic testing and treatment.

SYMPTOMS AND SIGNS

All HIV-associated respiratory diseases may present with similar respiratory symptoms including cough, dyspnea, and occasionally pleuritic chest pain. However, the character and duration of these symptoms may be useful to guide clinicians toward a particular diagnosis. For example, most patients with bacterial bronchitis or pneumonia present with cough productive of purulent sputum, whereas most patients with PCP have a dry, nonproductive cough.[1] Bacterial pneumonias caused by S pneumoniae and Haemophilus spp characteristically present abruptly with patients reporting 3 to 5 days of symptoms; however, PCP often presents with an insidious onset with patients noting 2 to 4 weeks of symptoms.[2]

Constitutional symptoms, such as fever, night sweats, and weight loss, may indicate the presence of a systemic or disseminated disease. Fever and weight loss may be the sole presenting complaints of disseminated mycobacterial or fungal disease or may be "B symptoms" associated with non-Hodgkin lymphoma (NHL).

Patients infected with HIV are predisposed to systemic dissemination of infections that originated in the lungs and the symptoms and signs associated with disseminated disease may dominate the clinical presentation. Bacterial pneumonia caused by S pneumoniae is often accompanied by bacteremia and septicemia in patients infected with HIV with CD4 counts less than 200 cells/μL and thus the clinical presentation may be that of sepsis and multiorgan system dysfunction. Similarly, tuberculosis (TB) is often accompanied by mycobacteremia in patients infected with HIV with CD4 counts less than 200 cells/μL, and patients infected with HIV with advanced HIV/AIDS are more likely to present with extrapulmonary TB and disseminated disease than patients uninfected with HIV.[3] Meningitis is a well-described acute presentation of TB and 43% to 65% of these patients are infected with HIV with CD4 counts less than 200 cells/μL.[4] In patients with tuberculous meningitis, clinical syndromes range from those mimicking typical bacterial meningitis to a nonspecific, subacute illness characterized by fever and headache.

Although the lungs are the portal of entry for Cryptococcus neoformans, patients are often minimally symptomatic until the infection has spread to the central nervous system (CNS). In a series of 106 patients with C neoformans infection, 84% presented with meningitis; cough or dyspnea was present in less than a third (N = 28; 31%).[5] The signs of extrapulmonary infection, including meningoencephalitis and cutaneous lesions (which resemble the lesions caused by molluscum contagiosum), should be recognized in attempting to establish a unifying diagnosis. Histoplasmosis may present with hypotension, hepatosplenomegaly, pancytopenia, hypoadrenalism, and necrotic skin and oral lesions.[6] Dissemination of coccidioidomycosis to extrapulmonary sites may result in cutaneous and soft tissue infection, lymph node involvement, osteomyelitis, arthritis, and meningitis.[7] Blastomycosis can disseminate into the skin, genitourinary tract, bone, and, rarely, the CNS.

CNS presentations typically dominate the presentations of Toxoplasma gondii and cytomegalovirus (CMV). For Toxoplasma, encephalitis and retinochoroiditis are frequent presentations, whereas CMV most often presents with retinitis, esophagitis, and colitis. In both cases, pulmonary involvement occurs in only a subset of patients.

Patients with human herpes virus-8 and Epstein-Barr virus–related malignancies tend to present with symptoms of systemic disease. Most commonly, patients with pulmonary Kaposi sarcoma (KS) have previously recognized cutaneous lesions or other visceral involvement; nonetheless, cutaneous involvement is absent in 5% to 23% of patients with symptomatic pulmonary KS.[8,9] The most common respiratory symptoms are progressive dyspnea, nonproductive cough, and fever. Patients with NHL typically present with "B symptoms" including fever, night sweats, and weight loss. Most of those with pulmonary involvement have respiratory symptoms, which vary depending on extent of parenchymal or pleural involvement. Patients with multicentric Castleman disease typically have fever and lymphadenopathy, splenomegaly, and hepatomegaly. Involvement of the respiratory system occurs in about one-third of patients and is characterized by lymphocytic interstitial pneumonitis.[10] The symptoms associated with primary effusion lymphoma (PEL) depend on the serosal surface affected; commonly affected serosal surfaces include the pleura (60%–90%); the pericardium (0%–30%); the peritoneum

(30%–60%); joint spaces; and, rarely, the meninges.[11,12] Most affected patients present with symptoms related to fluid accumulation, such as dyspnea (from pleural or pericardial effusions); abdominal distention (from ascites); or joint swelling.

Pulmonary manifestations of the immune reconstitution inflammatory syndrome (IRIS) depend on the underlying infectious, neoplastic, or autoimmune pathology.[13] The risk of IRIS is associated with the CD4 count at the start of ART, with a higher risk in patients infected with HIV with CD4 less than 50 cells/μL.[14] IRIS associated with TB (TB-IRIS) presents with fever, cough, dyspnea, lymph node enlargement, and new or worsening parenchymal opacities or new or enlarging pleural effusions on chest radiograph.[13,15] New or worsening tuberculous meningitis, granulomatous hepatitis, and subcutaneous or deep tissue abscesses are common extrapulmonary TB-IRIS presentations. Nontuberculous mycobacteria (eg, *Mycobacterium avium* complex) can also produce IRIS. In the lungs, these organisms commonly cause endobronchial disease; other manifestations include masses and cavitary lesions.[13,16] PCP-IRIS presents with symptoms seen in acute PCP including fever, dry nonproductive cough, and dyspnea, although development of organizing pneumonia has also been described.[16–18] Occasionally, PCP-IRIS is severe and patients develop acute respiratory failure.[19] Although paradoxic cryptococcal-IRIS predominantly affects the CNS, lung involvement is also well-described. Unlike TB-IRIS, which is rarely fatal, cryptococcal-IRIS has a mortality rate as high as 83%.[20–24] KS-associated IRIS usually presents with inflammation or enlargement of existing skin lesions, new skin lesions, and mucosal involvement; however, pulmonary deterioration is also common.[25] Pulmonary sarcoidosis can worsen in the setting of immune reconstitution and result in clinical and radiographic findings similar to those seen in patients uninfected with HIV.[26,27]

As extent of immunosuppression decreases in the era of ART, it is important to consider noninfectious pulmonary diseases in patients infected with HIV. Because of higher rates of tobacco and drug use in persons infected with HIV, and possibly because of HIV infection itself, COPD, lung cancer, and pulmonary arterial hypertension (PAH) are more common in persons infected with HIV.[28–31] Patients with COPD often complain of dyspnea and chronic cough; in the setting of an acute exacerbation these patients present with worsening shortness of breath, wheezing, and increased sputum production. Most patients with lung cancer complain of cough, especially those with endobronchial involvement; some also complain of hemoptysis, chest pain, and dyspnea caused by parenchymal or pleural involvement. Less frequent presentations of underlying lung cancer include superior vena cava syndrome and Pancoast syndrome. Superior vena cava syndrome typically causes a sensation of head fullness because of compression of the superior vena cava, whereas Pancoast syndrome is characterized by shoulder pain, Horner syndrome, and local tissue destruction caused by tumor at the apex of the lung. Most patients with PAH initially experience dyspnea, decreased exercise tolerance, and fatigue caused by an inability to increase cardiac output with exertion. As the PAH progresses and right ventricular failure develops, angina, syncope, and peripheral edema may develop.

CD4 COUNT

The CD4 count should be used to assess a patient's susceptibility to opportunistic infections and neoplasms (**Table 1**). Ideally, the CD4 count will have been obtained before the onset of

Table 1
CD4 count ranges for respiratory diseases

CD4 Count	Lower Respiratory Illness
Any	Acute bronchitis
	Bacterial pneumonia
	Tuberculosis
	Non-Hodgkin lymphoma
	Pulmonary embolus
	Bronchogenic carcinoma
	Chronic obstructive pulmonary disease
	Pulmonary arterial hypertension
≤500 cells/μL	Recurrent bacterial pneumonia
≤200 cells/μL	*Pneumocystis* pneumonia
	Cryptococcus neoformans pneumonia
	Sepsis secondary to bacterial pneumonia
	Disseminated or extrapulmonary tuberculosis
≤100 cells/μL	Pulmonary Kaposi sarcoma
	Toxoplasma pneumonitis
≤50 cells/μL	Disseminated *Histoplasma capsulatum*
	Disseminated *Coccidioides immitis*
	Aspergillus pneumonia
	Cytomegalovirus pneumonitis
	Disseminated nontuberculous mycobacterial pneumonia

pneumonia because the CD4 count is often decreased in the setting of an acute illness. Although bacterial pneumonia can occur at any CD4 count, Hirschtick and colleagues[32] in the Pulmonary Complications of HIV Infection Study (PCHIS) found that the risk of bacterial pneumonia was five times higher in subjects infected with HIV with CD4 counts less than 200 cells/μL compared with those with more than 500 cells/μL. Furthermore, the incidence of bacteremia is also more common in patients infected with HIV and correlates with the extent of immunosuppression; the lower the CD4 count, the higher the incidence of bacteremia. Redd and colleagues[33] reviewed the incidence of pneumococcal bacteremia at 10 San Francisco hospitals during a 4-year period. They estimated that the rate of bacteremia in patients with pneumococcal pneumonia increased 100-fold since the onset of the HIV epidemic. Virulent, hospital-acquired, pathogens are also more common in adults infected with HIV; surveys have found that *Pseudomonas aeruginosa* accounts for 16% to 67% of nosocomial pneumonias and CD4 counts less than 100 cells/μL predispose patients to this infection.[34-36] Similar to bacterial pneumonia, TB can occur at any CD4 count. As with bacterial pneumonia accompanied by bacteremia, the incidence of TB accompanied by mycobacteremia also correlates with the extent of immunosuppression; the lower the CD4 count, the higher the incidence of mycobacteremia.

After the CD4 count falls to less than or equal to 200 cells/μL, PCP becomes a common cause of respiratory complaints. Stansell and the PCHIS showed that 95% of 145 cases of PCP occurred in patients with CD4 counts less than 200 cells/μL.[37] *C neoformans* is also a frequent cause of pneumonia in patients with CD4 counts less than 200 cells/μL. In addition, at CD4 counts less than or equal to 100 cells/μL, *T gondii* pneumonitis and pulmonary KS become more common. A study of 64 patients infected with HIV with pulmonary toxoplasmosis diagnosed by bronchoalveolar lavage (BAL) reported a mean CD4 count of 40 cells/μL, with 82% having a CD4 count less than or equal to 50 cells/μL and only 4% had counts greater than 200 cells/μL.[38] Another study of 168 patients infected with HIV with pulmonary KS diagnosed by bronchoscopy reported a median CD4 count of 19 cells/μL; 68% of patients had counts less than or equal to 50 cells/μL, and only 4% of patients had counts greater than 200 cells/μL.[8]

At CD4 counts less than or equal to 50 cells/μL, patients become susceptible to CMV; *Aspergillus* spp; and disseminated endemic fungal diseases, such as histoplasmosis and coccidioidomycosis. Although it is important to use the CD4 count to assess a patient's susceptibility to certain opportunistic infections, astute clinicians realize that these infections may still occur at CD4 counts above established guidelines.

LABORATORY TESTS

Arterial blood gas analysis can be used to guide treatment decisions and is a useful prognostic tool. Patients with significant hypoxemia should be hospitalized. PCP patients with a Pao_2 less than or equal to 70 mm Hg or an alveolar-arterial oxygen gradient greater than or equal to 35 mm Hg should be treated with adjunctive corticosteroids.

The serum lactate dehydrogenase (LDH) level is often elevated in patients with PCP; however, this marker is nonspecific and can also be elevated in other pneumonias including TB and bacterial pneumonia and in neoplasms, such as NHL. The diagnostic accuracy of serum LDH was assessed in a retrospective analysis of 328 immunocompromised patients, 105 with and 193 without PCP.[39] In patients uninfected with HIV with PCP, the sensitivity of an elevated LDH was 63% and the specificity was 43%. In patients infected with HIV, the sensitivity was 100% and the specificity was 47%. The overall accuracy of LDH for the diagnosis of PCP was 52%, 51% in patients who are HIV negative, and 58% in patients who are HIV positive. The sensitivity of LDH in other published studies ranges from 83% to 100% with the lowest sensitivity seen in the outpatient setting.[1]

The degree of LDH elevation correlates with prognosis and response to treatment.[1,40,41] A high or rising serum LDH value despite PCP treatment correlates with a worse prognosis, a failure of therapy, and increased mortality. A low or declining serum LDH value on PCP treatment correlates with a better prognosis, a response to therapy, and decreased mortality. However, significant overlap in serum LDH levels between survivors and nonsurvivors precludes use of this laboratory value as an absolute predictor of mortality in individual patients.[40]

The white blood cell count is often elevated in patients with bacterial pneumonia. This white blood cell count elevation may be relative to the patient's baseline value in an individual whose baseline white blood cell count is below the normal range. Laboratory evidence of hepatic or bone marrow involvement may be a sign of extrapulmonary involvement from disseminated opportunistic infection or malignancy (eg, TB, NHL). The presence of these laboratory abnormalities may be important clues to the pulmonary diagnosis.

CHEST IMAGING

The chest radiographic appearance of pulmonary disease varies widely in patients infected with HIV and is dependent on the cause and severity of pulmonary disease and the degree of immuno-suppression. Although chest radiographs are the foundation of the evaluation of respiratory disease in persons infected with HIV and are the appropriate initial test for suspected pneumonia, chest computed tomography (CT) is often useful to identify and to more precisely define nodules, cavities, lymphadenopathy, and pleural fluid collections that may require drainage.[42,43]

Bacterial Pneumonia

Bacterial pneumonia most commonly presents with focal or multifocal areas of consolidation regardless of CD4 count (**Fig. 1**).[32,44] The typical chest radiographic appearance includes unilateral, lobar, or segmental consolidation; however, as immune function deteriorates, multilobar and bilateral radiographic disease becomes more common. Pleural effusions are present in 12% to 47% of patients with bacterial pneumonia[45,46] and empyemas develop in 2% to 6%.[47,48]

Similarly to their counterparts uninfected with HIV, S pneumoniae is the most common causative pathogen of bacterial pneumonia in patients with HIV. Rizzi and colleagues[49] described the chest radiographic appearance of pneumococcal lung disease in 57 patients infected with HIV, in whom

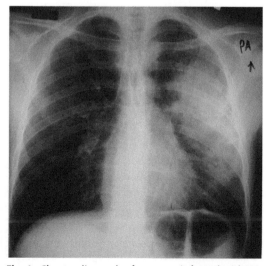

Fig. 1. Chest radiograph of a person infected with HIV with multilobar consolidation caused by *Streptococcus pneumoniae* detected in two blood cultures. (*Courtesy of* Laurence Huang, MD, San Francisco, CA.)

S pneumoniae was the sole respiratory pathogen isolated. Lobar consolidation was found in 40% of patients, multifocal distribution in 25%, and interstitial pattern of disease in 17.5%; pleural effusions were identified in 23% of patients, 62% of whom had CD4 counts less than 200 cells/μL.

Bacterial infections may also present with pulmonary nodules. Franquet and colleagues[50] reviewed 78 chest high-resolution CT (HRCT) scans of immunocompromised patients (25 of who had AIDS) with infectious pulmonary nodules. A total of 20 patients had bacterial infection and 95% of them had multiple pulmonary nodules greater than 10 mm in diameter. Nodules caused by bacterial pneumonia can cavitate; this is especially common with such pathogens as P aeruginosa and S aureus.[51] Less common bacterial causes of cavitary nodules or cavitary consolidation include Rhodococcus equi and Nocardia asteroides. R equi typically manifests as an area of consolidation limited to one lobe, usually an upper lobe, which may undergo cavitation with an air-fluid level.[52] The most common radiographic presentation of Nocardia is similar to TB and R equi, a lobar or multilobar consolidation with an upper lobe predominance and frequent cavitation.[53]

Tuberculosis

Pulmonary TB is commonly divided into primary infection and post primary infection. Primary infection refers to the development of active TB within 5 years after initial exposure; post primary infection refers to reactivation of latent TB. The radiographic appearance of pulmonary TB is largely dependent on the degree of immunosuppression.[54] Similar to immunocompetent persons, TB in patients infected with HIV with relatively intact immunity appears radiographically as opacity in the apical and posterior segments of the upper lobe and superior segment of the lower lobe. Cavitation is often present (**Fig. 2**). As immune function deteriorates (CD4 count <200 cells/μL), middle and lower lung involvement and disseminated disease (including a miliary pattern) become more common (**Fig. 3**). Cavitation is less common at this point because the host lacks the ability to mount an effective immune response against M tuberculosis. Mediastinal or hilar lymphadenopathy and pleural effusions are common in patients infected with HIV with low CD4 counts. Normal chest radiographic findings in patients infected with HIV with acid-fast bacillus smear-positive pulmonary TB have been reported in the range of 6% to 14%; most of these patients had CD4 cell counts less than 200 cells/μL.[55,56]

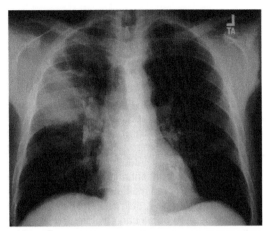

Fig. 2. Chest radiograph of a person infected with HIV, CD4 cell count greater than 200 cells/μL, revealing right upper lobe consolidation with areas of cavitation. Sputum acid-fast bacillus stain was positive and sputum cultures grew *Mycobacterium tuberculosis*. (*Courtesy of* Laurence Huang, MD, San Francisco, CA.)

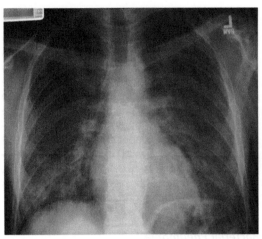

Fig. 4. Chest radiograph of a person infected with HIV, CD4 cell count less than 200 cells/μL, with bilateral, symmetric granular opacities caused by *Pneumocystis* pneumonia. Microscopic examination of bronchoscopy with bronchoalveolar lavage fluid demonstrated characteristic *Pneumocystis* cystic and trophic forms. (*Courtesy of* Laurence Huang, MD, San Francisco, CA.)

Pneumocystis Pneumonia

Classically, PCP presents with a bilateral, symmetric, perihilar or diffuse interstitial, reticular, or granular pattern on chest radiograph (**Fig. 4**).[57] These opacities typically begin in the perihilar region and then spread outward as the disease progresses. However, patients may also have minimal chest radiographic extent of disease or even normal chest radiographs.[58] When the clinical suspicion of PCP is high and radiographic disease is minimal, a chest HRCT is often helpful to rule out the presence of disease.[59] Infection with *Pneumocystis jirovecii* induces extensive ground-glass attenuation on chest HRCT (**Fig. 5**) and the absence of ground-glass attenuation rules out

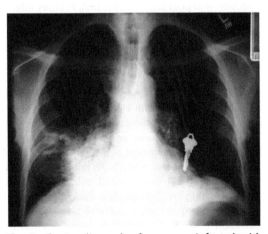

Fig. 3. Chest radiograph of a person infected with HIV, CD4 cell count less than 200 cells/μL, revealing right lower lung consolidation. Sputum acid-fast bacillus stains were negative but sputum cultures grew *Mycobacterium tuberculosis* that was mono-rifampin resistant. In this case, the key to the diagnosis of tuberculosis was knowledge of the patient's CD4 cell count and an understanding that tuberculosis can present with this pattern in individuals infected with HIV with advanced immunosuppression. (*Courtesy of* Laurence Huang, MD, San Francisco, CA.)

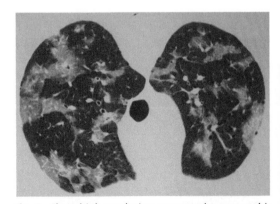

Fig. 5. Chest high-resolution computed tomographic (HRCT) scan of a person infected with HIV, CD4 cell count less than 200 cells/μL, with patchy ground-glass opacities caused by *Pneumocystis* pneumonia. Microscopic examination of induced sputum demonstrated characteristic *Pneumocystis* cystic and trophic forms. This individual's chest radiograph 1 day before chest HRCT was normal, demonstrating the increased sensitivity of chest HRCT compared with chest radiography for *Pneumocystis* pneumonia. (*Courtesy of* Laurence Huang, MD, San Francisco, CA.)

PCP.[59] The pattern of ground-glass is geographic in appearance with relatively normal secondary lobules adjacent to affected ones.

Other features of PCP include consolidation when the disease is severe, pneumatoceles that may be single or multiple in number and small or large in size, and pneumothorax. Pneumatoceles occur in up to one-third of patients with PCP. The presence of these thin-walled cysts predisposes patients to spontaneous pneumothoraces. Pleural effusions and intrathoracic lymphadenopathy are extremely uncommon chest radiographic presentations.

Cryptococcal Pneumonia

Cryptococcal pneumonia most often presents with a bilateral, reticular, or interstitial pattern on chest radiograph.[60] Other patterns of cryptococcal pneumonia include unilateral, reticular, or interstitial infiltrates; consolidation; nodular opacities; cavitation; pleural effusion; and intrathoracic adenopathy. Occasionally, patients with pulmonary cryptococcosis present with a mass-like cryptococcoma (**Fig. 6**).

Toxoplasma Pneumonia

Toxoplasma pneumonia most frequently presents with bilateral, reticular, or interstitial opacities on chest radiograph.[61] Occasionally, a reticulonodular or coarse nodular pattern is seen. Rarely, patients present with a chest radiographic picture of acute respiratory distress syndrome.

Viral Pneumonia

Unfortunately, it is often difficult to differentiate between viral and bacterial pneumonia based on diagnostic imaging.[62] In patients with viral pneumonia caused by typical respiratory pathogens, such as respiratory syncytial virus, adenovirus and influenza, chest CT scan findings can include bronchial wall thickening, ground-glass opacities (**Fig. 7**), multifocal consolidations, nodules or nodular opacities, and diffuse airspace disease.

KS, NHL, Multicentric Castleman Disease, and PEL

Although the gold standard for diagnosis of pulmonary KS remains direct visualization of typical endobronchial KS lesions by bronchoscopy (**Fig. 8**), there are certain patterns on chest imaging that are very suggestive.[63] On chest radiograph, bilateral, perihilar middle and lower lung zone infiltrates occur in most patients and coalescent nodular opacities are also common (**Fig. 9**). On CT, densities along the perivascular bundles (classically called "flame hemorrhages") are commonly seen as are pleural effusions. Nuclear scans can also be helpful diagnostic tools; KS does not take up gallium on scans but does seem to accumulate thallium. The presence of an abnormal chest radiograph, a negative gallium scan, and a positive thallium scan is suggestive of KS.[64] Thus, thallium and gallium scanning can be helpful in distinguishing KS from PCP and other infections.

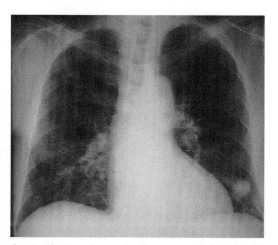

Fig. 6. Chest radiograph of a person infected with HIV, CD4 cell count less than 200 cells/μL, with left lower lobe lung mass that was initially concerning for lung cancer. CT-guided fine-needle aspiration revealed *Cryptococcus neoformans*. (*Courtesy of* Laurence Huang, MD, San Francisco, CA.)

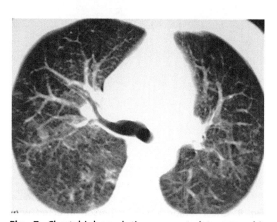

Fig. 7. Chest high-resolution computed tomographic scan of a person infected with HIV, CD4 cell count less than 50 cells/μL, with patchy ground-glass opacities caused by cytomegalovirus. The patient was initially thought to have *Pneumocystis* pneumonia but bronchoscopy with bronchoalveolar lavage was negative for *Pneumocystis* cystic and trophic forms. The patient then underwent video-assisted thoracoscopic surgical biopsy, which established the diagnosis of cytomegalovirus. (*Courtesy of* Laurence Huang, MD, San Francisco, CA.)

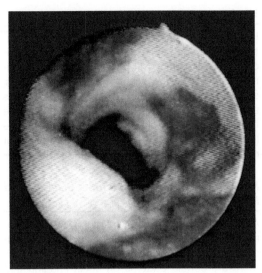

Fig. 8. Characteristic violaceous Kaposi sarcoma lesions seen in the trachea of a person infected with HIV, CD4 cell count less than 100 cells/µL. (*Courtesy of* Laurence Huang, MD, San Francisco, CA.)

Pulmonary NHL most often presents with single or multiple nodules, nodular opacities, or masses.[65] Lobar infiltrates and diffuse interstitial infiltrates have also been described. In patients

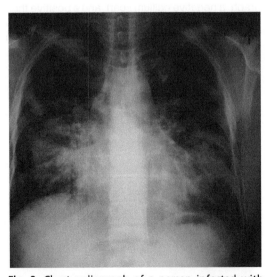

Fig. 9. Chest radiograph of a person infected with HIV, CD4 cell count less than 100 cells/µL, demonstrating the characteristic bilateral, middle and lower lung zone, perihilar or central distribution of abnormalities of pulmonary Kaposi sarcoma. This individual had no evidence of mucocutaneous Kaposi sarcoma and the diagnosis of pulmonary Kaposi sarcoma was established by bronchoscopy with visualization of multiple, characteristic Kaposi sarcoma lesions (see **Fig. 8**). (*Courtesy of* Laurence Huang, MD, San Francisco, CA.)

with Multicentric Castleman Disease and resultant lymphocytic interstitial pneumonitis, the main CT findings include poorly defined centrilobular nodules, thin-walled cysts, thickening of bronchovascular bundles, and interlobular septal thickening.[66] Chest radiographs and chest CTs in patients with primary effusion lymphoma show effusions (pleural or pericardial); slight serosal thickening; and the absence of parenchymal abnormalities, solid masses, or mediastinal enlargement.[11]

Noninfectious Pulmonary Disease

Appearance on imaging of COPD (**Fig. 10**), lung cancer, and PAH in patients infected with HIV mirrors that of their counterparts who are uninfected with HIV.[29–31]

DIAGNOSIS

In most cases, a confirmed microbiologic diagnosis is preferred to empiric therapy. A delayed or a missed diagnosis may have catastrophic consequences. That said, empiric therapy is usually indicated while a prompt diagnostic evaluation is undertaken.

Bacterial Pneumonia

Although bacteremia is 35 to 50 times more common in patients infected with HIV with bacterial

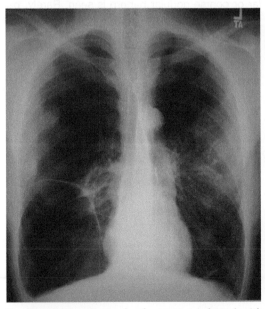

Fig. 10. Chest radiograph of a person infected with HIV with hyperinflation, flattened diaphragms, increased radiolucency of the lungs, and multiple, large bullae from severe chronic obstructive pulmonary disease. (*Courtesy of* Laurence Huang, MD, San Francisco, CA.)

pneumonia than patients uninfected with HIV, isolating the causative pathogen remains difficult. Hirschtick and colleagues[32] in PCHIS isolated the responsible pathogen in 33% of patients infected with HIV diagnosed with bacterial pneumonia. Blood cultures were positive in only 6.8% of patients; thus, most bacterial isolates came from either sputum or BAL cultures. The three most commonly identified organisms were S pneumoniae, S aureus, and Haemophilus influenzae. A study by Boulware and colleagues[67] suggests that urine pneumococcal C-polysaccharide antigen may be a useful diagnostic test in patients with pneumonia, especially in those with pneumonia caused by S pneumoniae. Among patients with pneumococcal pneumonia, this antigen had a sensitivity of 81%, a specificity of 98%, a positive predictive value of 98%, and a negative predictive value of 82%, independent of the person's HIV status. Despite low diagnostic yield of bacterial culture, blood and sputum cultures should be obtained in most patients infected with HIV because identifying the responsible pathogen can be used to guide antibiotic therapy.

Tuberculosis

Diagnosing pulmonary TB in subjects infected with HIV has been historically difficult because of the absence of rapid and sensitive diagnostic tools.[68] Acid-fast bacillus smear microscopy of expectorated sputum, a tool commonly used for the rapid diagnosis of pulmonary TB, has poor sensitivity (20%–50%)[69]; isolation of the organism in culture, the diagnostic gold standard, can take up to 8 weeks. Nevertheless, sputum should be collected for acid-fast bacillus smear and mycobacterial culture and blood mycobacterial cultures should be performed in patients infected with HIV with CD4 count less than 200 cells/μL.

A polymerase chain reaction (PCR) assay has been developed to rapidly detect M tuberculosis DNA and presence of rifampin resistance (Xpert MTB/RIF; Cepheid, Sunnyvale, CA).[70,71] In December 2010, the World Health Organization recommended Xpert MTB/RIF to be the initial screening test in patients with HIV and suspected TB. Using a single assay on a single unprocessed sputum sample, M tuberculosis complex–specific DNA was detected in 98% of smear-positive cases and in 72% of smear-negative cases using culture positivity as a reference standard.[70]

Pneumocystis Pneumonia

Patients with PCP most often present with a nonproductive cough and therefore diagnosis of PCP from sputum requires sputum induction.[72]

Analysis of induced sputum has a reported sensitivity ranging from 55% to 95%, with lower sensitivity reported in the earliest studies before routine centrifugation of sputum and higher sensitivity attributed to careful sample collection, concentration by centrifugation, and staining with fluorescent Pneumocystis antibodies.[73] In a San Francisco General Hospital and National Institutes of Health study, the use of sputum induction has led to definitive diagnoses in 80% to 95% of patients with PCP, thereby negating the need for bronchoscopy.[74]

Bronchoscopy with BAL is the gold standard for diagnosis of PCP with a sensitivity of up to 98%.[74,75] This procedure should be strongly considered in patients with a high suspicion of PCP and unrevealing induced sputum results or in medical facilities where induced sputum is unavailable or insensitive for diagnosis of PCP. Huang and colleagues[74] examined 992 cases of PCP diagnosed over a 4-year period and found only two cases that required transbronchial biopsy for final diagnosis; the remainder were diagnosed by either sputum induction or BAL (N = 800 and 190, accordingly). There is institutional variation in the sensitivity of sputum induction and bronchoscopy with BAL, thus the diagnostic protocol should be tailored to individual institutions.

1,3-β-D-glucan (BDG) is an element of the P jirovecii cyst wall (and the cell wall of most other fungal organisms) that has been studied as a marker of PCP infection. A meta-analysis that included 357 cases of PCP and 1723 control subjects (cases of invasive fungal infection were excluded) found that the average sensitivity and specificity of BDG were 94.8% (95% confidence interval, 90.8%–97.1%) and 86.3% (95% confidence interval, 81.7%–89.9%), respectively, and the area under the receiver operating characteristic curve was 0.965 (0.945–0.978).[76] Another study by the AIDS Clinical Trials Group Study A5164 Team found that median BDG in patients with PCP was 408 pg/mL, compared with 37 pg/mL in patients without PCP ($P<.001$); in this study the sensitivity of BDG (dichotomized at 80 pg/mL) was 92% and the specificity was 65%.[77] These findings suggest that BDG may be a clinically useful tool to identify patients with PCP, especially in clinical settings where bronchoscopy is unavailable. In some clinical centers, it may be a more sensitive test than induced sputum examination and could reduce the need for bronchoscopy and empiric therapy. In settings where other fungal pneumonias are common, however, the specificity of BDG may be low and diagnostic use may be limited.

Cryptococcal Pneumonia

Patients infected with HIV are predisposed to dissemination of fungal infections that originate in the lungs, thus fungal culture and occasionally biopsy of involved sites may be necessary. Cultures of cerebrospinal fluid, blood, BAL, and skin biopsies often yield a diagnosis of cryptococcosis. Serum cryptococcal antigen is positive in virtually all patients with HIV and pulmonary cryptococcal infection.[60] Because extrapulmonary disease is extremely common among patients infected with HIV with cryptococcal pneumonia, a positive serum cryptococcal antigen result should prompt investigation for disseminated disease with a work-up including fungal blood cultures, cerebral spinal fluid (CSF) CrAg, and CSF fungal cultures.

Histoplasmosis

Latent histoplasmosis can reactivate and disseminate in patients infected with HIV leading to involvement of extrapulmonary sites, such as the CNS, adrenal glands, mucocutaneous surfaces, and bone marrow. Tissue from these sites may be submitted for fungal culture in addition to blood, urine, and sputum and BAL cultures.[6] Urine *Histoplasma capsulatum* carbohydrate antigen is a valuable tool in diagnosis and in therapeutic monitoring of disseminated histoplasmosis.[78] Furthermore, a fourfold rise in antibody titer to *H capsulatum* can also be diagnostic in patients with acute and chronic pulmonary histoplasmosis.

Aspergillus

Aspergillus infection is rare in patients with HIV, but has been reported. Bronchoscopy with BAL is commonly used to make a diagnosis; however, the diagnostic yield of culture is low and results often take days to come back. Galactomannan antigen detection and real-time PCR assays of BAL fluid have been studied as adjunctive tests for the detection of invasive aspergillosis.[79] A study using a rabbit animal model of experimentally induced *Aspergillus fumigatus* infection confirmed the low sensitivity and high specificity of fungal culture (46% and 100%, respectively). In contrast, galactomannan antigen detection with enzyme immunoassay and quantitative PCR assays demonstrated higher sensitivities, with enzyme immunoassay being superior to PCR (100% and 80% sensitivity, respectively).[79] These findings are consistent with those reported in studies of galactomannan in BAL fluid in patients uninfected with HIV with invasive pulmonary aspergillosis.

Viral Pneumonia

Historically, viral pneumonia was diagnosed by culture or immunofluorescence microscopy of upper respiratory specimens (eg, nasopharyngeal aspirates) and lower respiratory samples (eg, induced sputum, tracheal aspirate, BAL fluid). Introduction of PCR has increased the ability to detect respiratory viruses, including those that are difficult to culture. Nasopharyngeal swabs have a higher sensitivity than throat swabs, but may be less sensitive than nasopharyngeal washes.[80] Transnasal nasopharyngeal flocked swabs also have high virus detection rates.[81] In general, PCR-based methods are between two and five times more sensitive than conventional diagnostic methods (culture, antigen detection, and serologic assays) for detection of respiratory viruses. This benefit applies particularly to adults and to the elderly, who might have a smaller nasopharyngeal viral load than children.

Establishing the diagnosis of CMV pneumonia in patients with AIDS is extremely difficult for several reasons. First, the clinical and radiographic findings overlap with other HIV-associated opportunistic pneumonias. Second, the virus may be cultured from pulmonary secretions in the absence of histologic evidence of disease. Third, CMV often coexists with other pulmonary pathogens.[82] Miles and colleagues[83] performed 120 BALs on 79 patients infected with HIV and detected CMV in 51.6% of cases; among 65 patients with PCP, CMV was detected in 40 (61.5%). In this study, there was no association between CMV detection and hypoxemia, abnormal chest radiograph, or increased mortality. Thus, the diagnosis of CMV pneumonitis cannot be based solely on detection of the virus in BAL fluid. To facilitate diagnosis, Waxman and colleagues[84] proposed the following diagnostic criteria for CMV pneumonia: (1) positive CMV cultures from both BAL and transbronchial biopsy specimens, (2) characteristic cytomegalic inclusion bodies from BAL and transbronchial biopsy specimens, and (3) absence of any other pulmonary pathogens. Unfortunately, although these diagnostic criteria improve the specificity of diagnosis, given the patchy nature of CMV-related pulmonary disease, sensitivity may be compromised.

Human Herpes Virus-8–associated Neoplasms: KS, Multicentric Castleman Disease, and PEL

The diagnosis of pulmonary KS is considered clinically confirmed if the characteristic endobronchial lesions of KS are seen at bronchoscopy.[8,85] Lung biopsy may be necessary to diagnose pulmonary KS if clinical, radiographic, or bronchoscopic picture is atypical. The diagnosis of multicentric

Castleman disease is made on tissue examination of a resected lymph node. These nodes are positive for human herpes virus-8 and 40% contain concurrent KS.[86] Pleural fluid cytology is almost always positive in PEL.

SUMMARY

The spectrum of HIV-associated pulmonary diseases is broad. Opportunistic infections, neoplasms, and, increasingly, noninfectious complications, such as COPD and lung cancer, are all major considerations. Thus, clinicians caring for persons infected with HIV must have a systematic approach. The approach begins with a thorough history and physical examination and often involves selected laboratory tests and a chest radiograph. Frequently, the clinical, laboratory, and chest radiographic presentation suggests a specific diagnosis or, at most, a few diagnoses, which then prompts specific diagnostic testing and treatment.

REFERENCES

1. Huang L, Stansell JD. AIDS and the lung. Med Clin North Am 1996;80:775–801.
2. Kovacs JA, Hiemenz JW, Macher AM, et al. *Pneumocystis carinii* pneumonia: a comparison between patients with the acquired immunodeficiency syndrome and patients with other immunodeficiencies. Ann Intern Med 1984;100:663–71.
3. Chaisson RE, Schecter GF, Theuer CP, et al. Tuberculosis in patients with the acquired immunodeficiency syndrome. Clinical features, response to therapy, and survival. Am Rev Respir Dis 1987; 136:570–4.
4. Jacob JT, Mehta AK, Leonard MK. Acute forms of tuberculosis in adults. Am J Med 2009;122:12–7.
5. Chuck SL, Sande MA. Infections with *Cryptococcus neoformans* in the acquired immunodeficiency syndrome. N Engl J Med 1989;321: 794–9.
6. Wheat LJ, Connolly-Stringfield PA, Baker RL, et al. Disseminated histoplasmosis in the acquired immune deficiency syndrome: clinical findings, diagnosis and treatment, and review of the literature. Medicine (Baltimore) 1990;69:361–74.
7. Fish DG, Ampel NM, Galgiani JN, et al. Coccidioidomycosis during human immunodeficiency virus infection. A review of 77 patients. Medicine (Baltimore) 1990;69:384–91.
8. Huang L, Schnapp LM, Gruden JF, et al. Presentation of AIDS-related pulmonary Kaposi's sarcoma diagnosed by bronchoscopy. Am J Respir Crit Care Med 1996;153:1385–90.
9. Cadranel J, Naccache J, Wislez M, et al. Pulmonary malignancies in the immunocompromised patient. Respiration 1999;66:289–309.
10. Mylona EE, Baraboutis IG, Lekakis LJ, et al. Multicentric Castleman's disease in HIV infection: a systematic review of the literature. AIDS Rev 2008;10: 25–35.
11. Nador RG, Cesarman E, Chadburn A, et al. Primary effusion lymphoma: a distinct clinicopathologic entity associated with the Kaposi's sarcoma-associated herpes virus. Blood 1996;88:645–56.
12. Simonelli C, Spina M, Cinelli R, et al. Clinical features and outcome of primary effusion lymphoma in HIV-infected patients: a single-institution study. J Clin Oncol 2003;21:3948–54.
13. Crothers K, Huang L. Pulmonary complications of immune reconstitution inflammatory syndromes in HIV-infected patients. Respirology 2009;14:486–94.
14. Muller M, Wandel S, Colebunders R, et al. Immune reconstitution inflammatory syndrome in patients starting antiretroviral therapy for HIV infection: a systematic review and meta-analysis. Lancet Infect Dis 2010;10:251–61.
15. Lawn SD, Wilkinson RJ, Lipman MC, et al. Immune reconstitution and "unmasking" of tuberculosis during antiretroviral therapy. Am J Respir Crit Care Med 2008;177:680–5.
16. Calligaro G, Meintjes G, Mendelson M. Pulmonary manifestations of the immune reconstitution inflammatory syndrome. Curr Opin Pulm Med 2011;17: 180–8.
17. Godoy MC, Silva CI, Ellis J, et al. Organizing pneumonia as a manifestation of *Pneumocystis jiroveci* immune reconstitution syndrome in HIV-positive patients: report of 2 cases. J Thorac Imaging 2008;23:39–43.
18. Mori S, Polatino S, Estrada-Y-Martin RM. *Pneumocystis*-associated organizing pneumonia as a manifestation of immune reconstitution inflammatory syndrome in an HIV-infected individual with a normal CD4+ T-cell count following antiretroviral therapy. Int J STD AIDS 2009;20:662–5.
19. Jagannathan P, Davis E, Jacobson M, et al. Life-threatening immune reconstitution inflammatory syndrome after *Pneumocystis* pneumonia: a cautionary case series. AIDS 2009;23:1794–6.
20. Lawn SD, Bekker LG, Myer L, et al. Cryptococcocal immune reconstitution disease: a major cause of early mortality in a South African antiretroviral programme. AIDS 2005;19:2050–2.
21. Kambugu A, Meya DB, Rhein J, et al. Outcomes of cryptococcal meningitis in Uganda before and after the availability of highly active antiretroviral therapy. Clin Infect Dis 2008;46:1694–701.
22. Murdoch DM, Venter WD, Feldman C, et al. Incidence and risk factors for the immune reconstitution inflammatory syndrome in HIV patients in

South Africa: a prospective study. AIDS 2008;22: 601–10.

23. Sungkanuparph S, Filler SG, Chetchotisakd P, et al. Cryptococcal immune reconstitution inflammatory syndrome after antiretroviral therapy in AIDS patients with cryptococcal meningitis: a prospective multicenter study. Clin Infect Dis 2009;49: 931–4.

24. Haddow LJ, Colebunders R, Meintjes G, et al. Cryptococcal immune reconstitution inflammatory syndrome in HIV-1-infected individuals: proposed clinical case definitions. Lancet Infect Dis 2010; 10:791–802.

25. Leidner RS, Aboulafia DM. Recrudescent Kaposi's sarcoma after initiation of HAART: a manifestation of immune reconstitution syndrome. AIDS Patient Care STDS 2005;19:635–44.

26. Morris DG, Jasmer RM, Huang L, et al. Sarcoidosis following HIV infection: evidence for CD4+ lymphocyte dependence. Chest 2003;124:929–35.

27. Foulon G, Wislez M, Naccache JM, et al. Sarcoidosis in HIV-infected patients in the era of highly active antiretroviral therapy. Clin Infect Dis 2004; 38:418–25.

28. Crothers K, Huang L, Goulet JL, et al. HIV infection and risk for incident pulmonary diseases in the combination antiretroviral therapy era. Am J Respir Crit Care Med 2011;183:388–95.

29. Morris A, George MP, Crothers K, et al. HIV and chronic obstructive pulmonary disease: is it worse and why? Proc Am Thorac Soc 2011;8:320–5.

30. Kirk GD, Merlo CA. HIV infection in the etiology of lung cancer: confounding, causality, and consequences. Proc Am Thorac Soc 2011;8:326–32.

31. Almodovar S, Hsue PY, Morelli J, et al. Pathogenesis of HIV-associated pulmonary hypertension: potential role of HIV-1 Nef. Proc Am Thorac Soc 2011;8:308–12.

32. Hirschtick RE, Glassroth J, Jordan MC, et al. Bacterial pneumonia in persons infected with the human immunodeficiency virus. Pulmonary Complications of HIV Infection Study Group. N Engl J Med 1995; 333:845–51.

33. Redd SC, Rutherford GW III, Sande MA, et al. The role of human immunodeficiency virus infection in pneumococcal bacteremia in San Francisco residents. J Infect Dis 1990;162:1012–7.

34. Meynard JL, Barbut F, Guiguet M, et al. Pseudomonas aeruginosa infection in human immunodeficiency virus infected patients. J Infect 1999;38: 176–81.

35. Manfredi R, Nanetti A, Ferri M, et al. Pseudomonas spp. complications in patients with HIV disease: an eight-year clinical and microbiological survey. Eur J Epidemiol 2000;16:111–8.

36. Sorvillo F, Beall G, Turner PA, et al. Incidence and determinants of Pseudomonas aeruginosa infection among persons with HIV: association with hospital exposure. Am J Infect Control 2001;29:79–84.

37. Stansell JD, Osmond DH, Charlebois E, et al. Predictors of Pneumocystis carinii pneumonia in HIV-infected persons. Pulmonary Complications of HIV Infection Study Group. Am J Respir Crit Care Med 1997;155:60–6.

38. Rabaud C, May T, Lucet JC, et al. Pulmonary toxoplasmosis in patients infected with human immunodeficiency virus: a French National Survey. Clin Infect Dis 1996;23:1249–54.

39. Vogel M, Weissgerber P, Goeppert B, et al. Accuracy of serum LDH elevation for the diagnosis of Pneumocystis jiroveci pneumonia. Swiss Med Wkly 2011;141:w13184.

40. Zaman MK, White DA. Serum lactate dehydrogenase levels and Pneumocystis carinii pneumonia. Diagnostic and prognostic significance. Am Rev Respir Dis 1988;137:796–800.

41. Garay SM, Greene J. Prognostic indicators in the initial presentation of Pneumocystis carinii pneumonia. Chest 1989;95:769–72.

42. Jasmer RM, Edinburgh KJ, Thompson A, et al. Clinical and radiographic predictors of the etiology of pulmonary nodules in HIV-infected patients. Chest 2000;117:1023–30.

43. Jasmer RM, Gotway MB, Creasman JM, et al. Clinical and radiographic predictors of the etiology of computed tomography-diagnosed intrathoracic lymphadenopathy in HIV-infected patients. J Acquir Immune Defic Syndr 2002;31:291–8.

44. Selwyn PA, Pumerantz AS, Durante A, et al. Clinical predictors of Pneumocystis carinii pneumonia, bacterial pneumonia and tuberculosis in HIV-infected patients. AIDS 1998;12:885–93.

45. Gil Suay V, Cordero PJ, Martinez E, et al. Parapneumonic effusions secondary to community-acquired bacterial pneumonia in human immunodeficiency virus-infected patients. Eur Respir J 1995;8:1934–9.

46. Afessa B, Green B. Bacterial pneumonia in hospitalized patients with HIV infection: the pulmonary complications, ICU support, and prognostic factors of hospitalized patients with HIV (PIP) Study. Chest 2000;117:1017–22.

47. Afessa B. Pleural effusion and pneumothorax in hospitalized patients with HIV infection: the pulmonary complications, ICU support, and prognostic factors of hospitalized patients with HIV (PIP) Study. Chest 2000;117:1031–7.

48. Miller RF, Howling SJ, Reid AJ, et al. Pleural effusions in patients with AIDS. Sex Transm Infect 2000;76:122–5.

49. Rizzi EB, Schinina V, Rovighi L, et al. HIV-related pneumococcal lung disease: does highly active antiretroviral therapy or bacteremia modify radiologic appearance? AIDS Patient Care STDS 2008; 22:105–11.

50. Franquet T, Muller NL, Gimenez A, et al. Infectious pulmonary nodules in immunocompromised patients: usefulness of computed tomography in predicting their etiology. J Comput Assist Tomogr 2003;27:461–8.

51. Aviram G, Fishman JE, Sagar M. Cavitary lung disease in AIDS: etiologies and correlation with immune status. AIDS Patient Care STDS 2001;15:353–61.

52. Muntaner L, Leyes M, Payeras A, et al. Radiologic features of *Rhodococcus equi* pneumonia in AIDS. Eur J Radiol 1997;24:66–70.

53. Kramer MR, Uttamchandani RB. The radiographic appearance of pulmonary nocardiosis associated with AIDS. Chest 1990;98:382–5.

54. Chamie G, Luetkemeyer A, Walusimbi-Nanteza M, et al. Significant variation in presentation of pulmonary tuberculosis across a high resolution of CD4 strata. Int J Tuberc Lung Dis 2010;14:1295–302.

55. Greenberg SD, Frager D, Suster B, et al. Active pulmonary tuberculosis in patients with AIDS: spectrum of radiographic findings (including a normal appearance). Radiology 1994;193:115–9.

56. Yoo SD, Cattamanchi A, Den Boon S, et al. Clinical significance of normal chest radiographs among HIV-seropositive patients with suspected tuberculosis in Uganda. Respirology 2011;16:836–41.

57. DeLorenzo LJ, Huang CT, Maguire GP, et al. Roentgenographic patterns of *Pneumocystis carinii* pneumonia in 104 patients with AIDS. Chest 1987;91:323–7.

58. Opravil M, Marincek B, Fuchs WA, et al. Shortcomings of chest radiography in detecting *Pneumocystis carinii* pneumonia. J Acquir Immune Defic Syndr 1994;7:39–45.

59. Gruden JF, Huang L, Turner J, et al. High-resolution CT in the evaluation of clinically suspected *Pneumocystis carinii* pneumonia in AIDS patients with normal, equivocal, or nonspecific radiographic findings. AJR Am J Roentgenol 1997;169:967–75.

60. Meyohas MC, Roux P, Bollens D, et al. Pulmonary cryptococcosis: localized and disseminated infections in 27 patients with AIDS. Clin Infect Dis 1995;21:628–33.

61. Pomeroy C, Filice GA. Pulmonary toxoplasmosis: a review. Clin Infect Dis 1992;14:863–70.

62. Miller WT Jr, Mickus TJ, Barbosa E Jr, et al. CT of viral lower respiratory tract infections in adults: comparison among viral organisms and between viral and bacterial infections. AJR Am J Roentgenol 2011;197:1088–95.

63. Gruden JF, Huang L, Webb WR, et al. AIDS-related Kaposi sarcoma of the lung: radiographic findings and staging system with bronchoscopic correlation. Radiology 1995;195:545–52.

64. Getz JM, Bekerman C. Diagnostic significance of Tl-201-Ga-67 discordant pattern of biodistribution in AIDS. Clin Nucl Med 1994;19:1117–8.

65. Eisner MD, Kaplan LD, Herndier B, et al. The pulmonary manifestations of AIDS-related non-Hodgkin's lymphoma. Chest 1996;110:729–36.

66. Do KH, Lee JS, Seo JB, et al. Pulmonary parenchymal involvement of low-grade lymphoproliferative disorders. J Comput Assist Tomogr 2005;29:825–30.

67. Boulware DR, Daley CL, Merrifield C, et al. Rapid diagnosis of pneumococcal pneumonia among HIV-infected adults with urine antigen detection. J Infect 2007;55:300–9.

68. Lawn SD, Zumla AI. Tuberculosis. Lancet 2011;378:57–72.

69. Getahun H, Harrington M, O'Brien R, et al. Diagnosis of smear-negative pulmonary tuberculosis in people with HIV infection or AIDS in resource-constrained settings: informing urgent policy changes. Lancet 2007;369:2042–9.

70. Boehme CC, Nabeta P, Hillemann D, et al. Rapid molecular detection of tuberculosis and rifampin resistance. N Engl J Med 2010;363:1005–15.

71. Boehme CC, Nicol MP, Nabeta P, et al. Feasibility, diagnostic accuracy, and effectiveness of decentralised use of the Xpert MTB/RIF test for diagnosis of tuberculosis and multidrug resistance: a multicentre implementation study. Lancet 2011;377:1495–505.

72. Huang L, Cattamanchi A, Davis JL, et al. HIV-associated *Pneumocystis* pneumonia. Proc Am Thorac Soc 2011;8:294–300.

73. Kovacs JA, Ng VL, Masur H, et al. Diagnosis of *Pneumocystis carinii* pneumonia: improved detection in sputum with use of monoclonal antibodies. N Engl J Med 1988;318:589–93.

74. Huang L, Hecht FM, Stansell JD, et al. Suspected *Pneumocystis carinii* pneumonia with a negative induced sputum examination. Is early bronchoscopy useful? Am J Respir Crit Care Med 1995;151:1866–71.

75. Golden JA, Hollander H, Stulbarg MS, et al. Bronchoalveolar lavage as the exclusive diagnostic modality for *Pneumocystis carinii* pneumonia. A prospective study among patients with acquired immunodeficiency syndrome. Chest 1986;90:18–22.

76. Karageorgopoulos DE, Qu JM, Korbila IP, et al. Accuracy of beta-D-glucan for the diagnosis of *Pneumocystis jirovecii* pneumonia: a meta-analysis. Clin Microbiol Infect 2013;19:39–49.

77. Sax PE, Komarow L, Finkelman MA, et al. Blood (1->3)-beta-D-glucan as a diagnostic test for HIV-related *Pneumocystis jirovecii* pneumonia. Clin Infect Dis 2011;53:197–202.

78. Wheat LJ, Kohler RB, Tewari RP. Diagnosis of disseminated histoplasmosis by detection of *Histoplasma capsulatum* antigen in serum and urine specimens. N Engl J Med 1986;314:83–8.

79. Francesconi A, Kasai M, Petraitiene R, et al. Characterization and comparison of galactomannan enzyme immunoassay and quantitative real-time PCR assay for detection of *Aspergillus fumigatus* in bronchoalveolar lavage fluid from experimental invasive pulmonary aspergillosis. J Clin Microbiol 2006;44:2475–80.

80. Lieberman D, Shimoni A, Keren-Naus A, et al. Identification of respiratory viruses in adults: nasopharyngeal versus oropharyngeal sampling. J Clin Microbiol 2009;47:3439–43.

81. Johansson N, Kalin M, Tiveljung-Lindell A, et al. Etiology of community-acquired pneumonia: increased microbiological yield with new diagnostic methods. Clin Infect Dis 2010;50:202–9.

82. Rodriguez-Barradas MC, Stool E, Musher DM, et al. Diagnosing and treating cytomegalovirus pneumonia in patients with AIDS. Clin Infect Dis 1996;23:76–81.

83. Miles PR, Baughman RP, Linnemann CC Jr. Cytomegalovirus in the bronchoalveolar lavage fluid of patients with AIDS. Chest 1990;97:1072–6.

84. Waxman AB, Goldie SJ, Brett-Smith H, et al. Cytomegalovirus as a primary pulmonary pathogen in AIDS. Chest 1997;111:128–34.

85. Meduri GU, Stover DE, Lee M, et al. Pulmonary Kaposi's sarcoma in the acquired immune deficiency syndrome. Clinical, radiographic, and pathologic manifestations. Am J Med 1986;81:11–8.

86. Oksenhendler E, Duarte M, Soulier J, et al. Multicentric Castleman's disease in HIV infection: a clinical and pathological study of 20 patients. AIDS 1996;10:61–7.

HIV-Associated Bacterial Pneumonia

Charles Feldman, MB BCh, DSc, PhD, FRCP[a],*,
Ronald Anderson, PhD[b]

KEYWORDS

- CD4 cell count • Community-acquired bacterial pneumonia • ART • HIV infection • Mortality
- Smoking • Treatment • Vaccination

KEY POINTS

- Community-acquired bacterial pneumonia (CAP) remains one of the most common opportunistic infections in patients who are infected with the human immunodeficiency virus (HIV), despite the use of cotrimoxazole prophylaxis and even the introduction of combination antiretroviral therapy (ART).
- The pathologic changes that occur in the immune system as a consequence of HIV infection explain the mechanisms associated with the increased risk of CAP.
- The clinical features of CAP in HIV-infected persons are similar to those in HIV-uninfected persons.
- Although the diagnostic workup of HIV-infected patients with CAP is similar to that of HIV-uninfected patients, use of the newer rapid laboratory techniques has expedited the diagnosis of these infections.
- Not only does the mortality remain high in HIV-infected persons with CAP but the occurrence of CAP is also associated with a permanent decline in lung function in these patients.
- Prevention of CAP remains critical and necessitates a comprehensive approach addressing, among many other factors, cigarette smoking cessation strategies, ART adherence, and immunization against those infections for which effective vaccinations are available.

INTRODUCTION

The respiratory tract is recognized to be the site most critically affected as a consequence of human immunodeficiency virus (HIV) infection/AIDS.[1] Although in the initial phase of the epidemic the lung was involved in almost 100% of the cases, currently, in the era of combination ART, it is involved in some 70% of the patients.[1] Pulmonary infections are the major component of these complications, with lower respiratory tract infections being 25-fold more common than in the general population. Respiratory infections in general, rather than only AIDS-related opportunistic infections, remain a major cause of morbidity and mortality and reason for hospital admission.[1] The spectrum of pathogens causing pulmonary infections in HIV-infected persons is vast, differs in various geographic areas, and has changed over the evolution of the epidemic because of the

Charles Feldman is supported by the National Research Foundation (NRF), South Africa.
[a] Division of Pulmonology, Department of Internal Medicine, Charlotte Maxeke Johannesburg Academic Hospital and Faculty of Health Sciences, University of the Witwatersrand, 7 York Road, Parktown, 2193, Johannesburg, South Africa; [b] Medical Research Council Unit for Inflammation and Immunity, Department of Immunology, Faculty of Health Sciences, University of Pretoria and Tshwane Academic Division of the National Health Laboratory Service, Pretoria, South Africa
* Corresponding author. Division of Pulmonology, Department of Internal Medicine, University of the Witwatersrand Medical School, 7 York Road, Parktown, 2193, Johannesburg, South Africa.
E-mail address: charles.feldman@wits.ac.za

Clin Chest Med 34 (2013) 205–216
http://dx.doi.org/10.1016/j.ccm.2013.01.006
0272-5231/13/$ – see front matter © 2013 Elsevier Inc. All rights reserved.

chestmed.theclinics.com

introduction of cotrimoxazole prophylaxis and ART.[1] The 3 most common infections, namely, tuberculosis (TB), bacterial pneumonia, and *Pneumocystis* pneumonia (PCP), have been documented to result in a worse course of HIV disease, as well as permanent impairment in lung function.[1]

EPIDEMIOLOGY, PATHOGENESIS, AND RISK FACTORS FOR BACTERIAL PNEUMONIA

Epidemiology

Although CAP is usually described as the most frequent pulmonary infection in HIV-infected individuals followed by PCP and TB, the relative prevalences of these 3 infections vary in different geographic regions.[1] In the early phases of the epidemic, PCP was the most common infection overall, but this has decreased considerably in incidence as a consequence of the use of cotrimoxazole prophylaxis initially, and subsequently the introduction of ART.[1] In Africa, for example, TB is the most common pulmonary infection, whereas in the United States and Western Europe, CAP is the most common.[1] Bacterial pneumonia is also the most common admission diagnosis in patients with HIV infection and occurs with a more than 10-fold increased risk of frequency.[1] The risk for the development of each of these infections is also influenced by the degree of immunosuppression of the patients, their demographic characteristics, their places of residence, their use of prophylaxis, and possibly genetic influences.[1]

Pathogenesis

The human lung, with its highly organized network of mediastinal lymph nodes, is a major target of HIV infection.[2,3] Relative to the gastrointestinal tract, however, the rate of immune attrition in the lungs is considerably slower.[4–6] There are several reasons for this, including (1) the mediastinal lymph nodes are the primary sites of T-cell antigen priming in the lung, with secondary bronchus-associated lymphoid tissue being much less prominent than that of the gut-associated secondary lymphoid tissue[4,7,8]; (2) the diversity and efficacy of the innate immune mechanisms of the airways[9]; (3) the relative resistance of lung CD4$^+$ T cells of the Th1[5] and Th17[6] subtypes, as well as alveolar macrophages,[10] to productive infection with and depletion by HIV; and (4) initiation of a vigorous anti-HIV response mediated by antigen-specific CD8$^+$ cytotoxic T cells, as well as natural killer (NK) cells and NKT cells.[3]

Spread of HIV to the lungs is achieved by several mechanisms including (1) infection of hematopoietic progenitor cells, especially those that differentiate into monocytes; these, in turn, mature into alveolar macrophages and myeloid dendritic cells (DCs) following trafficking to the lungs[11]; (2) capture of HIV by DC-specific intercellular adhesion molecule grabbing integrin (DC-SIGN) by monocytes and immature DCs, predominantly myeloid DCs, in blood[12,13]; (3) infection of these cells, as well as plasmacytoid DCs, with HIV via CD4/CCR5 interactions, albeit at low level[14,15]; and (4) acquisition of the integrins LFA-1 and VLA-4 by HIV during budding from infected cells, promoting attachment to and productive infection of vascular endothelial cells.[16,17]

In spite of the relative resistance of the lungs to HIV-mediated immune attrition, progressive infection inevitably affects negatively the numbers and functions of pulmonary CD4$^+$ T cells, and respiratory infections are the leading cause of mortality in HIV/AIDS. As is the case in other tissues, the CD4/CCR5 coexpressing T cells of the effector/memory phenotype are the most vulnerable.[2–5] HIV-mediated depletion of CD4$^+$ T cells is a direct consequence of both productive virus infection[18] and induction of Fas-mediated apoptosis in both HIV-infected and uninfected cells.[19] In addition to these direct mechanisms of HIV-induced T-cell depletion, increasing evidence has implicated chronic activation of plasmacytoid DCs as being an indirect mechanism of T-cell dysfunction and cytotoxicity.[20,21] In this setting, pulmonary plasmacytoid DCs interact with HIV via CD4, resulting in internalization of the virus. In the cell cytoplasm, viral RNA is recognized by the intracellular pathogen nucleic acid recognition receptors, Toll-like receptor (TLR)-7 and TLR-9,[20–23] and possibly by the more recently described cytoplasmic pathogen nucleic acid sensors.[24] This recognition leads, in turn, to excessive and sustained production of (1) type I interferon (IFN), especially IFN-α; (2) the tryptophan catabolizing enzyme, indoleamine 2,3-dioxygenase; and (3) the cytokine, transforming growth factor β (TGF-β), all of which contribute to immune dysfunction.[20,25–33] These immunosuppressive mechanisms are summarized in **Table 1**. With respect to TGF-β-mediated profibrotic activity, extensive fibrosis of the T-cell zone of lymphoid tissue has been proposed to be a significant factor in the failure of T-cell reconstitution after initiation of ART, despite viral suppression.[33]

Pneumococcal pneumonia

The striking association of HIV infection with increased susceptibility for development of bacterial CAP, due in particular to *Streptococcus pneumoniae* (pneumococcus), is well recognized and has been the subject of several recent reviews.[3,34–36] This risk increases significantly with advanced

Table 1
Mechanisms by which HIV-mediated chronic activation of plasmacytoid dendritic cells contributes to dysfunction and depletion of T cells

Mechanism	Consequence	References
Excessive production of IFN-α	Apoptosis of CD4$^+$ and CD8$^+$ T cells	25–28
Increased activity of indoleamine 2,3-dioxygenase	Acquisition of a tolerogenic phenotype with resultant suppression of T-cell responses	20
Acquisition of expression of CCR7	Enables migration of HIV-infected, activated plasmacytoid dendritic cells to lymphoid tissue	25
Increased synthesis of the cytokine TGF-β	Promotes (1) the generation of immunosuppressive CD4$^+$, CD25$^+$, and Foxp3$^+$ regulatory T cells and (2) collagen deposition in lymphatic tissues, resulting in disruption of architecture and failure to maintain T-cell populations	29–33

disease and associated immunosuppression and is further increased when HIV infection is associated with other risk factors.

The adaptive immune responses operative against the pneumococcus are extremely vulnerable to HIV-mediated suppression. Foremost among these are (1) the production of IgG and secretory IgA antibodies with opsonophagocytic and adherence-neutralizing properties, respectively, directed against capsular polysaccharides, and (2) the generation of CD4$^+$ T cells of the Th1 and Th17 subtypes, which target various protein antigens, resulting in production of the cytokines IFN-γ and interleukin (IL)-17A, respectively. IFN-γ promotes the activation of alveolar macrophages and neutrophil influx, whereas IL-17A promotes recruitment and activation of monocytes and neutrophils (reviewed in[37,38]). In the case of the former, the production and reactivity of capsular antibodies are compromised as a consequence of (1) depletion of CD154-expressing memory helper T cells of the Th1 and Th2 subtypes, which provide help to antibody producing B cells,[39] and (2) loss of antigen-specific memory B cells with advancing disease.[3] Progressive loss of Th1 and Th17 cells results from the mechanisms described in the preceding section. In addition, HIV-associated neutropenia and monocytopenia, as well as dysfunction of several of the protective activities of these cells, including chemotaxis to bacterial proteins, and antimicrobial activity, are potential contributors to predisposition to pneumococcal disease.[40,41]

Cigarette smoking may cause further impairment of innate and adaptive immune host defenses by compromising the protective activities of the mucociliary escalator, as well as those of alveolar macrophages and pulmonary T cells, underscoring the interactions between HIV infection and smoking in promoting colonization of the airways by the pneumococcus, a prerequisite for future development of invasive pneumococcal disease (reviewed in[42]). These various mechanisms that predispose HIV-infected patients to severe pneumococcal disease are shown in **Table 2**.

Table 2
HIV-mediated alterations in innate and adaptive immune mechanisms that predispose to severe pneumococcal disease

Abnormality	Mechanism	References
Decreased production and reactivity of anticapsular antibodies of the IgA and IgG classes, as well as antibodies to pneumococcal protein surface adhesins	Decreased numbers of Th1 and Th2 effector/memory cells, as well as antigen-specific T cells	37,38
Decreased mobilization and activation of neutrophils/monocytes/alveolar macrophages	Decreased production of IL-17 and IFN-γ due to loss of Th1 and Th17 cells, as well as to intrinsic defects in these cells	10,37–40
Decreased production of neutrophils and monocytes in the bone marrow	Dysfunction of progenitor cells	40,41

Haemophilus influenzae

Although less common than the pneumococcus, *H. influenzae*, usually nontypeable, is a major etiologic agent of pneumonia in HIV-infected individuals, being most evident in advanced disease when the total circulating CD4$^+$ T-cell count declines to less than 100 cells/µL.[43] The risk for development of invasive disease is around 100 times higher than that of HIV-uninfected persons of comparable age.[44]

Risk Factors

HIV infection is, by itself, a risk factor for pneumonia, and the incidence in infected persons is greater than in uninfected individuals, although the exact mechanisms are uncertain.[35,45] Although bacterial pneumonia can occur throughout the course of HIV infection, the stage of HIV infection is the most consistent risk factor.[46] The frequency of CAP has an inverse relationship with CD4 cell count, occurring most commonly when the CD4 cell count decreases; the median CD4 cell count when pneumonia occurs is often near 200 cells/mm^3,[1] although CAP becomes particularly more common in cases with a CD4 cell count less than 200 cells/mm^3.[47]

Among the specific risk factors for CAP in HIV-infected individuals are cigarette and illicit drug smoking and injection drug use (IDU). Cigarette smoking is associated with an increased risk of up to 5-fold.[1,46–48] Studies have suggested that cigarette smoking is associated with poorer virological and immunologic responses to ART, and this may explain, at least partly, why patients on ART have an ongoing increased risk of pneumonia.[34,49,50] Furthermore, smoking may also accelerate the progression to AIDS.[49,51] Numerous studies attest to the negative impact of cigarette smoking and the positive benefit of smoking cessation.[34,35,47,52,53] Additional risk factors for CAP include increased age; increased viral load and previous pneumonia; underlying comorbid conditions, including alcoholism, cirrhosis, asthma, cardiovascular disease, renal conditions, and sickle cell disease; malnutrition; and lower socioeconomic circumstances (**Box 1**).[46]

Effective control of the HIV viral load has a significant positive impact on decreasing the risk of pneumonia.[1] Few reports have documented the impact of ART on the occurrence of pneumonia.[1] There have been some reports suggesting that ART does decrease the prevalence, being particularly beneficial in patients with a CD4 cell count less than 200 cells/mm^3 and more effective with continuous rather than intermittent therapy,[1,52] but rates of pneumonia in patients on ART may still

> **Box 1**
> **Risk factors for bacterial CAP in HIV-infected patients**
>
> - Cigarette and illicit drug smoking
> - Injection drug abuse
> - Older age
> - Detectable HIV viral load
> - Lower CD4 cell count, especially less than 200 cells/µL
> - Previous pneumonia
> - Underlying comorbid conditions (including cardiovascular disease, renal disease, respiratory diseases, hepatic cirrhosis, and alcoholism)
> - Lower socioeconomic status
> - Potential genetic factors

be higher than in the general population.[35,54,55] One study documented a persistent high burden of invasive pneumococcal disease in HIV-infected adults, despite a stable prevalence of HIV and an increased rollout of ART.[56]

ETIOLOGY OF COMMUNITY-ACQUIRED BACTERIAL PNEUMONIA

An etiologic diagnosis is obtained in some 35% to 75% of HIV-infected patients with bacterial CAP.[35,46] In general, the bacterial cause of CAP is similar in HIV-infected and HIV-uninfected individuals (**Box 2**). Polymicrobial infections do occur, and coinfections with common bacterial pathogens and opportunistic pathogens, such as *Pneumocystis jirovecii* and even *Mycobacterium*

> **Box 2**
> **Bacterial cause of community-acquired pneumonia in HIV-infected persons**
>
> - Most common
>   - *S. pneumoniae*
>   - *H. influenzae*
> - Frequent
>   - *Staphylococcus aureus*
>   - *Klebsiella pneumoniae*
> - Less common
>   - Atypical pathogens
> - Uncommon/unusual infections
>   - *Rhodococcus equi*
>   - *Pseudomonas aeruginosa*

tuberculosis, have been described.[57] Bacteremia is more commonly noted with bacterial pneumonias, and relapses or recurrent infections have also been documented in HIV-infected patients.[1]

Streptococcus pneumoniae

S. pneumoniae is by far the most common cause of bacterial pneumonia in HIV-infected individuals, being implicated in some 20% of cases overall, 40% of cases in which a microbiological diagnosis is made, and 70% of cases with bacteremic pneumonias.[1,46,48] In several studies, such infections have been associated with an increased risk of bacteremia, and rates of invasive pneumococcal disease have been reported to be up to 100-fold higher than those of HIV-uninfected persons.[3,34–36,46,48]

Although recurrent infections are also commonly noted, there has been some data, although conflicting, suggesting that ART has not had a major impact on the incidence of CAP, and particularly invasive pneumococcal infections, as indicated elsewhere.[1,34] Thus, even in the post-combination ART era, the risk for development of invasive disease remains extremely high, being about 35-fold higher than that of the HIV-uninfected population.[3] There have also been conflicting data on the impact of prior pneumococcal vaccination on the subsequent risk for pneumococcal infections.[1]

Haemophilus influenzae

This pathogen is said to account for approximately 10% to 15% of cases of bacterial pneumonia of known microbiological cause.[1,46] It is more frequent among patients with advanced HIV disease and usually presents as a subacute infection.[1,43] Radiographic presentation is commonly a diffuse pulmonary infiltrate.[1,43] The mortality rate is not higher with this form of pneumonia than that occurring in the general population.[43]

Staphylococcus aureus

This pathogen is said to be the third most common cause of bacterial CAP,[1] accounting for some 5% of cases.[54] This infection is most common among persons with IDU, and such infections are associated with endocarditis, with or without septic pulmonary emboli, even in patients without prior evidence of cardiac valvular disease.[1] Recent viral, especially influenza, infection is also a risk factor for *S. aureus.*[45] HIV-infected persons are also at increased risk for community-acquired methicillin-resistant *S. aureus.*[58] When infections with *S. aureus* are suspected or proved, specific therapy needs to be initiated, but despite appropriate

treatment this infection is associated with a high mortality rate.[59]

Gram-Negative Pathogens

Gram-negative organisms currently account for approximately 5% of pneumonias in HIV-infected persons, particularly due to *P. aeruginosa.*[46,60] Both community-acquired and nosocomial pneumonia infections occur in HIV-infected patients, although infections other than pneumonia are also found.[60] In the precombination ART era, *P. aeruginosa* was a common cause of CAP, whereas currently, some studies have suggested that much fewer infections are caused by this microorganism.[1,60] Because pseudomonal infections occur especially among patients with advanced immunosuppression (CD4 cell counts <50 cells/mm^3), it follows that after the introduction of combination ART, these infections have become much less frequent.[1,51] The mortality rate for pneumonia caused by this microorganism is higher than that for the other, more common, bacterial pathogens.[60,61]

Atypical Pathogens

Although *Legionella* infections are uncommon, they seem to occur most often in patients with AIDS compared with the general population and may possibly be associated with a more severe clinical course and a worse prognosis.[1,62,63] Infections with *Mycoplasma pneumoniae* and *Chlamydia pneumoniae* seem to be uncommon causes of pneumonia in HIV-infected individuals, but there are no studies systematically evaluating their exact role.[1,45,51]

Other Infections

Several other, less common, bacterial infections also occur. For example, *R. equi* can cause pneumonia in HIV-infected persons, especially in cases with advanced immunosuppression, and this pathogen typically causes an infection with an indolent course, with clinical and even radiological features (eg, cavitation) mimicking those of pulmonary TB.[1,51,64] For the treatment of both these infections, early initiation of ART and the use of combination antimicrobial agents is recommended, which needs tailoring according to the antimicrobial sensitivity patterns of the cultured isolates.[1,64]

Moraxella catarrhalis may also cause pneumonia in HIV-infected patients, especially in those cases with a low CD4 cell count and/or coexisting respiratory diseases, and may be associated with considerable morbidity.[65] *Nocardia* is an aerobic actinomycete that can cause infections, including pneumonia, usually in association with immuno-suppression, including HIV infection.[66,67] The clinical course is often chronic, although dissemination can occur and be associated with a high mortality rate.[67] The diagnosis is frequently delayed, and a high index of suspicion is required.[67] Treatment with antimicrobial agents with proved synergy is recommended for initial therapy.[67]

CLINICAL PRESENTATION

In general, the clinical presentation of bacterial CAP in HIV-infected patients is similar to that occurring in cases that are not HIV infected.[1,35,45] Patients usually present with the typical features of a cough productive of sputum, fever, rigors, and chest pain together with focal consolidations in the lung.[45] Clinical differences noted include the facts that more cases are women, that the patients are younger and more likely to be drug users, and that they have a higher frequency of respiratory symptoms.[68] Presentation with pneumonia may be the first manifestation of underlying HIV infection; thus, particularly in young patients with pneumonia and no apparent risk factors, HIV infection should be considered.[45] There is a spectrum of disease severities, as in HIV-uninfected patients, and the commonly used severity of illness scoring indices, such as the Pneumonia Severity Index and the CURB-65 score, seem to be of equivalent value in predicting severity and/or outcome.[48] Pneumonia most commonly presents on radiograph as a lobar or segmental consolidation, although patchy consolidation may sometimes occur and occasionally the presentation is as a diffuse reticulonodular infiltrate, particularly in the case of H. influenzae infection that may mimic PCP.[1,51] Cavitation may be seen in the presence of P. aeruginosa, S. aureus, and R. equi infections.[1,45] Some studies have indicated a higher prevalence of complicated parapneumonic effusions with either S. pneumoniae or S. aureus in HIV-infected individuals.[45]

LABORATORY DIAGNOSIS OF BACTERIAL PNEUMONIA IN HIV/AIDS

Although the principles of laboratory diagnosis of pulmonary infection in the setting of HIV/AIDS are based on conventional microbiological, immunologic, radiological, and histologic strategies, interpretation is often complicated in advanced disease with atypical presentation. Furthermore, diagnostic strategies must be comprehensive and consider evaluation for other potential causes of pneumonia in addition to bacterial causes. For example, in the case of HIV/M. tuberculosis coinfection, acid-fast bacilli sputum positivity and cavitation and upper lobe infiltrates are less common in patients with severe immunosuppression,[69] necessitating the acquisition of more sensitive procedures for the rapid detection of mycobacterium tuberculosis (MTB) in smear-negative sputum or other body fluids. One of the most promising of these is the GeneXpert MTB/RIF (Cepheid, Sunnyvale, CA, USA), an automated molecular diagnostic procedure that has a reported sensitivity and specificity for the detection of mycobacterial DNA in sputum of 86% and greater than 97%, respectively.[70] IFN-γ-release assays have limited utility in the diagnosis of active TB in HIV-infected patients with advanced disease in a high prevalence setting such as sub-Saharan Africa.[71]

In the case of the pneumococcus, second only to M. tuberculosis as the major cause of opportunistic pneumonia in HIV-infected patients in the developing world,[69] confirmation of invasive disease has been improved by the acquisition of improved laboratory diagnostic procedures. Foremost among these are (1) quantitative real-time polymerase chain reaction procedures for the detection of pneumococcal DNA in biologic fluids and (2) the BinaxNOW (Binax Inc, Scarborough, ME, USA) S. pneumoniae immunochromatographic procedure, which detects the C-polysaccharide antigen in urine with good sensitivity and specificity in adult patients with invasive disease.[72]

Laboratory diagnosis of opportunistic pneumonia caused by P. jirovecii, the third most frequently encountered respiratory pathogen in HIV-infected patients in the developing world, is based on detection of the organism and/or its DNA using microscopy with specialized stains or molecular procedures, respectively.[69]

Multiplex, molecular analytical procedures for the detection of bacterial and fungal DNA in biologic fluids have become available. However, these are largely untested in the setting of advanced HIV infection in which interpretation may be complicated by the complexity of the lung microbiome, as well as by leakage of microbial nucleic acid from the gastrointestinal tract (GIT).[3,73] Additional in-depth discussions of the diagnostic evaluation of nonbacterial causes of pneumonia are covered in greater detail in accompanying articles in this issue of Clinics in Chest Medicine.

TREATMENT OF BACTERIAL CAP IN HIV-INFECTED PERSONS

Controversy exists regarding the appropriate diagnostic and treatment algorithms for patients with pulmonary infections in HIV-infected patients overall.[1] Although some have suggested that an aggressive invasive initial diagnostic approach should be followed, it is more commonly recommended that patients should initially be treated empirically. This approach should be based on epidemiologic evidence and current clinical and radiological features together with an aggressive noninvasive diagnostic approach. Thereafter, invasive techniques should be undertaken in patients not responding to initial therapy in whom the initial noninvasive diagnostic workup has not been helpful.[1] One such approach is illustrated in **Fig. 1**.[74] Although it is often recommended that

a CD4 cell count be performed as part of the diagnostic workup and may be helpful in indicating likely microbial cause, this is potentially of limited value, because several infections, including pneumococcal pneumonia, are associated with a transient and often substantial decrease in the CD4 cell count[1,34,75]; this is reinforced by at least one additional study indicating that the outcome of HIV-infected patients with CAP is not predicted by the CD4 cell count (or even HIV RNA levels) after adjusting for confounders.[76] However, others have suggested that the CD4 cell count should be

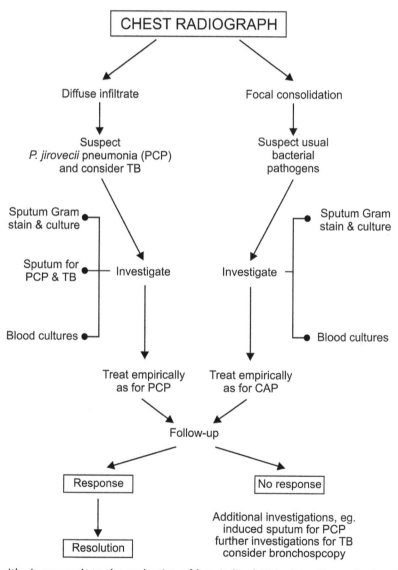

Fig. 1. An algorithmic approach to the evaluation of hospitalized HIV-seropositive patients with community-acquired pneumonia, based on the chest radiographic features. This approach needs to be considered in conjunction with the clinical features. (*Reproduced from* Feldman C. Bacterial pneumonia in the HIV-seropositive patient. CME 2001;19:390–4; with permission.)

considered as a crucial factor in the decision as to whether to admit HIV-infected patients with bacterial CAP to the hospital (**Fig. 2**).[35]

The treatment of bacterial CAP in HIV-infected patients is generally similar to that of patients not infected with HIV.[1,35,45] Antibiotic treatment should be directed at the most common bacterial pathogens and be modified according to subsequent microbiological findings.[1] Usual recommended treatment is the use of either a β-lactam–macrolide combination or fluoroquinolone monotherapy.[35,45,48] A large prospective multicenter international observational study of antibiotic treatment in patients with invasive pneumococcal disease (predominantly due to pneumonia) showed a positive impact of combination antibiotic therapy on outcome, even in the subset of patients who were HIV infected.[34] One consideration with the use of fluoroquinolones in areas where TB is common is that empiric use of these agents in patients suspected as having CAP, but who actually have TB, may potentially be associated with masking of the TB diagnosis and/or development of drug resistance in tuberculous microorganisms.[45]

OUTCOMES OF BACTERIAL PNEUMONIA

Although studies have indicated that the mortality of HIV-infected patients with bacterial pneumonia may reach 30%, most have indicated that mortality is in the range of 10% to 15%.[1] In the post-combination ART era, there seems to have been a decrease in mortality, most probably because infections with certain microbial pathogens (eg, gram-negative microorganisms) have become less common.[1] One area that has been particularly controversial, both in all-cause CAP and specifically in pneumococcal pneumonia, is whether the outcome is worse in HIV-infected versus HIV-uninfected persons.[1] Some studies have suggested that the outcome is no different,[1,77–79] whereas more recent studies in both all-cause CAP and pneumococcal pneumonia have suggested

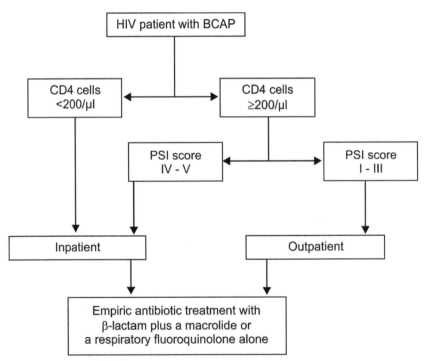

In HIV-infected patients with BCAP, CD4 cell count should be evaluated. Patients with a CD4 cell count of <200 cells/μl should be always hospitalized, whereas those with a CD4 count of at least 200 cells/μl could be managed according to PSI. Both inpatients and outpatients should start empiric antibiotic therapy with a β-lactam and a macrolide or a respiratory fluoroquinolone alone. BCAP, bacterial community-acquired pneumonia; PSI pneumonia severity index.

Fig. 2. Proposed flowchart for the management of HIV-infected patients with bacterial community-acquired pneumonia. (*Reproduced from* Maddedu G, Fiori ML, Mura MS. Bacterial community-acquired pneumonia in HIV-infected patients. Curr Opin Pulm Med 2010;16:201–7; with permission.)

that the mortality rate for CAP is higher in HIV-infected patients.[1,35,68] In one of these studies, which was in patients with bacteremic pneumococcal pneumonia, when cases were stratified according to age and severity of illness, HIV-infected patients had a higher mortality rate with a significant trend for increasing mortality in those with lower CD4 cell counts.[35,68] For this reason, some investigators have suggested that the CD4 cell count should be used as an indicator of the need for hospital admission of cases, as mentioned previously.[35]

Both bacterial pneumonia and PCP have been found to be associated with a more rapid decline in the immune status of HIV-infected persons.[2] Furthermore, a decline in lung function occurs (as measured by the forced expiratory volume in 1 s [FEV_1], the forced vital capacity [FVC], FEV_1/FVC ratio, and the diffusing capacity of the lung for carbon monoxide), which persists following infection.[80] This condition highlights the importance of the prevention of opportunistic infections in HIV-infected persons.

PREVENTION OF BACTERIAL CAP
General Measures

Given the considerable impact of bacterial CAP on HIV-infected patients, aggressive strategies should be implemented for the prevention of such infections. This strategy should be a comprehensive approach and include efforts to reduce drug and alcohol abuse, initiate and assist with smoking cessation strategies, and initiate either ART in those fulfilling the criteria for treatment or ART adherence support programs for those already on treatment.[48] These efforts should be combined with appropriate vaccination where available.

Immunoprophylaxis

Pneumococcal vaccine
As mentioned earlier, those infected with HIV are at extremely high risk for development of invasive pneumococcal disease, which persists, albeit at lesser magnitude, following implementation of ART. Pneumococcal vaccination strategies are clearly a priority in the setting of HIV infection, and the current status of these has been covered in several recent reviews.[34–36,38] In summary, early studies undertaken in various geographic regions in the pre/early combination ART period using the 23-valent pneumococcal polysaccharide vaccine were largely inconclusive with respect to efficacy. More recent studies undertaken in the postcombination ART era have, however, established major determinants of vaccine efficacy to

be timing of immunization, particularly in relation to concomitant initiation of ART; degree of immunosuppression; viral load; and presence of other risk factors, especially cigarette smoking.[34–36] According to Hibberd, as reported in UpToDate, the current recommendation of the Centers for Disease Control, National Institutes of Health, and the HIV Medicine Association of the Infectious Diseases Society of America with respect to pneumococcal immunization is "to administer pneumococcal vaccine to adults and children with CD4 counts of >200 μL/blood as soon as HIV infection is diagnosed, providing that they have not had the vaccine during the previous five years."[81,82] In those with CD4 counts of less than 200 cells/μL who had been previously immunized, revaccination could be considered when the CD4 count increases to 200 cells/μL or higher following implementation of ART.[81,82] To sustain efficacy, a single revaccination is recommended after 5 years for HIV-infected patients.[81,83]

Future prospects with respect to improved efficacy of immunization include the development of novel conjugate vaccines that use highly conserved, broadly serotype-unrestricted, recombinant surface and subsurface pneumococcal protein antigens as carriers of capsular polysaccharides.[37] Ideally, these should confer much broader coverage than current vaccines in the setting of induction of both cell-mediated (Th1/Th17-based) and humoral protective immune responses.[37,38]

Haemophilus influenzae vaccine
Most cases of severe H. influenzae infection in HIV-infected persons that occur with advanced immunosuppression involve nontypeable strains of this pathogen.[42] Accordingly, immunization of adults, unlike children, with H. influenzae type B (Hib) conjugate vaccine is not recommended,[80,82] although this situation may change with the development of novel vaccines based on conserved surface proteins.[84] In the case of children, both HIV-infected and HIV-uninfected, high rates of Hib conjugate vaccine failure have raised concerns about current immunization schedules.[85]

REFERENCES

1. Benito N, Moreno A, Miro JM, et al. Pulmonary infections in HIV-infected patients: an update in the 21st century. Eur Respir J 2012;39:730–45.
2. Morris A, Crothers K, Beck JM, et al. An official ATS workshop report: emerging issues and current controversies in HIV-associated pulmonary diseases. Proc Am Thorac Soc 2011;8:17–26.

3. Segal LN, Methé BA, Nolan A, et al. HIV-1 and bacterial pneumonia in the era of antiretroviral therapy. Proc Am Thorac Soc 2011;8:282–7.

4. Schacker T. The role of secondary lymphatic tissue in immune deficiency of HIV infection. AIDS 2008; 22(Suppl 3):S13–8.

5. Brenchley JM, Knox KS, Asher AI, et al. High frequencies of polyfunctional HIV-specific T cells are associated with preservation of mucosal CD4 T cells in bronchoalveolar lavage. Mucosal Immunol 2008;1:49–58.

6. Brenchley JM, Paiardini M, Knox KS, et al. Differential Th 17 CD4 T-cell depletion in pathogenic and nonpathogenic lentiviral infections. Blood 2008; 112:2826–35.

7. Lefrançois L, Puddington L. Intestinal and pulmonary mucosal T cells: local heroes fight to maintain the status quo. Annu Rev Immunol 2006;24:681–704.

8. Moyron-Quiroz J, Rangel-Moreno J, Carragher DM, et al. The function of local lymphoid tissues in pulmonary immune responses. Adv Exp Med Biol 2007;590:55–68.

9. Parker D, Prince A. Innate immunity in the respiratory epithelium. Am J Respir Cell Mol Biol 2011;45: 189–201.

10. Collini P, Noursadeghi M, Sabroe I, et al. Monocyte and macrophage dysfunction as a cause of HIV-1 induced dysfunction of innate immunity. Curr Mol Med 2010;10:727–40.

11. Alexaki A, Wigdahl B. HIV-1 infection of bone marrow hematopoietic progenitor cells and their role in trafficking and viral dissemination. PLoS Pathog 2008;4(12):e1000215.

12. van Kooyk Y, Geijtenbeek TB. DC-SIGN: escape mechanism for pathogens. Nat Rev Immunol 2003; 3:697–709.

13. Da Silva RC, Segat L, Crovella S. Role of DC-SIGN and L-SIGN receptors in HIV-1 vertical transmission. Hum Immunol 2011;72:305–11.

14. Coleman CM, Wu L. HIV interactions with monocytes and dendritic cells: viral latency and reservoirs. Retrovirology 2009;6:51.

15. Pritschet K, Donhauser N, Schuster P, et al. CD4- and dynamin-dependent endocytosis of HIV-1 into plasmacytoid dendritic cells. Virology 2012;423: 152–64.

16. Liao Z, Roos JW, Hildreth JE. Increased infectivity of HIV type 1 particles bound to cell surface and solid phase ICAM-1 and VCAM-1 through acquired adhesion molecules LFA-1 and VLA-4. AIDS Res Hum Retroviruses 2000;16:355–66.

17. Conaldi PG, Serra C, Dolei A, et al. Productive HIV-1 infection of human vascular endothelial cells requires cell proliferation and is stimulated by combined treatment with interleukin-1 beta plus tumor necrosis factor-alpha. J Med Virol 1995;47: 355–63.

18. Mattapallil JJ, Douek DC, Hill B, et al. Massive infection and loss of memory CD4+ T cells in multiple tissues during acute SIV infection. Nature 2005; 434:1093–7.

19. Li Q, Duan L, Estes JD, et al. Peak SIV replication in resting memory CD4+ T cells depletes gut lamina propria CD4+ T cells. Nature 2005;434:1148–52.

20. Boasso A, Shearer GM. Chronic innate immune activation as a cause of HIV-1 immunopathogenesis. Clin Immunol 2008;126:235–42.

21. Borrow P, Shattock RJ, Vyakarnam A. Innate immunity against HIV: a priority target for HIV prevention research. Retrovirology 2010;7:84.

22. Masten BJ, Olson GK, Tarleton CA, et al. Characterization of myeloid and plasmacytoid dendritic cells in human lung. J Immunol 2006;177:7784–93.

23. Schmidt B, Ashlock BM, Foster H, et al. HIV-infected cells are major inducers of plasmacytoid dendritic cell interferon production, maturation and migration. Virology 2005;343:256–66.

24. Barber GN. Cytoplasmic DNA innate immune pathways. Immunol Rev 2011;243:99–108.

25. Herbeuval JP, Hardy AW, Boasso A, et al. Regulation of TNF-related apoptosis-inducing ligand on primary CD4+ T cells by HIV-1: role of type I IFN-producing plasmacytoid dendritic cells. Proc Natl Acad Sci U S A 2005;102:13974–9.

26. Herveual JP, Grivel JC, Boasso A, et al. CD4+ T-cell death induced by infectious and non-infectious HIV-1: role of type 1 interferon-dependent, TRAIL/DR5-mediated apoptosis. Blood 2005;106:3524–31.

27. Fraietta J, Mueller Y, Do D, et al. Type 1 interferon increases the sensitivity of human immunodeficiency virus (HIV)-specific CD8+ T lymphocytes to CD95/Fas-mediated apoptosis [abstract]. J Immunol 2010;184:42.22.

28. Langlois RA, Legge KL. Plasmacytoid dendritic cells enhance mortality during lethal influenza infections by eliminating virus-specific CD8 T cells. J Immunol 2010;184:4440–6.

29. Labidi-Galy SI, Sisirak V, Meeus P, et al. Quantitative and functional alterations of plasmacytoid dendritic cells contribute to immune tolerance in ovarian cancer. Cancer Res 2011;71:5423–34.

30. Dumitriu IE, Dunbar DR, Howie SE, et al. Human dendritic cells produce TGF-beta 1 under the influence of lung carcinoma cells and prime the differentiation of CD4+CD25+Foxp3+ regulatory T cells. J Immunol 2009;182:2795–807.

31. Zeng M, Smith AJ, Wietgrefe SW, et al. Cumulative mechanisms of lymphoid tissue fibrosis and T cell depletion in HIV-1 and SIV infections. J Clin Invest 2011;121:998–1008.

32. Zeng M, Paiardini M, Engram JC, et al. Critical role for CD4 T cells in maintaining lymphoid tissue structure for immune cell homeostasis and reconstitution. Blood 2012;120(9):1856–67.

33. Nies-Kraske E, Schacker TW, Condoluci D, et al. Evaluation of the pathogenesis of decreasing CD4(+) T cell counts in human immunodeficiency virus type 1-infected patients receiving successfully suppressive antiretroviral therapy. J Infect Dis 2009; 199:1648–56.

34. Feldman C. Pneumonia associated with HIV infection. Curr Opin Infect Dis 2005;18:165–70.

35. Madeddu G, Fiori ML, Mura MS. Bacterial community-acquired pneumonia in HIV-infected patients. Curr Opin Pulm Med 2010;16:201–7.

36. Raju R, Peters BS, Breen RA. Lung infections in the HIV-infected adult. Curr Opin Pulm Med 2012;18: 253–8.

37. Anderson R, Feldman C. Key virulence factors of Streptococcus pneumoniae and non-typeable Haemophilus influenzae: roles in host defence and immunisation. South Afr J Epidemiol Infect 2011; 26:6–12.

38. Malley R, Anderson PW. Serotype-independent pneumococcal experimental vaccines that induce cellular as well as humoral immunity. Proc Natl Acad Sci U S A 2012;109:3623–7.

39. Glennie SJ, Sepako E, Mzinza D, et al. Impaired T cell memory response to Streptococcus pneumoniae precedes CD4 T cell depletion in HIV-infected Malawian adults. PLoS One 2011;6(9):e25610.

40. Kuritzkes DR. Neutropenia, neutrophil dysfunction, and bacterial infection in patients with human immunodeficiency virus disease: the role of granulocyte colony-stimulating factor. Clin Infect Dis 2000;30: 256–60.

41. Engelich G, Wright DG, Hartshorn K. Acquired disorders of phagocyte function complicating medical and surgical illness. Clin Infect Dis 2001; 33:2040–8.

42. Feldman C, Anderson R. Antibiotic resistance of pathogens causing community-acquired pneumonia. Semin Respir Crit Care Med 2012;33:232–43.

43. Cordero E, Pachón J, Rivero A, et al. Haemophilus influenzae pneumonia in human immunodeficiency virus-infected patients. Clin Infect Dis 2000;30: 461–5.

44. Steinhart R, Reingold AL, Taylor F, et al. Invasive Haemophilus influenzae infections in men with HIV infection. JAMA 1992;268:3350–2.

45. Huang L, Crothers K. HIV-associated opportunistic pneumonias. Respirology 2009;14:474–85.

46. Feikin DR, Feldman C, Schuchat A, et al. Global strategies to prevent bacterial pneumonia in adults with HIV disease. Lancet 2004;4:445–55.

47. Hirschtick RE, Glassroth J, Jordan MC, et al. Bacterial pneumonia in persons infected with the human immunodeficiency virus. N Engl J Med 1995;333: 845–51.

48. Madeddu G, Fois AG, Pirina P, et al. Pneumococcal pneumonia: clinical features, diagnosis and management in HIV-infected and HIV noninfected patients. Curr Opin Pulm Med 2009;15:236–42.

49. Feldman JG, Minkoff H, Schneider MF, et al. Association of cigarette smoking with HIV prognosis among women in the HAART Era: a report from the Women's Interagency HIV Study. Am J Public Health 2006;96:1060–5.

50. Wolff AF, O'Donnell AE. Pulmonary manifestations of HIV infection in the era of highly active antiretroviral therapy. Chest 2001;120:1888–93.

51. Rosen MJ. Pulmonary complications of HIV infection. Respirology 2008;13:181–90.

52. Gordin FM, Roediger MP, Girard PM, et al. Pneumonia in HIV-infected persons. Increased risk with cigarette smoking and treatment interruptions. Am J Respir Crit Care Med 2008;178:630–6.

53. Bénard A, Mercié P, Alioum A, et al. Bacterial pneumonia among HIV-infected patients: decreased risk after tobacco smoking cessation. ANRS CO3 Aquitaine Cohort, 2000-2007. PLoS One 2010;5:e8896.

54. Hull MW, Phillips P, Montaner JS. Changing global epidemiology of pulmonary manifestations of HIV/ AIDS. Chest 2008;134:1287–98.

55. Siemieniuk RA, Gregson DB, Gill MJ. The persisting burden of invasive pneumococcal disease in HIV patients: an observational cohort study. BMC Infect Dis 2011;11:314.

56. Nunes MC, von Gottberg A, de Gouveia L, et al. Persistent high burden of invasive pneumococcal disease in South African HIV-infected adults in the era of an antiretroviral treatment program. PLoS One 2011;6:e27929.

57. Schleicher GK, Feldman C. Dual infection with Streptococcus pneumoniae and Mycobacterium tuberculosis in HIV-seropositive patients with community acquired pneumonia. Int J Tuberc Lung Dis 2003;7:1207–8.

58. Popovich KJ, Weinstein RA, Aroutcheva A, et al. Community-associated methicillin-resistant Staphylococcus aureus and HIV: intersecting epidemics. Clin Infect Dis 2010;50:979–87.

59. Levine SJ, White DA, Fels AO. The incidence and significance of Staphylococcus aureus in respiratory cultures from patients infected with the human immunodeficiency virus. Am Rev Respir Dis 1990; 141:89–93.

60. Fujitani S, Sun HY, Yu VL, et al. Pneumonia due to Pseudomonas aeruginosa: part I: epidemiology, clinical diagnosis, and source. Chest 2011;139: 909–19.

61. Manfredi R, Nanetti A, Ferri M, et al. Pseudomonas spp. complications in patients with HIV disease: an eight-year clinical and microbiological survey. Eur J Epidemiol 2000;16:111–8.

62. Pedro-Botet ML, Sabrià M, Sopena N, et al. Legionnaires disease and HIV infection. Chest 2003;124: 543–7.

63. Pedro-Botet ML, Sopena N, García-Cruz A, et al. *Streptococcus pneumoniae* and *Legionella pneumophila* pneumonia in HIV-infected patients. Scand J Infect Dis 2007;39:122–8.

64. Topino S, Galati V, Grilli E, et al. *Rhodococcus equi* infection in HIV-infected individuals: case reports and review of the literature. AIDS Patient Care STDS 2010;24:211–22.

65. Manfredi R, Nanetti A, Valentini R, et al. *Moraxella catarrhalis* pneumonia during HIV disease. J Chemother 2000;12:406–11.

66. Minero MV, Marin M, Cercenado E, et al. Nocardiosis at the turn of the century. Medicine 2009;88:250–61.

67. Menéndez R, Cordero PJ, Santos M, et al. Pulmonary infection with *Nocardia* species: a report of 10 cases and review. Eur Respir J 1997;10:1542–6.

68. Feldman C, Klugman KP, Yu VL, et al. Bacteraemic pneumococcal pneumonia: impact of HIV on clinical presentation and outcome. J Infect 2007;55:125–35.

69. Feldman C, Anderson R. Respiratory infections in specific populations: HIV patients. In: Blasi F, Dimopolous G, editors. Textbook of Respiratory and Critical Care Infections, in press.

70. Scott LE, McCarthy K, Gous N, et al. Comparison of Xpert MTB/RIF with other nucleic acid technologies for diagnosing pulmonary tuberculosis in a high HIV prevalence setting: a prospective study. PLoS Med 2011;8(7):e1001061.

71. Cattamanchi A, Ssewenyana I, Davis JL, et al. Role of interferon-gamma release assays in the diagnosis of pulmonary tuberculosis in patients with advanced HIV infection. BMC Infect Dis 2010;10:75.

72. Smith MD, Sheppard CL, Hogan A, et al. Diagnosis of *Streptococcus pneumoniae* infection in adults with bacteremia and community-acquired pneumonia: clinical comparison of pneumococcal PCR and urinary antigen detection. J Clin Microbiol 2009;47:1046–9.

73. Streubens MJ. Detection of microbial DNAemia: does it matter for sepsis management? Intensive Care Med 2010;36:193–5.

74. Feldman C, Brink AJ, Richards G, et al, Working Group of the South African Thoracic Society. Management of community-acquired pneumonia in adults. S Afr Med J 2007;97:1296–306.

75. Schleicher GK, Hopley MJ, Feldman C. CD4 T-lymphocyte subset counts in HIV-seropositive patients during the course of community-acquired pneumonia caused by *Streptococcus pneumoniae*. Clin Microbiol Infect 2004;10:587–9.

76. Bordon J, Kapoor R, Martinez C, et al. CD4+ cell counts and HIV-RNA levels do not predict outcomes of community-acquired pneumonia in hospitalized HIV-infected patients. Int J Infect Dis 2011;15:e822–7.

77. Malinis M, Myers J, Bordon J, et al. Clinical outcomes of HIV-infected patients hospitalized with bacterial community-acquired pneumonia. Int J Infect Dis 2010;14:e22–7.

78. Feldman C, Glatthaar M, Morar R, et al. Bacteremic pneumococcal pneumonia in HIV-seropositive and HIV-seronegative adults. Chest 1999;116:107–14.

79. Kohli R, Lo Y, Homel P, et al. Bacterial pneumonia, HIV therapy, and disease progression among HIV-infected women in the HIV Epidemiologic Research (HER) Study. Clin Infect Dis 2006;43:90–8.

80. Morris AM, Huang L, Bacchetti P, et al. Permanent declines in pulmonary function following pneumonia in human immunodeficiency virus-infected persons. Am J Respir Crit Care Med 2000;162:612–6.

81. Hibberd PL. Immunizations in HIV-infected patients. In: UpToDate® 2012. Available at: http://www.uptodate.com/contents/immunizations-in-hiv-infected-patients. Accessed May 24, 2012.

82. Kaplan JE, Benson C, Holmes KH, et al. Guidelines for prevention and treatment of opportunistic infections in HIV-infected adults and adolescents: recommendations from CDC, the National Institutes of Health, and the HIV Medicine Association of the Infectious Diseases Society of America. MMWR Recomm Rep 2009;58(RR-4):1–207.

83. Advisory Committee on Immunization Practices. Recommended adult immunization schedule: United States, 2009. Ann Intern Med 2009;150:40–4.

84. Murphy TF. Current and future prospects for a vaccine for nontypeable *Haemophilus influenzae*. Curr Infect Dis Rep 2009;11:177–82.

85. Crowther-Gibson P, Cohen C, Klugman KP, et al. Risk factors for multidrug-resistant invasive pneumococcal disease in South Africa, 2003-2008: the pre-vaccine era in a high HIV prevalence setting. Antimicrobial Agents Chemother 2012;56(10):5088–95.

Human Immunodeficiency Virus–Associated Tuberculosis
Update on Prevention and Treatment

Kerry L. Dierberg, MD, MPH[a], Richard E. Chaisson, MD[b],*

KEYWORDS

- Tuberculosis • Human immunodeficiency virus • HIV-associated tuberculosis

KEY POINTS

- Tuberculosis (TB) is the leading cause of opportunistic infection and mortality among human immunodeficiency virus (HIV)-infected persons.
- All HIV-infected patients should be screened for TB and treated for latent TB infection if there is no evidence of active TB disease. In low-burden areas, preventive therapy should be targeted at those with documented latent TB infection.
- All patients with HIV-associated TB should receive standard anti-TB therapy and early initiation of antiretroviral therapy.
- Treatment of HIV-associated TB is often complicated by development of immune reconstitution inflammatory disease.
- Coadministration of TB treatment and antiretroviral therapy can be complicated by overlapping drug toxicities and drug-drug interactions.

INTRODUCTION

Tuberculosis (TB) continues to be one of the leading causes of death from infectious disease worldwide, and is the leading opportunistic infection and cause of mortality among people with human immunodeficiency virus (HIV) infection.[1,2] People with HIV infection are at increased risk for reactivation of latent TB infection and acquisition of new TB infection in comparison with HIV-uninfected persons and are less likely to present with classic clinical or radiographic findings of TB.[3–7] In addition, treatment of HIV-related TB is complicated by overlapping drug toxicities and drug-drug interactions between antiretroviral therapy and anti-TB therapy, as well as the risk for development of immune reconstitution inflammatory disease.

Screening for symptoms of TB in all people with HIV infection, use of isoniazid preventive therapy for those with latent TB infection, earlier diagnosis and treatment of active TB disease, and early initiation of antiretroviral therapy are essential for controlling the spread of TB. This review provides an overview and updates on the prevention and treatment of TB in HIV-infected persons.

EPIDEMIOLOGY

Based on World Health Organization (WHO) reports, there were 8.7 million new cases of TB

[a] Division of Infectious Diseases, Department of Medicine, Johns Hopkins University School of Medicine, 1550 Orleans Street, Baltimore, MD 21287, USA; [b] Center for Tuberculosis Research, Division of Infectious Diseases, Department of Medicine, Johns Hopkins University School of Medicine, 1550 Orleans Street, 1M.08, Baltimore, MD 21287, USA
* Corresponding author.
E-mail address: rchaiss@jhmi.edu

Clin Chest Med 34 (2013) 217–228
http://dx.doi.org/10.1016/j.ccm.2013.02.003
0272-5231/13/$ – see front matter © 2013 Elsevier Inc. All rights reserved.

and 1.4 million deaths from TB worldwide in 2011. The largest burden of TB was in Asia and Africa, which accounted for 59% and 26% of all cases, respectively. Among the 22 high-burden countries, 26% of all incident cases were in India and 12% were in China, followed by South Africa (6%) and Pakistan (5%). Approximately 3.7% of all new TB cases and 20% of previously treated cases have multidrug-resistant TB (MDR TB, characterized by resistance to isoniazid and rifampin), with more than 60% of these cases in India, China, and Russia. It is estimated that 9% of the MDR TB cases are extensively drug-resistant TB (XDR TB; MDR TB with additional resistance to fluoroquinolones and injectable agents).[2]

It is estimated that 1.1 million (13%) of all TB cases are coinfected with HIV, and approximately 80% of these cases are in Africa. Of the 1.4 million deaths globally from TB in 2011, approximately 400,000 were HIV-associated TB deaths. HIV testing for all TB patients is recommended; however, this remains a significant challenge for many TB programs. In 2011, it is estimated that approximately 40% of all notified TB cases had HIV testing, which is a substantial increase from 3.1% in 2004, but this remains insufficient given the growing burden of TB-HIV coinfection.[2]

TB and HIV continue to be leading causes of morbidity and mortality in women and children.[1,2,8] In 2011, an estimated 2.9 million and 500,000 cases of the 8.7 million incident cases occurred in women and children, respectively. There were an estimated 500,000 million deaths among women attributable to TB in 2011, and approximately 40% of these also had HIV infection, making TB a greater killer of women than complications of childbirth.[2]

In the United States the rates of TB have continued to decline, with a total of 10,521 new cases (incidence 3.4 per 100,000) reported to the US Centers for Disease Control and Prevention (CDC) in 2011. However, foreign-born persons and racial/ethnic minorities continue to be affected disproportionately, with rates 12 times greater than in United States–born persons. The highest incidence of TB was reported in persons from Mexico (21.3%), the Philippines (11.5%), Vietnam (8.2%), India (7.6%), and China (5.6%). Of the 81% of TB cases with a documented HIV test, 7.9% tested HIV positive.[9]

HIV infection continues to be the most important biological risk factor for developing TB. Other classic risk factors for developing TB include poverty, overcrowding, and malnutrition. However, it is also known that smoking doubles a person's risk for developing TB infection. Alcohol consumption, diabetes, and immunosuppressive therapy with steroids, tumor necrosis factor antagonists, or other immune-modulating medications also increase risk for TB.[1]

PREVENTION
Screening for TB

HIV-infected persons are at increased risk for developing TB disease both from recent infection and from reactivation of latent infection. The risk of reactivation of latent TB is approximately 5%–10% per year for HIV-infected persons, compared with a 10% lifetime risk for HIV-uninfected persons.[4] In countries with generalized HIV epidemics, TB is a common presenting sign of HIV infection, and in areas with low rates of HIV infection the prevalence of HIV is substantially higher in people with TB than in the general population. Based on these risks, the WHO recommends integrated TB and HIV services. Specifically, all people with active TB disease should be tested for HIV. If they are HIV-infected, they should receive trimethoprim-sulfamethoxazole prophylaxis and be assessed for the need for antiretroviral therapy.[4,10,11] All HIV-infected patients should be screened for symptoms of TB (intensified case finding) and then evaluated with specific diagnostic studies if symptoms are present. In high-burden settings, patients without active TB should receive isoniazid preventive therapy (IPT), as well as antiretroviral therapy, to reduce TB risk. In low-burden settings such as the United States, IPT or other preventive regimens should be targeted at those with latent TB infection as documented by a positive tuberculin skin test or positive interferon-γ release assay (IGRA). Screening should be performed at the time of HIV diagnosis and regularly thereafter, especially in settings where the TB burden is high.[1,12] The CDC also recommends that all HIV-infected persons in the United States be screened for active and latent TB at the time of diagnosis of HIV, and then yearly based on risk of TB exposure.[4]

Standardized TB screening for all HIV-infected patients provides the opportunity to diagnose and treat active disease earlier, and to identify patients who are eligible for IPT. HIV-infected persons may present with classic symptoms of TB, including cough, fever, night sweats, and weight loss; however, many will have minimal symptoms, making the diagnosis of active TB difficult. In addition, because extrapulmonary TB is extremely common in HIV-infected individuals, clinical presentations may vary greatly. This problem continues to be a significant obstacle to screening HIV patients for TB and for uptake of IPT.

Despite recommendations that all HIV-infected patients be screened for TB, the best symptom-screening criteria remain unclear. In 2011, Getahun and colleagues published the results of a meta-analysis aimed at developing a standardized TB symptom-screening rule for HIV-infected persons.[8] Based on the results of this study, the best screening rule was the presence of any 1 of the following symptoms: current cough (any duration), fever, night sweats, or weight loss. The overall sensitivity and specificity of this rule was 78.9% and 49.6%, respectively, with a high negative predictive value (90%–97%), suggesting that the absence of these 4 symptoms is effective for excluding active TB and identifying people eligible for IPT.[12,13] These screening criteria have also been shown to be effective for HIV-infected pregnant women.[14]

However, as suggested by the sensitivity of just less than 80%, the use of WHO-recommended symptom screening will still miss approximately 20% of TB cases among HIV patients.[5]

Diagnostic testing for TB is challenging, particularly in resource-limited areas, and sputum acid-fast smears have extremely low sensitivity in the setting of HIV infection. Culture using liquid media such as the Mycobacterial Growth Indicator Tube (MGIT; Becton Dickinson, Franklin Lakes, NJ) increases sensitivity to greater than 95% but culture is expensive and time-consuming, and requires Biosafety Level 3 laboratory facilities. Recently, rapid molecular diagnostic assays have been introduced, which can detect *Mycobacterium tuberculosis* in sputum and other specimens in as little as 90 minutes, and which can also detect gene mutations associated with drug resistance. The Xpert MTB/RIF (Cepheid, Sunnyvale, CA) is a cartridge-based system that has high sensitivity (70%–90%) for *M tuberculosis* and detects rifampin resistance with greater than 95% accuracy.[15,16] Several line-probe nucleic acid amplification assays also detect *M tuberculosis* and several forms of drug resistance, including MDR and XDR, in as little as 2 hours. Details of these diagnostic methods are beyond the scope of this article, and the reader is referred to a recent review of this topic.[17–19]

A tuberculin skin test (TST) or IGRA can be helpful in diagnosing latent TB infection, but neither is 100% sensitive or specific and HIV-infected patients may have false-negative results.[4] The QuantiFERON-TB Gold In-tube (QGIT) and the T-SPOT.TB IGRAs have been approved by the US Food and Drug Administration (FDA) and the WHO for the diagnosis of latent TB infection; however, the WHO does not recommend use of these tests in low-income and middle-income countries.[20] Studies have not demonstrated increased accuracy of IGRAs for the diagnosis of latent TB, and discordance in test results between IGRAs and TST have been demonstrated. However, IGRAs are less likely to be false positive in persons who have previously received bacillus Calmette-Guérin vaccination.[21,22]

Treatment of Latent TB Infection

Several studies have demonstrated the benefit of isoniazid preventive therapy for latent TB infection, with 44% to 58% reduction in the risk of TB.[12,23,24] A Cochrane systematic review of 12 trials, published in 2010, demonstrated that IPT reduced the risk of active TB by 64% in HIV-infected participants with a positive TST, but only by 14% in TST negative individuals.[23]

Several recent studies have focused on the optimal regimen and treatment duration for latent TB in HIV-infected persons. Prior studies have demonstrated a 32% to 64% reduction in TB risk with 6 to 9 months of isoniazid or isoniazid plus rifampin for 3 months.[23,24]

A randomized controlled trial conducted in South Africa demonstrated no significant differences in rates of TB or death in HIV-infected adults treated for latent TB infection with rifapentine (900 mg) plus isoniazid (900 mg) once weekly for 3 months, rifampin (600 mg) plus isoniazid (900 mg) twice weekly for 3 months, or isoniazid (300 mg/d) continuously for up to 6 years, compared with a control regimen of isoniazid daily for 6 months. A large study in mostly HIV-seronegative individuals also found that once-weekly rifapentine and isoniazid for 12 weeks was noninferior to 9 months of daily isoniazid for treating latent TB infection, and this regimen has been endorsed by the CDC.[24]

The use of continuous IPT is an appealing option for high-burden settings, as it theoretically should also protect patients from disease caused by reinfection. In the study by Martinson and colleagues,[24] the as-treated analysis found that the risk of TB and death was significantly reduced while participants took isoniazid, but this benefit was lost if treatment was discontinued. In a randomized, double-blind trial conducted in Botswana comparing 6 months versus 36 months of isoniazid in patients with HIV, a significantly lower risk of TB was seen with 36 months of isoniazid, although this benefit was found only in those who were TST positive. The lack of benefit for TST-negative patients is puzzling, as prevention of disease attributable to new infections should accrue to all patients in this high-burden setting; however, it is possible that TST-positive individuals are at higher risk of reinfection than TST-negative persons, therefore continuous isoniazid therapy is protective for this population in particular.[25]

IPT has been shown to be safe and effective in reducing the risk of TB in HIV-infected mothers. TB during pregnancy and the postpartum period is associated with increased maternal mortality, TB in the infant, and vertical transmission of HIV, therefore screening for latent TB and use of IPT is essential as a part of maternal health care.[8,26]

The CDC currently recommends the following treatment regimens for latent TB in HIV-infected individuals[4,9,27]:

- Isoniazid daily for 9 months (recommendation strength: AII)
- Isoniazid daily for 6 months (recommendation strength: CI)
- Rifampin daily for 4 months (recommendation strength: BIII), or rifapentine plus isoniazid once weekly for 3 months (recommendation strength: BI) in antiretroviral therapy–naive patients only[28]

Antiretroviral Therapy

Studies have shown that antiretroviral therapy reduces risk of developing TB and death in HIV-infected persons; however, the risk continues to remain higher than in HIV-uninfected persons. A recent meta-analysis found that antiretroviral therapy was associated with reductions in rates of TB ranging from 57% to 84%, depending on the CD4 cell count at which treatment began. The HIV Prevention Trials Network (HPTN) 052 trial of early initiation of antiretroviral therapy to prevent HIV transmission in discordant couples also demonstrated that individuals randomized to early antiretroviral therapy had a 50% reduction in the risk of TB, emphasizing the benefits of earlier treatment of HIV infection.[29] Protection against TB is further optimized when IPT is combined with antiretroviral therapy; synergistic protection was found in one study of South African patients who received both IPT and antiretrovirals when compared with the protection afforded by either treatment alone.[8,30,31] A recently completed trial of patients with advanced HIV infection who were receiving antiretroviral therapy showed a greater than 50% reduction in rates of TB for patients randomized to receive isoniazid versus those randomized to placebo.[32]

CLINICAL MANIFESTATIONS OF HIV-ASSOCIATED TB

TB continues to be the leading opportunistic infection and cause of mortality among people with HIV infection, and is often the presenting condition for patients with undiagnosed HIV.[1,2,11] People with HIV infection who acquire new TB infections have a greatly increased likelihood of progression to active disease, and rates of mortality attributable to TB are higher in HIV-infected persons than in HIV-uninfected individuals.[11]

Pulmonary TB

Pulmonary TB is the most common form of TB in both HIV-infected and HIV-uninfected individuals. HIV-infected persons may present with classic symptoms of pulmonary TB, including cough, hemoptysis, fever, weight loss, and night sweats; however, HIV-infected persons frequently present with minimal or atypical symptoms, making the diagnosis of TB more difficult for clinicians. Patients with a CD4 cell count > 350 cells per mm^3 are more likely than patients with advanced immunosuppression to have a similar presentation to HIV-uninfected individuals.[3–5,7]

Several studies have also demonstrated that HIV-infected persons are more likely to have "nonclassic" or atypical findings on chest radiograph when compared with HIV-uninfected persons, including noncavitary infiltrates, miliary disease, pleural effusions, or normal chest radiographs.[6,7,33] Patients with HIV-associated TB are more likely to have smear-negative disease, likely due in part to the lack of cavitary lung disease.[7,11,34]

The combination of atypical or minimal symptoms and radiologic findings and the increased likelihood of having a negative sputum acid-fast bacilli smear often results in a delay in diagnosis of HIV-associated TB and delay in initiation of treatment. Most HIV patients with subclinical TB will eventually develop symptoms of the disease, though often when the disease is much more advanced. HIV-infected patients with subclinical TB who are started on antiretroviral therapy are also likely to present with symptoms of TB as their immune system recovers, which is referred to as "unmasking" immune reconstitution inflammatory syndrome (IRIS).[35–37] Screening of patients beginning antiretroviral therapy for active TB using culture, Xpert MTB/RIF, or other sensitive diagnostic modalities can identify those with subclinical disease, allowing for earlier initiation of anti-TB therapy and preventing IRIS.

Drug-Resistant TB

MDR TB is TB that is resistant to isoniazid and rifampicin, and XDR TB is MDR TB that is also resistant to a fluoroquinolone and at least 1 injectable agent (capreomycin, kanamycin, amikacin).

Mortality rates are high for HIV-infected patients who develop drug-resistant TB, with rates up to 90% for those infected with XDR TB. Based on WHO guidelines, all HIV-infected patients diagnosed with TB should have drug susceptibility testing (DST) at the start of TB therapy. Clinicians should have a high index of suspicion for drug-resistant TB if the patient remains sputum-smear negative or is clinically failing first-line anti-TB treatment.

Extrapulmonary TB

Patients with HIV are more likely than HIV-uninfected individuals to develop extrapulmonary disease and disseminated TB disease, especially at lower CD4 counts.[11,38] More than half of all patients with HIV-related TB who undergo a thorough workup have extrapulmonary disease, most of whom also have pulmonary TB. In patients with prominent pulmonary symptoms and signs, extrapulmonary manifestations of TB may be overlooked.

The most common forms of extrapulmonary disease in patients with HIV infection are TB lymphadenitis, pleural TB, TB meningitis, and disseminated TB with bacteremia. Other sites of disease in HIV-associated TB include the abdomen (peritoneum, gastrointestinal tract, liver, kidneys), bone and joint, pericardium, genitourinary system, and soft tissues.[11]

TREATMENT OF HIV-ASSOCIATED TB

The WHO, the US Public Health Service, and the Department of Health and Human Services all recommend that all HIV-infected individuals diagnosed with TB should receive anti-TB treatment and antiretroviral therapy; in resource-limited settings, the WHO also recommends that all patients receive trimethoprim-sulfamethoxazole (TMP-SMX) prophylaxis, whereas United States and European guidelines restrict this recommendation to patients with CD4 cell counts < 200 cells/mm^3.[11] Details on use of antiretroviral therapy are provided here.

Pulmonary TB

Based on current guidelines, the treatment of HIV-associated pulmonary TB is the same as for HIV-uninfected individuals. Patients with pulmonary TB should receive 2 months of intensive therapy with a standard 4-drug regimen (isoniazid, rifampin, pyrazinamide, and ethambutol), followed by 4 months of continuation therapy with a 2-drug regimen (isoniazid and rifampin). All patients should receive pyridoxine (vitamin B$_6$) 50 mg daily

to prevent peripheral neuropathy associated with isoniazid.[3,11]

Several studies have demonstrated lower recurrence rates in HIV-infected patients with TB when treated for a longer duration. A study conducted in the former Zaire that compared 6 months versus 12 months of rifampicin-based therapy demonstrated lower recurrence rates in those treated for 12 months, although longer therapy did not improve survival.[39] A randomized controlled trial evaluating standard 6-month therapy compared with 6 months of therapy, followed by isoniazid preventive therapy, showed a significant impact of secondary isoniazid therapy on the risk of TB recurrence.[40] It is unclear whether the reduced recurrence rates in these studies were due to decreased relapse or reinfection, but it is likely that prolonged isoniazid controls disease because of reinfection in high-burden settings, as rates of recurrence in patients treated in the United States do not appear to be elevated.[41] These findings suggest that longer duration of therapy, or standard 6-month therapy followed by isoniazid preventive therapy, may be indicated in high-TB burden settings where the risk of reinfection is high, and the WHO recommends use of IPT in patients with HIV previously treated for TB.[42] Risk of recurrence is also decreased by treatment with antiretroviral therapy. A study in Brazil found that use of antiretroviral therapy reduced recurrent TB by 50%.[43]

Extrapulmonary TB

As with pulmonary TB, current guidelines recommend using the same treatment regimens and duration for HIV-associated extrapulmonary TB as for extrapulmonary TB in HIV-uninfected individuals.[3,11] Patients with TB meningitis or pericardial TB should also receive corticosteroid therapy. Specific treatment guidelines are based on the site of disease, and are summarized in **Table 1**.

Drug-Resistant TB

All patients with HIV-related TB should have DST performed at the time of TB diagnosis, if possible.[3] For patients diagnosed with TB who do not have baseline DST, susceptibility testing should be performed at the time of clinical failure or relapse, given the high mortality rates from MDR TB and XDR TB in HIV-infected patients.[11] Choice of an MDR TB or XDR TB regimen should be guided by DST results whenever possible. For patients diagnosed with Xpert MTB/RIF who are found to have resistance to rifampin, additional susceptibility testing for both first-line and second-line drugs must be performed.

Table 1
Management of HIV-associated TB

Site of Disease	First-Line Anti-TB Regimen[a]	Duration of Treatment (mo)[b]	Use of Steroids	Other Recommendations[c]
Pulmonary	Induction phase: H R Z E	2	No	
	Continuation phase: H R	4	No	
Pleural	Induction phase: H R Z E	2	No	Thoracentesis for symptomatic relief; surgical debridement for empyema
	Continuation phase: H R	4	No	
Lymphadenitis	Induction phase: H R Z E	2	No	Excision of large or fluctuant lymph nodes may be required
	Continuation phase: H R	4	No	
Meningitis	Induction phase: H R Z Sm	2	Yes	Dexamethasone 12 mg/kg × 3 wk, followed by taper over 3–5 wk
	Continuation phase: H R	7–10	Yes	Poor CNS penetration of ethambutol, so replaced by streptomycin; fluoroquinolones (moxifloxacin or levofloxacin) can also be used. HAART should be delayed due to increased risk of TB IRIS
Pericardium	Induction phase: H R Z E	2	Yes	Prednisone (11 wk): 60 mg/d × 4 wk, 30 mg/d × 4 wk, 15 mg/d × 2 wk, then 5 mg/d × 1 wk
	Continuation phase: H R	4	Yes	Surgery may be required if constrictive pericarditis develops
Bone/joint	Induction phase: H R Z E	2	No	Surgical decompression of spinal disease in cases of cord compression or spinal instability
	Continuation phase: H R	7	No	
Abdominal (peritonitis, enteritis)	Induction phase: H R Z E	2	No	
	Continuation phase: H R	4	No	
Urogenital (renal, GU tract)	Induction phase: H R Z E	2	No	Surgery may be indicated for obstructive uropathy
	Continuation phase: H R	4	No	
Disseminated	Induction phase: H R Z E	2	No	
	Continuation phase: H R	4	No	

Abbreviations: CNS, central nervous system; E, ethambutol; GU, genitourinary; H, Isoniazid; HAART, highly active antiretroviral therapy; IRIS, immune reconstitution inflammatory syndrome; R, rifampin; Sm, streptomycin; Z, pyrazinamide.
  [a] All patients with pulmonary and extrapulmonary TB should receive pyridoxine, 50 mg daily.
  [b] Duration of therapy may be extended in cases of slow clinical response.
  [c] Directly observed therapy recommended for treatment of all forms of TB. Trimethoprim-sulfamethoxazole recommended throughout course of TB treatment in all HIV-infected patients. Timing of HAART initiation based on CD4 cell count and site of disease.
  Data from Blumberg HM, Burman WJ, Chaisson RE, et al. American Thoracic Society/Centers for Disease Control and Prevention/Infectious Diseases Society of America: treatment of tuberculosis. Am J Respir Crit Care Med 2003;167(4):603–62; and WHO treatment of tuberculosis: guidelines for national programmes. 2012. Available at: http://www.who.int/tb/publications/tb_treatmentguidelines/en/index.html. Accessed December 29, 2012.

Directly observed therapy (DOT) is recommended for all patients receiving treatment for HIV-associated TB. If possible, patients should receive daily treatment under DOT, as studies have demonstrated decreased relapse rates in patients receiving daily therapy in comparison with intermittent therapy.[11,44] The WHO now recommends daily treatment under DOT for all patients with HIV-associated TB.[11]

Trimethoprim-sulfamethoxazole (TMP-SMX) is currently recommended by the WHO for all HIV-infected individuals at the time of TB diagnosis and throughout the duration of TB treatment. Studies have demonstrated decreased mortality in HIV-infected TB patients. TMP-SMX is known to prevent *Pneumocystis jirovecii* pneumonia, and may reduce risk for bacterial infections such as gastrointestinal tract disease and malaria.[11,45]

TB in Pregnancy

TB in women poses special challenges but is critically important, as transmission of HIV and TB to the fetus and poor obstetric and perinatal outcomes are common when TB is not recognized and properly treated.[3,8,11,26] The WHO currently recommends treatment with standard regimens as listed in **Table 1**, including use of pyrazinamide. However, pyrazinamide is not recommended in the United States owing to limited safety data regarding its use in pregnancy, although its use is warranted when clinicians determine that the benefits outweigh the risks.[3] Streptomycin should be avoided in pregnant women because of the known risk of ototoxicity in the fetus.[11,46] All infants born to mothers with TB should receive IPT once active TB is ruled out.[11] Both the WHO and CDC recommend breastfeeding if the mother is on first-line anti-TB therapy.[3,11,26]

ROLE OF ANTIRETROVIRAL THERAPY IN THE TREATMENT OF HIV-ASSOCIATED TB

Because TB is a clinical manifestation of immunodeficiency and independently increases the risk of HIV progression and death, highly active antiretroviral therapy (HAART) is recommended for all HIV-infected individuals diagnosed with TB, regardless of CD4 cell count.[11,47–54] Several recent studies have helped provide guidance on the best timing for initiation of HAART after TB treatment is started. The SaPIT trial in South Africa demonstrated significantly lower mortality for patients who received integrated TB and HIV therapy, in comparison with delaying HAART until TB therapy was completed. The CAMELIA study showed that Cambodian patients with advanced HIV infection (median CD4 count 25 cells/mm^3) had a 34%

lower risk of dying if HAART was initiated within 2 weeks of starting TB therapy rather than starting antiretroviral therapy at 8 weeks. The STRIDE and SaPIT studies both found that immediate initiation of HAART (within 2 weeks), in comparison with later initiation (8 weeks), substantially lowered the risk of death or developing a new AIDS diagnosis in patients with CD4 counts < 50 cells/mm^3, but there was no benefit for patients with higher CD4 counts. Based on the results of these trials, the US Department of Health and Human Services (DHHS) recommends initiating HAART based on the following guidelines[55]:

- If CD4 cell count is < 50 cells/mm^3, initiate HAART within 2 weeks of starting TB therapy.
- If CD4 cell count is 50 cells/mm^3 or more and patients have clinical disease of major severity (including low Karnofsky score, low body mass index, low hemoglobin, low albumin, organ system dysfunction, or extent of disease), initiate HAART within 2 to 4 weeks.
- If CD4 cell count is > 50 cells/mm^3 but without severe clinical disease, initiation of HAART can be delayed but should be started within 8 to 12 weeks of starting TB therapy.

For patients with TB meningitis, HAART should not be started within 2 weeks of initiating TB treatment, regardless of CD4 cell count, because of the increased risk for central nervous system IRIS and associated poor outcomes, including death. For these patients, HAART should be delayed for up to 8 weeks.[56]

While the early initiation of HAART in patients with HIV-associated TB has been shown to significantly reduce mortality and progression of HIV disease, it has also been associated with IRIS. TB IRIS is most common in the first 3 months after initiation of HAART and in patients with a CD4 cell count lower than 100 cells/mm^3 at the time HAART is initiated.[4,11,35,36,52,54]

IRIS often presents with fever, new or worsening pulmonary infiltrates, new or worsening serositis, enlarged lymph nodes, or apparent worsening of disease at another site. IRIS is a diagnosis of exclusion, and other causes of these symptoms, such as another opportunistic infection, malignancy, or TB treatment failure, should be ruled out before making this diagnosis. Diagnostic criteria for IRIS developed by an international working group of experts have been published, and are shown in **Box 1**.[37]

Up to one-third of all patients receiving combined therapy for TB and HIV will develop IRIS, although most patients have only mild to moderate symptoms and the condition is rarely fatal.[57] Management of IRIS depends on clinical symptomatology, and is directed at reducing inflammation and drainage of abscesses or fluid collections. Some patients can be managed with nonsteroidal anti-inflammatory agents, but many patients will require corticosteroid treatment for improvement in symptoms. A randomized placebo-controlled trial conducted in South Africa demonstrated that treatment with prednisone 1.5 mg/kg/d for 2 weeks, followed by 0.75 mg/kg/d for 2 weeks, significantly improved symptoms and reduced the need for invasive procedures or hospitalization.[58] Although most patients can be managed with corticosteroids alone, the exception is patients with TB meningitis, who have increased risk of central nervous system IRIS and severe adverse events and death associated with early initiation of HAART.[56] Treatment in this situation may require an increased dosage of corticosteroids, intracranial pressure management with frequent lumbar punctures, and neurosurgical intervention.

Drug-Drug Interactions

Treatment of HIV-related TB is complicated by overlapping drug toxicities and by drug-drug interactions between antiretroviral therapy and anti-TB therapy. The most important drug interactions to consider occur between rifamycins and antiretroviral medications, including nonnucleoside reverse transcriptase inhibitors (NNRTIs) and protease inhibitors. Drug-drug interactions also occur with use of integrase inhibitors and with CCR5 receptor antagonists.[59–62]

The rifamycins (rifampin, rifabutin, and rifapentine) are CYP450 enzyme inducers, which can increase the metabolism of drugs cleared by this pathway. Cotreatment of TB and HIV requires close attention to selection and dosing of rifamycins and antiretrovirals (**Table 2**).[59] Rifampin has been shown to increase the clearance of NNRTIs, including efavirenz and nevirapine.[4,59–61] Rifampin decreases exposure to nevirapine by approximately 50%, and results in higher rates of virologic failure than when the drug is used without rifampin. Exposure to efavirenz is reduced by 20% to 25% by coadministration of rifampin, but virologic outcomes are not affected. Some authorities recommend increasing the efavirenz dosage from 600 to 800 mg daily when coadministered with rifampin, but clinical and virologic data do not support this advice, and patients treated with standard dosages of efavirenz while taking rifampin-based TB therapy do not have compromised outcomes.

Conversely, rifampin coadministration with protease inhibitors results in 80% to 98% reductions in exposure, and compromise antiretroviral therapy. Therefore, rifabutin is the preferred rifamycin with protease inhibitor-based regimens, as it is only a very weak inducer of CYP450 isoenzymes. Boosted protease inhibitor regimens using ritonavir increase serum concentrations of rifabutin and can lead to clinically important toxicity, including uveitis. Consequently, dosing of rifabutin during protease inhibitor–based HAART needs to be adjusted; previous guidelines recommended a dosage of 150 mg every other day, but more recent data support use of a dosage of 150 mg daily or 300 mg every other day to ensure adequate exposure to the anti-TB effect of rifabutin and prevent the development of rifampin-resistant TB.[59]

Table 2
Management of drug interactions between HIV medications and rifamycins used in TB treatment

HIV Medication	Rifampin vs Rifabutin[a]	Interaction	Recommendation
Protease Inhibitors (with ritonavir)			
Lopinavir, fosamprenavir, atazanavir, saquinavir, indinavir, darunavir, and tipranavir	Rifabutin	Modest decreases in PI exposure; ritonavir increases rifabutin exposure, potentially resulting in toxicity	Decrease rifabutin dose to 150 mg every other day; usual PI and ritonavir dose; rifampin not recommended
NNRTIs			
Efavirenz (EFV)	Rifampin	Rifampin reduces efavirenz exposure by ~25%	No change in dosing; some recommend increasing EFV dose to 800 mg
	Rifabutin	Efavirenz increases rifabutin clearance by 30%–40%	Increase rifabutin dose to 450–600 mg daily (or 600 mg 3 times weekly)
Etravirine (ETV)	Rifabutin	Bidirectional interaction	Use rifabutin 300 mg daily; rifampin or rifapentine not recommended; if ETV given with ritonavir-boosted PI, do not use rifabutin
Rilpivirine (RVP)	Rifabutin	Rifabutin decreases RVP AUC by 46%	Contraindicated; rifampin also contraindicated
Nevirapine (NVP)	Rifabutin	Rifampin reduces nevirapine AUC by 37%–58% and Cmin by 37%–68%	Coadminister at usual doses; avoid rifampin due to increased virologic failure
Integrase Inhibitor			
Raltegravir (RAL)	Rifabutin	Rifabutin reduces RAL trough by 20%, but RAL AUC is not affected	Administer rifabutin 300 mg daily with RAL 400 mg twice daily Rifampin not recommended, but if used give RAL 800 mg twice daily and monitor virologic response closely
Coreceptor Inhibitor			
Maraviroc (MVC)	Rifabutin	Modest impact of rifabutin on MVC exposure likely	Administer MVC 300 mg twice daily and rifabutin 300 mg daily; rifampin not recommended but if used, increase MVC to 600 mg twice daily

Additional information is available at http://www.cdc.gov/tb/publications/guidelines/TB_HIV_Drugs/default.htm.

Abbreviations: AUC, area under the curve; Cmax, maximum plasma concentration of drug; Cmin, minimum concentration of drug; NNRTI, nonnucleoside reverse transcriptase inhibitors; PI, protease inhibitor.

[a] Rifapentine should not be used when coadministered with antiretroviral medications unless in the context of a clinical trial.

Data from CDC TB managing drug interactions in the treatment of HIV-related tuberculosis. 2012. Available at: http://www.cdc.gov/tb/publications/guidelines/TB_HIV_Drugs/default.htm. Accessed December 31, 2012; and Sterling TR, Pham PA, Chaisson RE. HIV infection-related tuberculosis: clinical manifestations and treatment. Clin Infect Dis 2010;50(Suppl 3):S223–30.

SUMMARY

Given the increased risk of TB disease and associated high mortality in patients with HIV infection, clinicians should have a high index of suspicion for TB in patients with HIV, even in patients with minimal or atypical symptoms. Aggressive diagnostic efforts using sensitive assays should be applied to HIV-infected individuals with signs or symptoms of TB. Treatment of latent TB infection, early initiation of antiretroviral therapy, and early treatment of active TB disease are essential in reducing the burden of HIV-associated TB and preventing further TB transmission.

REFERENCES

1. Lawn SD, Zumla AI. Tuberculosis. Lancet 2011; 378(9785):57–72.
2. WHO global tuberculosis report. 2012. Available at: http://www.who.int/tb/publications/global_report/en/. Accessed December 29, 2012.
3. Blumberg HM, Burman WJ, Chaisson RE, et al. American Thoracic Society/Centers for Disease Control and Prevention/Infectious Diseases Society of America: treatment of tuberculosis. Am J Respir Crit Care Med 2003;167(4):603–62.
4. Kaplan JE, Benson C, Holmes KH, et al. Guidelines for prevention and treatment of opportunistic infections in HIV-infected adults and adolescents: recommendations from CDC, the National Institutes of Health, and the HIV Medicine Association of the Infectious Diseases Society of America. MMWR Recomm Rep 2009;58(RR-4):1–207 [quiz: CE1–4].
5. Bassett IV, Wang B, Chetty S, et al. Intensive tuberculosis screening for HIV-infected patients starting antiretroviral therapy in Durban, South Africa. Clin Infect Dis 2010;51(7):823–9.
6. Geng E, Kreiswirth B, Burzynski J, et al. Clinical and radiographic correlates of primary and reactivation tuberculosis: a molecular epidemiology study. JAMA 2005;293(22):2740–5.
7. Chamie G, Luetkemeyer A, Walusimbi-Nanteza M, et al. Significant variation in presentation of pulmonary tuberculosis across a high resolution of CD4 strata. Int J Tuberc Lung Dis 2010;14(10):1295–302.
8. Getahun H, Sculier D, Sismanidis C, et al. Prevention, diagnosis, and treatment of tuberculosis in children and mothers: evidence for action for maternal, neonatal, and child health services. J Infect Dis 2012;205:S216–27.
9. Centers for Disease Control and Prevention (CDC). Trends in tuberculosis—United States, 2011. MMWR Morb Mortal Wkly Rep 2012;61(11):181–5.
10. Fujiwara PI, Dlodlo RA, Ferroussier O, et al. Implementing collaborative TB-HIV activities: a programmatic guide. 2012. Available at: http://www.theunion. org/index.php/en/resources/technical-publications/ item/2091-implementing-collaborative-tb-hiv-activities- a-programmatic-guide. Updated 2012.
11. WHO Treatment of tuberculosis: Guidelines for national programmes. 2012. Available at: http:// www.who.int/tb/publications/tb_treatmentguidelines/ en/index.html. Accessed December 29, 2012.
12. WHO WHO three 'I's meeting: Intensified case finding, isoniazid preventive therapy and TB infection control for people living with HIV. 2012. Available at: http://www.who.int/hiv/pub/tb/3is_mreport/ en/index.html. Accessed December 29, 2012.
13. Getahun H, Kittikraisak W, Heilig CM, et al. Development of a standardized screening rule for tuberculosis in people living with HIV in resource constrained settings: individual patient data meta-analysis. PLoS Med 2011;8(1). Available at: http:// www.plosmedicine.org/. Accessed December 29, 2012.
14. Gupta A, Chandrasekhar A, Gupte N, et al. Symptom screening among HIV-infected pregnant women is acceptable and has high negative predictive value for active tuberculosis. Clin Infect Dis 2011;53(10):1015–8.
15. Boehme CC, Nicol MP, Nabeta P, et al. Feasibility, diagnostic accuracy, and effectiveness of decentralised use of the Xpert MTB/RIF test for diagnosis of tuberculosis and multidrug resistance: a multicentre implementation study. Lancet 2011;377(9776): 1495–505.
16. Lawn SD, Brooks SV, Kranzer K, et al. Screening for HIV-associated tuberculosis and rifampicin resistance before antiretroviral therapy using the Xpert MTB/RIF assay: a prospective study. PLoS Med 2011;8(7):e1001067.
17. Dorman SE. New diagnostic tests for tuberculosis: Bench, bedside, and beyond. Clin Infect Dis 2010; 50(S3):S173–7. Available at: www.refworks.com.
18. Pai M, Ramsay A, O'Brien R. Evidence-based tuberculosis diagnosis. PLoS Medicine 2008;5(7):e156.
19. Reid MJ, Shah NS. Approaches to tuberculosis screening and diagnosis in people with HIV in resource-limited settings. Lancet Infect Dis 2009; 9(7):408.
20. World Health Organization. Use of tuberculosis interferon-gamma release assays (IGRAs) in low and middle-income countries: policy statement. Available at: http://www.who.int/tb/features_archive/ policy_statement_igra_oct2011.pdf. Accessed January 1, 2013.
21. Rangaka MX, Wilkinson KA, Glynn JR, et al. Predictive value of interferon-gamma release assays for incident active tuberculosis: a systematic review and meta-analysis. Lancet Infect Dis 2012;12(1): 45–55.
22. Mahan CS, Johnson DF, Curley C, et al. Concordance of a positive tuberculin skin test and an

interferon gamma release assay in bacille Calmette-Guerin vaccinated persons. Int J Tuberc Lung Dis 2011;15(2):174–8, i.

23. Akolo C, Adetifa I, Shepperd S, et al. Treatment of latent tuberculosis infection in HIV infected persons. Cochrane Database Syst Rev 2010;(1):CD000171.

24. Martinson NA, Barnes GL, Moulton LH, et al. New regimens to prevent tuberculosis in adults with HIV infection. N Engl J Med 2011;365(1):11–20.

25. Samandari T, Agizew TB, Nyirenda S, et al. 6-Month versus 36-month isoniazid preventive treatment of tuberculosis in adults with HIV infection in Botswana: a randomised, double-blind, placebo-controlled trial. Lancet 2011;377(9777):1588–98.

26. Mathad JS, Gupta A. Tuberculosis in pregnant and postpartum women: epidemiology, management, and research gaps. Clin Infect Dis 2012;55(11):1532–49.

27. Targeted tuberculin testing and treatment of latent tuberculosis infection. American Thoracic Society. MMWR Recomm Rep 2000;49(RR-6):1–51.

28. Sterling TR, Villarino ME, Borisov AS, et al. Three months of rifapentine and isoniazid for latent tuberculosis infection. N Engl J Med 2011;365(23): 2155–66.

29. Cohen MS, Chen YQ, McCauley M, et al. Prevention of HIV-1 infection with early antiretroviral therapy. N Engl J Med 2011;365(6):493–505.

30. Golub JE, Pronyk P, Mohapi L, et al. Isoniazid preventive therapy, HAART and tuberculosis risk in HIV-infected adults in South Africa: a prospective cohort. AIDS 2009;23(5):631–6.

31. Suthar AB, Lawn SD, del Amo J, et al. Antiretroviral therapy for prevention of tuberculosis in adults with HIV: a systematic review and meta-analysis. PLoS Med 2012;9(7):e1001270.

32. Rangaka MX, Boulle A, Wilkinson RJ, et al. Randomized controlled trial of isoniazid preventive therapy in HIV-infected persons on antiretroviral therapy. Clin Infect Dis 2012;55(12):1698–706.

33. Pepper T, Joseph P, Mwenya C, et al. Normal chest radiography in pulmonary tuberculosis: implications for obtaining respiratory specimen cultures. Int J Tuberc Lung Dis 2008;12(4):397–403.

34. Getahun H, Harrington M, O'Brien R, et al. Diagnosis of smear-negative pulmonary tuberculosis in people with HIV infection or AIDS in resource-constrained settings: informing urgent policy changes. Lancet 2007;369(9578):2042–9.

35. Manabe YC, Breen R, Perti T, et al. Unmasked tuberculosis and tuberculosis immune reconstitution inflammatory disease: a disease spectrum after initiation of antiretroviral therapy. J Infect Dis 2009; 199(3):437–44.

36. Lawn SD, Wilkinson RJ, Lipman MC, et al. Immune reconstitution and "unmasking" of tuberculosis during antiretroviral therapy. Am J Respir Crit Care Med 2008;177(7):680–5.

37. Meintjes G, Lawn SD, Scano F, et al. Tuberculosis-associated immune reconstitution inflammatory syndrome: case definitions for use in resource-limited settings. Lancet Infect Dis 2008; 8(8):516–23.

38. Chaisson RE, Schecter GF, Theuer CP, et al. Tuberculosis in patients with the acquired immunodeficiency syndrome. Clinical features, response to therapy, and survival. Am Rev Respir Dis 1987; 136(3):570–4.

39. Perriens JH, St Louis ME, Mukadi YB, et al. Pulmonary tuberculosis in HIV-infected patients in Zaire. A controlled trial of treatment for either 6 or 12 months. N Engl J Med 1995;332(12):779–84.

40. Fitzgerald DW, Desvarieux M, Severe P, et al. Effect of post-treatment isoniazid on prevention of recurrent tuberculosis in HIV-1-infected individuals: a randomised trial. Lancet 2000;356(9240): 1470–4.

41. Nahid P, Gonzalez LC, Rudoy I, et al. Treatment outcomes of patients with HIV and tuberculosis. Am J Respir Crit Care Med 2007;175(11):1199–206.

42. Churchyard GJ, Fielding K, Charalambous S, et al. Efficacy of secondary isoniazid preventive therapy among HIV-infected Southern Africans: time to change policy? AIDS 2003;17(14):2063–70.

43. Golub JE, Durovni B, King BS, et al. Recurrent tuberculosis in HIV-infected patients in Rio de Janeiro, Brazil. AIDS 2008;22(18):2527–33.

44. Chang KC, Leung CC, Yew WW, et al. Dosing schedules of 6-month regimens and relapse for pulmonary tuberculosis. Am J Respir Crit Care Med 2006; 174(10):1153–8.

45. Harries AD, Zachariah R, Lawn SD. Providing HIV care for co-infected tuberculosis patients: a perspective from Sub-Saharan Africa. Int J Tuberc Lung Dis 2009;13(1):6–16.

46. Bothamley G. Drug treatment for tuberculosis during pregnancy: safety considerations. Drug Saf 2001; 24(7):553–65.

47. Santoro-Lopes G, de Pinho AM, Harrison LH, et al. Reduced risk of tuberculosis among Brazilian patients with advanced human immunodeficiency virus infection treated with highly active antiretroviral therapy. Clin Infect Dis 2002;34(4):543–6.

48. Girardi E, Sabin CA, d'Arminio Monforte A, et al. Incidence of tuberculosis among HIV-infected patients receiving highly active antiretroviral therapy in Europe and North America. Clin Infect Dis 2005; 41(12):1772–82.

49. Lawn SD, Myer L, Bekker LG, et al. Burden of tuberculosis in an antiretroviral treatment programme in Sub-Saharan Africa: impact on treatment outcomes and implications for tuberculosis control. AIDS 2006;20(12):1605–12.

50. Hung CC, Chen MY, Hsiao CF, et al. Improved outcomes of HIV-1-infected adults with tuberculosis

in the era of highly active antiretroviral therapy. AIDS 2003;17(18):2615–22.

51. Abdool Karim SS, Naidoo K, Grobler A, et al. Timing of initiation of antiretroviral drugs during tuberculosis therapy. N Engl J Med 2010;362(8):697–706.

52. Abdool Karim SS, Naidoo K, Grobler A, et al. Integration of antiretroviral therapy with tuberculosis treatment. N Engl J Med 2011;365(16):1492–501.

53. Blanc FX, Sok T, Laureillard D, et al. Earlier versus later start of antiretroviral therapy in HIV-infected adults with tuberculosis. N Engl J Med 2011;365(16):1471–81.

54. Havlir DV, Kendall MA, Ive P, et al. Timing of antiretroviral therapy for HIV-1 infection and tuberculosis. N Engl J Med 2011;365(16):1482–91.

55. United States Department of Health and Human Services. Guidelines for the use of antiretroviral agents in HIV-1-infected adults and adolescents. 2012. Available at: http://www.aidsinfo.nih.gov/contentfiles/lvguidelines/adultandadolescentgl.pdf. Accessed December 31, 2012.

56. Torok ME, Yen NT, Chau TT, et al. Timing of initiation of antiretroviral therapy in human immunodeficiency virus (HIV)–associated tuberculous meningitis. Clin Infect Dis 2011;52(11):1374–83.

57. Muller M, Wandel S, Colebunders R, et al. Immune reconstitution inflammatory syndrome in patients starting antiretroviral therapy for HIV infection: a systematic review and meta-analysis. Lancet Infect Dis 2010;10(4):251–61.

58. Meintjes G, Wilkinson RJ, Morroni C, et al. Randomized placebo-controlled trial of prednisone for paradoxical tuberculosis-associated immune reconstitution inflammatory syndrome. AIDS 2010;24(15):2381–90.

59. CDC TB managing drug interactions in the treatment of HIV-related tuberculosis. 2012. Available at: http://www.cdc.gov/tb/publications/guidelines/TB_HIV_Drugs/default.htm. Accessed December 31, 2012.

60. Boulle A, Van Cutsem G, Cohen K, et al. Outcomes of nevirapine- and efavirenz-based antiretroviral therapy when coadministered with rifampicin-based antitubercular therapy. JAMA 2008;300(5):530–9.

61. Manosuthi W, Sungkanuparph S, Tantanathip P, et al. A randomized trial comparing plasma drug concentrations and efficacies between 2 nonnucleoside reverse-transcriptase inhibitor-based regimens in HIV-infected patients receiving rifampicin: the N2R study. Clin Infect Dis 2009;48(12):1752–9.

62. Sterling TR, Pham PA, Chaisson RE. HIV infection-related tuberculosis: clinical manifestations and treatment. Clin Infect Dis 2010;50(Suppl 3):S223–30.

Pneumocystis Pneumonia Associated with Human Immunodeficiency Virus

Robert F. Miller, MBBS, FRCP[a],*, Laurence Huang, MD[b],
Peter D. Walzer, MD, MSc[c]

KEYWORDS

- *Pneumocystis jirovecii* • Pneumocystis pneumonia • AIDS • HIV • Lung • Diagnosis

KEY POINTS

- Pneumocystis pneumonia (PCP) is caused by the yeastlike fungus *Pneumocystis.*
- Despite the widespread availability of specific anti-*Pneumocystis* prophylaxis and of combination antiretroviral therapy (ART), PCP remains a common AIDS-defining presentation in the United States and in Europe.
- PCP is increasingly recognized among persons living in Africa.
- *Pneumocystis* cannot be cultured and bronchoalveolar lavage is the gold standard diagnostic test to diagnose PCP.
- Use of adjunctive biomarkers for diagnosis requires further evaluation.
- Trimethoprim-sulfamethoxazole remains the preferred first-line treatment regimen. In the era of ART, mortality from PCP is approximately 10% to 12%. The optimal time to start ART in a patient with PCP remains uncertain.

INTRODUCTION

Different species of the ascomycetous yeastlike fungus *Pneumocystis* asymptomatically infect/colonize numerous healthy mammalian hosts and in immune-compromised mammals (including humans) can cause a potentially life-threatening pneumonia (Pneumocystis pneumonia [PCP]). The organism is host obligate and species specific: it cannot be grown outside the host and organisms from 1 host cannot infect other mammalian hosts.[1] Thus, *Pneumocystis jirovecii* is the cause of PCP in humans, whereas *Pneumocystis carinii* is the cause of PCP in rats.

Pneumocystis was identified in 1909 by Carlos Chagas, who mistakenly described it as part of the life cycle of the protozoan parasite *Trypanosoma cruzii*. It was first recognized as a human pathogen when it was described as the cause of interstitial plasma cell pneumonia among premature/malnourished infants in European orphanages immediately after World War II. In the 1960s and 1970s, descriptions of PCP were mainly in children with congenital immunodeficiency and also in adults and children with acquired immunologic deficits resulting from malignancy (specifically, glioma and acute leukemia) or its treatment (with glucocorticoids and purine analogues). The advent of organ transplantation and iatrogenic immunosuppression in the 1960s was associated with reports of PCP among this patient population.

Dr Huang is supported by NIH K24 HL087713, R01 HL090335, and U01 HL098964.
[a] Research Department of Infection and Population Health, University College London, London WC1E 6JB, UK; [b] Division of Pulmonary and Critical Care Medicine and HIV/AIDS Division, San Francisco General Hospital, University of California San Francisco, 995 Potrero Avenue, San Francisco, CA 94110, USA; [c] Division of Infectious Diseases, Department of Internal Medicine, University of Cincinnati College of Medicine, 231 Albert Sabin Way, Cincinnati, OH 45267-0560, USA
* Corresponding author.
E-mail address: robert.miller@ucl.ac.uk

Clin Chest Med 34 (2013) 229–241
http://dx.doi.org/10.1016/j.ccm.2013.02.001

In 1981, PCP was reported in 15 previously healthy men who had sex with other men (MSM) or who were injection drug users and heralded the advent of the global pandemic of human immunodeficiency virus [HIV]/AIDS.[2,3] Despite the availability of prophylaxis and of combination antiretroviral therapy (ART) PCP remains an important clinical presentation among HIV-infected persons.[4]

EPIDEMIOLOGY OF HIV-ASSOCIATED PCP

Before the onset of the AIDS epidemic, PCP was uncommon in the United States; between November 1967 and December 1970, 194 patients were reported to the Centers for Disease Control (CDC),[5] and in the 1970s, fewer than 100 cases per year were seen in the United States. During the early years of the AIDS epidemic, PCP accounted for two-thirds of AIDS-defining illness in patients in the United States, and an estimated 75% of HIV-infected patients developed PCP during their lifetime[6,7]; rates of PCP were as high as 20 per 100 person-years among those with CD4 cell counts less than 200 cells/μL.[7,8]

The first substantial decline in the incidence of PCP occurred after the introduction of anti-*Pneumocystis* prophylaxis in 1989.[9] In the United States, because of an increasing incidence of AIDS from 1989 to 1992, absolute numbers of reported cases of PCP as an AIDS-defining illness remained stable, but the percentage with PCP declined, from 53% in 1989% to 42% in 1992.[7]

The advent of ART resulted in further declines in rates of PCP and other opportunistic infections (OIs).[7,10,11] Several large, multicenter studies have tracked the incidence and epidemiologic features of PCP in the era of ART. Data from the ASD (Adult and Adolescent Spectrum of HIV Disease) study showed a marked reduction in incidence of all OIs in 1996 and 1997, when ART first became widely available; from 1992 to 1995, cases of PCP declined by 3.4% per year, and from 1996 to 1998 declined by 21.5% per year.[7,11] The Multicenter AIDS Cohort Study also showed a marked reduction in OIs after introduction of ART.[12]

In Europe, the EuroSIDA study[13,14] has examined changes in incidence of AIDS-defining disease before and after ART was introduced (1994–1998) and found results similar to those in the United States. The incidence of PCP in EuroSIDA fell from 4.9 cases per 100 person-years before March 1995 to 0.3 cases per 100 person-years after March 1998.

Despite these improvements, data from the Hospital Outpatient Study show that PCP remains the second most common AIDS-defining OI in the United States; in 1994 to 1997, the incidence was 29.9 per 1000 person-years, and decreased to 7.7 and 3.9 per 1000 person-years in 1998 to 2002 and 2003 to 2007, respectively.[15] In the United Kingdom, PCP was the commonest AIDS-defining illness in the decade 2001 to 2010.[16]

In the United States, Western Europe, and Australasia, PCP still occurs among HIV-infected persons despite the availability of ART and anti-*Pneumocystis* prophylaxis. The Multicenter AIDS Cohort Study examined use of PCP prophylaxis among HIV-infected adults who developed PCP during 1999 to 2001.[12] More than 43% of PCP cases occurred in persons not receiving medical care, most of who were likely not known to be HIV-infected, and a further 41% were prescribed prophylaxis but were either nonadherent with PCP prophylaxis, or PCP developed despite prophylaxis adherence. Possible explanations for PCP in this latter group include decreased efficacy of prophylaxis among those with low CD4 counts and development of drug-resistant *Pneumocystis*. An additional 9.6% were under medical care but did not receive prophylaxis, based on current recommendations (ie, CD4 count >200 cell/μL, or >14% of total lymphocyte count).[17]

In the pre-ART era, the greatest risk factor for PCP in an HIV-infected person was a CD4 cell count less than 200 cells/μL; this remains an important risk factor in the ART era. The more the CD4 count decreases lower than 200 cells/μL, the greater the risk for PCP.[18] Those who develop PCP despite receipt of ART usually have a low CD4 count. In the ASD study, the CD4 count among persons developing PCP while receiving ART was low (median = 29 cells/μL), and was also similarly low among those not taking ART (median = 13 cells/μL).[11] The prospective pan-European EuroSIDA study reported that the median CD4 count was 30 cells/μL among persons developing PCP while receiving ART and was similar among those not receiving ART who developed PCP.[8] Patients without improvement in their CD4 count after starting ART remain at risk for PCP. One recent study showed that approximately 5% of HIV-infected persons have a CD4 count greater than 200 cells/μL at presentation with PCP.[19]

Other potential clinical risk factors for development of PCP include gender, race or ethnicity, and risk factor for HIV acquisition. Men are more likely than women to develop PCP[17]; 1 study reported that African Americans have a lower risk for PCP than white persons[17] but this finding has not been replicated.[10] MSM seem to be at equal risk, when compared with other risk-exposure groups.[10]

PCP still occurs frequently among HIV-infected patients in many parts of the developing world.[20] Studies from Thailand show that the prevalence of PCP is up to 40%.[21] Central and South America also report large numbers of PCP cases. One Brazilian study found that 55% of HIV-infected persons with respiratory symptoms had PCP,[22] and a study from Mexico reported a 24% PCP prevalence.[23]

By contrast, PCP has until recently been believed to be rare in African adults. However, high rates of anti-Pneumocystis antibodies among African children suggest that exposure to the organism is common, and PCP is a common cause of pneumonia among children in sub-Saharan Africa.[24] PCP might have been underreported in Africa for several reasons. Limited local diagnostic resources, including lack of trained clinical and laboratory personnel and expensive equipment, mean that invasive investigations such as induced sputum and bronchoalveolar lavage (BAL) are less commonly performed, and reliance on empiric therapy for HIV-infected persons with presumed PCP potentially results in underestimation of the true incidence of PCP. Many HIV-infected African adults may not reach a stage at which they would be susceptible to PCP, because these populations have high rates of tuberculosis and bacterial pneumonia, which may result in death at higher CD4 counts. Environmental factors, such as temperature and seasonality, might also contribute to a low rate of PCP in Africa. The population may be more resistant to development of PCP; HIV-infected African Americans have been shown to have lower rates of PCP than white Americans[18]; or P jirovecii strains isolated in Africa may be less virulent, a possibility that can be answered only by large-scale molecular epidemiologic studies.

As the AIDS epidemic progresses in Africa, most, but not all, studies suggest that the incidence of PCP is increasing[20,24–27]; however, it is unclear whether this increase results from changes in incidence of PCP or from improvements in detection techniques.

PATHOGENESIS

Studies in animal models have shown that Pneumocystis is communicable via the airborne route. Young animals acquire Pneumocystis infection soon after birth and have an important role in spreading infection. Molecular epidemiologic studies in humans support the findings from these experimental models.[28,29] The incubation period

from inhalation to presentation with PCP in humans is believed to be approximately 4 to 8 weeks.

Most healthy adults do not have detectable Pneumocystis in respiratory specimens,[30,31] but several groups of individuals, both HIV-infected and uninfected, including those with chronic obstructive pulmonary disease (COPD), and pregnant women may become colonized with Pneumocystis, thus increasing the potential number of persons affected.[32–34] Pneumocystis colonization may increase the risk for progression to PCP among HIV-infected and uninfected persons. Persons colonized with Pneumocystis may also transmit infection to others who have minor or significant immune suppression and act as an infectious reservoir. Long-term colonization of asymptomatic HIV-infected and uninfected (eg, COPD) hosts may result in pulmonary inflammation and progressive impairment of lung function.[33,35,36]

After inhalation, Pneumocystis eludes the upper airway defenses and deposits in alveoli, where it adheres tightly to alveolar type I cells and provokes a host inflammatory response.[36] In most hosts with an intact immune system, the organism is rapidly coughed out. If the host has any underlying minor immune suppression/HIV-associated immunodeficiency, colonization with Pneumocystis ensues.[34,35] If the host then becomes more immune compromised, by progression of HIV, or by additional therapeutic immune suppression, then Pneumocystis propagates within the alveoli, and slowly floods the alveoli out. At the same time, disruption of the alveolar-capillary membrane, with ventilation-perfusion abnormalities similar to the changes seen in acute respiratory distress syndrome, also occur and manifest as impaired gas exchange. These events culminate in presentation with PCP.

CLINICAL MANIFESTATIONS

The clinical presentation of PCP among HIV-infected patients is nonspecific and can be mimicked by a variety of infectious and noninfectious causes. Patients typically present with a triad of progressive exertional dyspnea, nonproductive cough, and fever of several days' or weeks' duration, which is often associated with an inability to take in a maximum inspiration (not because of pain).[37,38] Although a productive cough and chest tightness may occur, purulent sputum should raise suspicion of bacterial infection. Hemoptysis is not a feature. Among HIV-infected persons, symptoms are usually of longer duration than among non-HIV-infected, medically immunosuppressed patients.[39] HIV-infected patients frequently have prolonged prodromal periods with subtle clinical manifestations developing over 3 to 8 weeks; however, some individuals present with a fulminant deterioration of symptoms over 7 to 10 days, or less. On physical examination, varying degrees of respiratory distress (tachycardia, central cyanosis) may be evident as well as stigmata of immune suppression, including oral hairy leukoplakia, molluscum contagiosum, seborrheic dermatitis, and cutaneous Kaposi sarcoma (KS). Auscultation of the chest is usually normal; rarely, fine end-inspiratory crackles may be heard.

DIAGNOSIS
Noninvasive Investigations

Chest radiology
In early PCP, the chest radiograph may be normal; with later presentations, and with more severe disease, diffuse perihilar interstitial infiltrates are seen (**Fig. 1**). These appearances may progress to diffuse bilateral air space (alveolar) consolidation resembling pulmonary edema or acute respiratory distress syndrome. With delayed presentation or untreated severe disease, there may be confluent alveolar shadowing (white-out) throughout both lungs, with sparing of the costophrenic angles and apices (**Fig. 2**). The chest radiographic appearances in PCP may change rapidly from normal at presentation to markedly abnormal over a period of only 2 to 3 days (**Fig. 3**). Atypical radiographic features include cystic air space and pneumatocele formation, unilateral consolidation, lobar infiltrates, nodules, mediastinal lymphadenopathy, pleural effusions, and upper zone infiltrates resembling tuberculosis (**Fig. 4**).

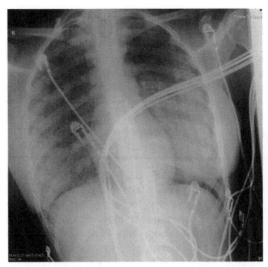

Fig. 2. Chest radiograph showing severe PCP. The patient is intubated and mechanically ventilated; there is a left-sided pneumothorax.

Although the chest radiograph is a sensitive way of detecting PCP, it is nonspecific; these typical and atypical radiographic appearances are also seen in other fungal, mycobacterial, and bacterial infections, and in noninfectious conditions, such as interstitial pneumonitis and pulmonary KS. With treatment of PCP, improvements in the chest radiographic appearances are not usually apparent for 7 to 10 days. After clinical recovery, some radiographs show residual fibrosis or postinfectious bronchiectasis.

High-resolution chest computed tomography
High-resolution computed tomography (HRCT) of the chest may be useful in the symptomatic patient with suspected PCP who has a normal or equivocal chest radiograph. Patches of ground-glass shadowing are typical for PCP but also occur in viral (eg, cytomegalovirus, influenza A) or fungal pneumonia and in occult alveolar hemorrhage (**Fig. 5**). Chest HRCT may be used to rule out the diagnosis of PCP; the absence of ground-glass opacities strongly argues against the presence of PCP.

Arterial blood gases
In patients presenting early with PCP, even although the arterial oxygen tension (Pao$_2$) may be normal or near normal, respiratory alkalosis with hypocarbia (indicating hyperventilation) is often detected; hypoxia may occur with progression of the PCP. The alveolar-arterial oxygen gradient (A-ao$_2$) is widened in more than 90% of patients with PCP, but this finding, although suggestive, is nonspecific, because both hypoxemia and a widened A-ao$_2$ gradient also occur in

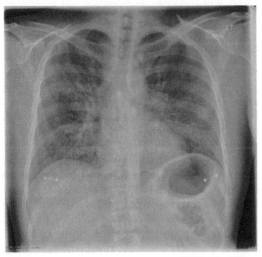

Fig. 1. Chest radiograph showing bilateral diffuse interstitial infiltrates.

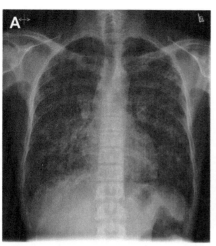
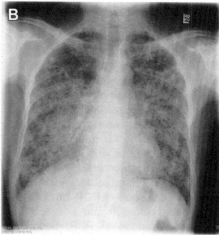

Fig. 3. (*A*) Chest radiograph on admission with PCP. (*B*) Chest radiograph [same patient as (*A*)], after an interval of 3 days, showing marked deterioration in radiographic abnormalities.

bacterial and mycobacterial infection, nonspecific interstitial pneumonitis, and pulmonary KS.

Exercise oximetry
Among HIV-infected patients who have respiratory symptoms, a normal or near-normal chest radiograph and normal resting Pao$_2$ values, exercise-induced arterial desaturation is a sensitive and specific method of detecting PCP. A normal exercise test (without desaturation) virtually excludes the diagnosis.

Pulmonary function testing
Data from the North American Pulmonary Complications of HIV Infection Study suggest that HIV-infected individuals who have rapid rates of

decline in D$_{LCO}$ (carbon monoxide diffusion in the lung) are at an increased risk for development of PCP.[18] A normal D$_{LCO}$ in an individual who has respiratory symptoms but a normal or unchanged chest radiograph makes the diagnosis of PCP unlikely.

Serum lactate dehydrogenase
An increased serum lactate dehydrogenase (LDH) level is highly suggestive of PCP in an HIV-infected patient with subacute respiratory symptoms.[40] However, an increased serum LDH is nonspecific, because it is also found in other pulmonary diseases, including pulmonary embolism, nonspecific interstitial pneumonitis, and fungal, bacterial, and mycobacterial pneumonia, as well as in extrapulmonary disease, such as multicentric Castleman disease and lymphoma.

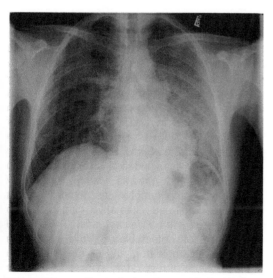

Fig. 4. Chest radiograph showing atypical radiologic appearances; asymmetric infiltrates.

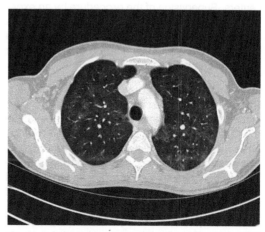

Fig. 5. Computed tomography showing widespread changes of ground-glass shadowing.

Serum (1–3) β-ᴅ-glucan

Measurement of the fungal cell wall component (1–3) β-ᴅ-glucan (BG) in serum has been used as an adjunctive diagnostic tool for diagnosis of PCP.[41,42] BG levels are higher among both HIV-infected and HIV-uninfected patients with PCP, when compared with symptomatic patients with confirmed alternative diagnoses, including aspergillosis and histoplasmosis. False-positive results occur in bacterial pneumonia, patients undergoing hemodialysis, and those who have recently received intravenous immunoglobulin. The serum BG assay seems to be a promising adjunctive noninvasive test for diagnosis of PCP, but further validation is needed before it can be used to monitor treatment response in PCP, because despite clinical recovery, reductions in BG titer are both delayed and unpredictable.[43]

Plasma/serum S-adenosylmethionine

Pneumocystis has been reported to lack S-adenosylmethionine synthetase, is unable to metabolize S-adenosylmethionine (SAM, or Adomet), and so scavenges this from the human host. It was hypothesized that HIV-infected persons with PCP would have low serum/plasma SAM levels. Whereas measurement of plasma SAM levels enabled discrimination between PCP and other causes of pneumonia in some studies,[44] 1 study showed overlapping serum SAM levels.[45] This assay lacks clinical diagnostic usefulness.

Invasive Investigations

Sputum induction

Pneumocystis is rarely identified in spontaneously expectorated sputum. Induced sputum, obtained by inhalation of an aerosol of hypertonic saline is a useful screening technique. The diagnostic yield from this technique varies considerably between centers. Supervision of the procedure by an experienced nurse or respiratory therapist increases the yield; a negative result for Pneumocystis from sputum induction should prompt referral for bronchoscopy.

Fiber-optic bronchoscopy

Fiber-optic bronchoscopy with BAL has a high diagnostic yield, greater than 90% for detection of PCP. Transbronchial biopsy adds little to diagnosis, and is associated with complications, including pneumothorax and hemorrhage. Treatment should never be deferred in an HIV-infected person with suspected PCP pending results of bronchoscopy, because significant clinical deterioration may occur. The yield for diagnosis of PCP from BAL fluid is not reduced for up to 14 days after starting treatment.

Video-assisted thoracoscopic biopsy

Video-assisted thoracoscopic biopsy is occasionally performed in HIV-infected patients with suspected PCP and who have negative results from 2 or more bronchoscopies, and among patients whose clinical course is at variance with laboratory-confirmed PCP.

Histologic diagnosis

Pneumocystis cannot reliably be cultured ex vivo, and so diagnosis of PCP is by microscopic visualization of the organism in induced sputum, BAL fluid, or lung tissue. Histopathologically, PCP is characterized by the presence of a foamy, vacuolated exudate filling alveoli. With late presenting or severe disease, there may be interstitial fibrosis, edema, and development of hyaline membranes. Hypertrophy of type II alveolar cells, inferring tissue repair, is frequently seen.

Several histologic stains have been used to identify Pneumocystis. Stains that identify the wall of the cystic form (methenamine silver, toluidine blue O, and cresyl violet) are widely used, because they require minimal laboratory expertise and are easily interpreted, and stains that show the nuclei of all Pneumocystis developmental stages (Diff-Quik or Wright-Giemsa) can provide a rapid diagnosis (within minutes) but require laboratory expertise. Other reagents, including Papanicolaou and calcofluor white, a chemiluminescent agent, are used by some laboratories.

Use of Pneumocystis-specific monoclonal antibodies and immunofluorescence stains has greater diagnostic sensitivity than histologic stains, but is more expensive and requires specific laboratory expertise.

Molecular detection tests

Detection of Pneumocystis-specific DNA using the polymerase chain reaction (PCR) in BAL fluid and induced sputum is superior to histologic staining for diagnosis of PCP. Pneumocystis DNA may also be detected in oropharyngeal wash (OPW) samples in HIV-infected persons presenting with PCP. The specificity and clinical significance of molecular detection assays is impaired by the finding of Pneumocystis DNA in respiratory samples (BAL fluid, induced sputum, or OPW) from HIV-infected patients without respiratory symptoms, and in symptomatic persons without PCP with confirmed alternative diagnosis who are colonized with Pneumocystis. The clinical significance of detectable P jirovecii DNA in a respiratory sample from an HIV-infected person in the absence of respiratory symptoms or other confirmatory tests (representing colonization) is unclear.

Although PCR is not licensed for diagnosis, several clinical laboratories in the United States and Europe use this method applied to invasive (BAL and induced sputum) and noninvasive sampling techniques (OPW) for diagnosis of PCP.[46–48]

Empirical therapy

Empirical therapy for HIV-infected patients presenting with symptoms and chest radiographic and arterial blood gas abnormalities typical of PCP is used in health care settings that lack diagnostic facilities. This strategy is possible if a patient with a CD4 less than 200 cells/μL (or stigmata of immune suppression) has typical radiologic abnormalities, is not receiving *Pneumocystis* prophylaxis or ART, and has a low probability of other (opportunistic) infections, such as tuberculosis.[38]

Treatment

An assessment of the severity of the pneumonia, using the results of arterial blood gas estimations, enables decisions to be made about choice of therapy; some drugs are unproved or ineffective in severe disease. When breathing room air, Pao_2 greater than 70 mm Hg (>9.3 kPa) indicates mild PCP, and 70 mm Hg or less (<9.3 kPa) indicates moderate to severe PCP. Alternatively, an A-ao$_2$ gradient less than 35 mm Hg, 35 to 45 mm Hg, and greater than 45 mm Hg (>6 kPa) indicates mild, moderate, and severe PCP, respectively. Severity stratification also identifies patients who will benefit from adjunctive glucocorticoids.

Patients with glucose 6-phosphate dehydrogenase deficiency should not receive trimethoprim/sulfamethoxazole (TMP-SMX), dapsone, or primaquine as these medications increase the risk of hemolysis.

Trimethoprim-sulfamethoxazole

Trimethoprim-sulfamethoxazole (TMP-SMX) [Bactrim, Bactrimel, cotrimoxazole, Cotrim, Septra, Septrin, Sulfatrim,Trisul] (20 mg/kg daily of TMP and 100 mg/kg daily of SMX) given in 2 to 4 divided doses orally or intravenously is first-choice therapy for PCP of all grades of severity; this drug combination acts by inhibiting folic acid metabolism. In HIV-infected patients, treatment is given for 21 days because shorter courses are associated with treatment failure. In patients with moderate or severe disease, TMP-SMX is typically given intravenously for the first 7 to 10 days, then orally; in patients with mild disease, oral TMP-SMX may be given throughout. This treatment regimen is effective in 70% to 80% of patients. Adverse reactions to TMP-SMX, which are usually first evident at 6 to 14 days of treatment, are common and include neutropenia and anemia in 40% of patients

or less, rash in 25%, fever in more than 30%, and abnormal liver function tests in approximately 10%.[49,50]

Coadministration of folic or folinic acid does not reduce or prevent hematologic toxicity and may be associated with increased therapeutic failure. Dose reduction of TMP-SMX, to 75% of the dose given earlier, is associated with a reduced toxicity profile but may be associated with reduced efficacy. It is not clear why there is such a high frequency of adverse reactions to TMP-SMX among HIV-infected patients compared with patients immunosuppressed by other causes, but it may be caused by HIV-induced changes in acetylator status, accumulation of toxic metabolites such as hydroxylamines, or to glutathione deficiency.

Alternative therapy

Several other treatments are available if TMP-SMX is not tolerated by the patient or if treatment fails.[17]

Clindamycin and primaquine

This combination was originally used only to salvage patients with mild and moderately severe PCP failing TMP-SMX or intravenous pentamidine. It is now used as alternative therapy in patients with PCP of all severity. Clindamycin (Cleocyin, Daclin) 450 to 600 mg 4 times daily is combined with primaquine 15 to 30 mg daily (orally). Clindamycin is usually given intravenously for the first 7 to 10 days, then orally in moderate and severe disease; the treatment may be given orally throughout in patients with mild disease. The mechanism of action of this combination is not known. Clindamycin-primaquine is as effective as TMP-SMX or dapsone-trimethoprim (see later discussion) when given as initial treatment of patients with PCP of mild and moderate severity and may be superior to intravenous pentamidine when used in patients intolerant of, or who are failing treatment with, TMP-SMX.[51] Almost two-thirds of patients develop a rash and approximately one-quarter develop diarrhea (both caused by clindamycin). Analysis of stool for detection of *Clostridium difficile* is indicated if diarrhea occurs. Methemoglobinemia (caused by primaquine) occurs in up to 40% of patients, but this is less likely if 15 mg rather than 30 mg of primaquine is used.

Dapsone with trimethoprim

Among patients with mild or moderate severity PCP, a combination of oral dapsone (Axzone) (100 mg per day) and TMP (20 mg/kg daily) is as effective as TMP-SMX (doses as outlined earlier) and is better tolerated. Rash, nausea and vomiting, mild hyperkalemia (caused by trimethoprim, in ≤50%) and asymptomatic methemoglobinemia (caused by dapsone) are common side effects. This combination has not shown efficacy in severe PCP.

Atovaquone

Oral atovaquone (Mepron) is a hydroxynaphthoquinolone that acts against *Plasmodia* by inhibiting electron transport. At a dose of 750 mg twice daily, it is ineffective in patients with severe PCP and less effective than either oral TMP-SMX or intravenous pentamidine for treatment of mild and moderate severity PCP, but is better tolerated than either drug. Adverse reactions include fever, rash, nausea and vomiting, constipation, and abnormal liver function tests.

Parenteral pentamidine

Intravenous pentamidine (Pentacarinat, Pentam 300, pentamidine isethionate for injection) is now only rarely used in mild and moderately severe PCP. It continues to be used in patients with severe PCP. Its mode of action against *Pneumocystis* is unknown. It is given at a dose of 3 to 4 mg/kg daily, by intravenous infusion over at least 1 hour. Compared with TMP-SMX, intravenous pentamidine has almost equivalent efficacy but greater toxicity; up to 60% of patients develop increases in the serum creatinine level; approximately half develop leukopenia. Hypotension, nausea, and vomiting occur in up to a quarter of patients; hypoglycemia occurs in approximately 20%; cardiac dysrhythmias (torsade de pointes) pancreatitis, hypocalcemia, and hypomagnesemia are also described. Autopsy data suggest that it takes at least 5 days for intravenous pentamidine to reach therapeutic concentrations in the lung. Using a dose of 3 mg/kg daily is associated with fewer adverse drug reactions, but data showing equivalent efficacy with the 4-mg/kg dose are lacking. There are no therapeutic advantages to combining TMP-SMX and intravenous pentamidine and this combination has a higher toxicity profile.

Caspofungin

Caspofungin (Cancidas) is an echinocandin that inhibits (1–3) BG synthase and is effective against *Aspergillus* and *Candida* spp. Several case reports and small case series show that caspofungin as monotherapy or combined with other therapy may be effective in patients with PCP who are not responding or tolerating first-line therapy. Caspofungin has not been prospectively evaluated against TMP-SMX or other regimens as first-line therapy.

Nebulized (aerosolized) pentamidine

Nebulized (aerosolized) pentamidine has no role in treatment of PCP.

Adjunctive corticosteroids

In HIV-infected patients with moderate and severe PCP, adjunctive therapy with corticosteroids has been shown to reduce the likelihood of respiratory failure (by half) and death (by one-third). Corticosteroids probably act by reducing the intrapulmonary inflammatory response of the body to *Pneumocystis*. It is recommended that glucocorticoids are given to HIV-infected patients with proved or suspected PCP who have a Pao_2 of 70 mm Hg or greater (<9.3 kPa) or an A-ao_2 greater than 35 mm Hg (>4.7 kPa).[17]

Corticosteroid treatment should begin at the start of specific anti-*Pneumocystis* therapy. In some patients, treatment begins on an empiric basis and the diagnosis should be confirmed as soon as practical. Regimens include oral prednisolone 40 mg twice daily for 5 days, thereafter 40 mg once daily for days 6 to 10, and then 11 further days of 20 mg daily and intravenous methylprednisolone at 75% of these doses.[17] There is no evidence that adjunctive corticosteroids are of benefit in patients with mild PCP. Patients receiving adjunctive corticosteroids should be monitored for hyperglycemia.

General management

In the first few days of treatment, HIV-infected patients with PCP may experience deterioration in their clinical condition, with worsening of the chest radiograph and oxygenation. This situation is believed to arise either from the host inflammatory response to dying *Pneumocystis*, or to *Pneumocystis*-induced changes in surfactant leading to worsening of lung injury.

Patients with mild PCP may be treated as outpatients with oral TMP-SMX under close supervision of a physician. Patients with moderate and severe PCP should be treated with intravenous TMP-SMX, or with clindamycin with primaquine, and adjunctive corticosteroids. Patients who are not responding by 5 to 7 days should be candidates to switch to alternative therapy. Before ascribing deterioration to treatment failure and considering a change in therapy, alternative causes should be evaluated (**Table 1**). In addition, it is important to perform bronchoscopy if the diagnosis is empirical, and to treat any codisease already detected in BAL fluid.

All hypoxemic patients with PCP should receive supplemental oxygen therapy via nasal cannula or a tight-fitting face mask in order to maintain the Pao_2 60 mm Hg or greater (≥8.0 kPa). If an inspired

Table 1
Causes of deterioration in an HIV-infected adult receiving treatment of PCP

Cause	Explanation
Severe progressive PCP	
Iatrogenic	Pulmonary edema caused by intravenous fluid overload when giving TMP-SMX
	Immune reconstitution inflammatory syndrome after early initiation of ART
Side effects of therapy	Anemia (eg, TMP-SMX)
	Methemoglobinemia (eg, dapsone, primaquine)
Inadequate therapy	Incorrect dosage or oral route of administration
	Adjuvant glucocorticoids not given for moderate or severe PCP
After bronchoscopy	Sedation
	Pneumothorax
Pneumothorax	Spontaneous
	Associated with mechanical ventilation
Codisease in lung	Bacterial infection
	Pulmonary KS
	Intercurrent pulmonary embolism
Incorrect diagnosis	Empiric diagnosis of PCP and correct diagnosis is another disease (eg, bacterial pneumonia)

oxygen concentration of 60% fails to maintain the Pao_2 60 mm Hg or greater ($\geq$8.0 kPa), referral to the intensive care unit (ICU) for mechanical ventilation should be considered. The prognosis of patients with severe PCP with respiratory failure has improved in recent years, as a consequence of general improvements in ICU management of respiratory failure.[52,53]

Prognosis

Over the last 20 years, the outcome for HIV-infected persons with PCP has improved. This improvement is likely because of a combination of earlier detection of disease, timely institution of treatment, and more effective management of complications. In the ART era, mortality from PCP is 9.7% to 11.6%.[19,54,55] Several clinical and laboratory features have been shown to predict a poor outcome among HIV-infected patients with PCP. Prognostic factors at presentation include increasing patient age, lack of knowledge of HIV status, presentation with a second or subsequent episode of PCP, evidence of poor oxygenation (Pao_2 <53 mm Hg [<7.0 kPa] or an A-aO_2 gradient >30 mm Hg] >4.0 kPa]), marked chest radiographic abnormalities, peripheral blood leukocytosis (white blood cell count >10.8 $\times$ 10^9/L), a low hemoglobin (<12 g/dL), a low serum albumin (<3.5 g/L), and increased serum LDH enzyme levels (>300 IU/L). After admission and investigation, identification in BAL fluid of a copathogen (viral, eg, CMV, or bacterial), greater than 5% neutrophilia or increased interleukin 8 levels, evidence of

fibrosis and edema on transbronchial biopsy, and increased serum LDH enzyme levels that do not decrease despite treatment, identification of comorbidity (eg, non-Hodgkin lymphoma), presence of pulmonary KS, or admission to the ICU, a high APACHE II (Acute Physiology and Chronic Health Evaluation) score, need for mechanical ventilation, or development of a pneumothorax are also predictive of a poor outcome.

Several prognostic scores have been derived from factors present at or soon after an HIV-infected person's presentation with PCP; scores based on wasting, A-ao$_2$ gradient, and serum albumin[56]; age, injection drug use, A-ao$_2$ gradient, serum albumin and serum bilirubin[57]; age, hemoglobin, Pao_2, pulmonary KS, and comorbidity[58] all associate with mortality. The potential value of such prognostic scores lies in their ability to identify those at greatest risk of death and to inform clinicians about which patients can safely be managed in an outpatient setting. Although these prognostic scores have been derived from large cohorts of HIV-infected patients with PCP in the United States or United Kingdom, none has been validated in other US/UK cohorts or in developing-world settings.[56–58]

Starting ART in a patient with PCP

The optimal time to initiate ART in a person with PCP remains to be determined; some clinicians start ART immediately, whereas others prefer to see a clinical response to PCP treatment. One randomized trial of patients with OI, in which approximately two-thirds of patients had PCP, showed that ART when initiated early (within 2 weeks) and compared with therapy deferred until 4 weeks or more after initiation of treatment of the OI was associated with a significant reduction in progression to AIDS/mortality, but no increased risk of immune reconstitution inflammatory syndrome.[59,60] Although this study supports early ART, it does not show whether immediate treatment at time of PCP diagnosis or waiting for a response to PCP treatment (usually within 4–7 days) is a better strategy. The study excluded those with severe laboratory abnormalities and required patients to be able to take oral medication (mechanically ventilated patients were not studied), inferring possible selection bias in favor of less sick patients. By contrast, marked respiratory deterioration from ART, if initiated early, has also been reported.[61]

Prophylaxis

With progressive immunosuppression and decreases in CD4 counts, HIV-infected individuals are at increased risk of developing PCP. Primary prophylaxis, to prevent a first episode of PCP, is given when the CD4 lymphocyte count decreases less than 200 cells/μL or the CD4/total lymphocyte ratio is less than 1:5 (or <14%), to patients with HIV-related constitutional symptoms such as unexplained fever (>100°F) of 2 weeks or more in duration, or oral *Candida* regardless of CD4 count, and to patients with other AIDS-defining diagnoses, such as KS. Secondary prophylaxis is given in order to prevent a recurrence of PCP.

One double-strength (DS) TMP-SMX tablet (containing 160 mg of TMP and 800 mg of SMX) once daily is the first-choice regimen for both primary and secondary prophylaxis. Lower doses, 1 DS TMP-SMX 3 times weekly or 1 single-strength TMP-SMX tablet (containing 80 mg of TMP and 400 mg of SMX) once daily, may be equally effective and have fewer adverse drug reactions. Rash, with or without fever, occurs in 20% of patients or less. Desensitization should be attempted in those unable to tolerate TMP-SMX. Alternatively, other less effective agents are available for prophylaxis, including nebulized pentamidine (Nebupent), 300 mg (delivered via a Respirgard II nebulizer [Southwest Medical, Phoenix, AZ]) once per month (once per fortnight in HIV-infected patients with CD4 counts <50 cells/μL), dapsone 100 mg once daily (or 50 mg twice daily), dapsone 50 mg once daily with pyrimethamine 75 mg once weekly and leucovorin 25 mg once weekly, or dapsone 200 mg with 75 mg pyrimethamine and 25 mg leucovorin (all once weekly), and oral atovaquone 750 mg twice daily, with or without pyrimethamine 75 mg once daily and leucovorin 25 mg once daily.[17]

Discontinuing prophylaxis

The widespread availability and uptake of ART in North America, Europe, and Australasia has been associated with marked reductions in incidence of many OIs, including PCP, hospital admissions, and mortality from HIV infection. In most patients, within a few weeks of starting ART, there are rapid decreases in plasma HIV RNA and, in parallel, increases in CD4 counts. The CDC/National Institutes of Health/Infectious Diseases Society of America recommend that primary prophylaxis against PCP may be discontinued in HIV-infected persons who respond to ART with an increase in CD4 counts to more than 200 cells/μL, sustained for at least 6 months.[17] Many of these patients also have reduction in HIV RNA to lower than the limit of detection. Withdrawal of secondary prophylaxis may be carried out, using these criteria. If, despite ART, the CD4 lymphocyte count decreases less than 200 cells/μL or the plasma HIV RNA load increases, then prophylaxis should be reinstituted using the criteria for primary prophylaxis. Close patient monitoring is needed to detect any such changes rapidly.

Recent data accrued from a cohort study, a retrospective review, and a case series show a low incidence of PCP among patients who discontinue or never start PCP prophylaxis, who received ART and had CD4 counts between 100–200 cells/μL and plasma HIV viral loads less than 50 to 400 copies/mL.[62–64] Although these data support discontinuation of primary PCP prophylaxis in certain patients with CD4 counts between 100 and 200 cells/μL, with some experts recommending this approach for their patients, this intervention has not yet been widely adopted.[17]

SUMMARY

The yeastlike fungus *Pneumocystis* causes PCP, which, despite the widespread availability of specific anti-*Pneumocystis* prophylaxis and of combination ART, remains a common AIDS-defining presentation in the United States and in Europe, and is increasingly recognized among persons living in Africa. *Pneumocystis* cannot be cultured and the gold standard diagnostic test to diagnose PCP is BAL. Use of adjunctive biomarkers such as serum (1–3) BG for diagnosis requires further evaluation. Recommended first-line treatment is with TMP-SMX. Mortality from PCP in the era of ART is approximately 10% to 12%. The optimal time to start ART in a patient with PCP remains uncertain.

REFERENCES

1. Cushion MT. Are members of the fungal genus *Pneumocystis* (a) commensals; (b) opportunists; (c) pathogens; or (d) all of the above? PLoS Pathog 2010;6:e1001009.

2. Gottlieb MS, Schroff R, Schanker HM, et al. *Pneumocystis carinii* pneumonia and mucosal candidiasis in previously healthy homosexual men: evidence of a new acquired cellular immunodeficiency. N Engl J Med 1981;305:1425–31.

3. Masur H, Michelis M, Greene J, et al. An outbreak of community-acquired *Pneumocystis carinii* pneumonia–initial manifestation of cellular immune dysfunction. N Engl J Med 1981;305:1431–8.

4. Huang L, Cattamanchi A, Davies JL, et al, on behalf of the International HIV-associated opportunistic pneumonias (IHOP) study, the lung HIV study. HIV-associated *Pneumocystis* pneumonia. Proc Am Thorac Soc 2011;8:294–300.

5. Walzer PD, Perl DP, Krogstad DJ, et al. *Pneumocystis carinii* pneumonia in the United States. Epidemiologic, diagnostic, and clinical features. Ann Intern Med 1974;80:83–93.

6. Hay JW, Osmond DH, Jacobson MA. Projecting the medical costs of AIDS and ARC in the United States. J Acquir Immune Defic Syndr 1988;1:466–85.

7. Morris A, Lundgren JD, Masur H, et al. Current epidemiology of *Pneumocystis pneumonia*. Emerg Infect Dis 2004;10:1713–20.

8. Phair J, Muñoz A, Detels R, et al. The risk of *Pneumocystis carinii* pneumonia among men infected with human immunodeficiency virus type 1. Multicenter AIDS Cohort Study. N Engl J Med 1990;322:161–5.

9. Jones JL, Hanson DL, Dworkin MS, et al. Surveillance for AIDS-defining opportunistic illnesses, 1992-1997. MMWR CDC Surveill Summ 1999;48:1–22.

10. Kaplan JE, Hanson DL, Navin TR, et al. Risk factors for primary *Pneumocystis carinii* pneumonia in human immunodeficiency virus-infected adolescents and adults in the United States: reassessment of indications for chemoprophylaxis. J Infect Dis 1998;178:1126–32.

11. Kaplan JE, Hanson D, Dworkin MS, et al. Epidemiology of human immunodeficiency virus-associated opportunistic infections in the United States in the era of highly active antiretroviral therapy. Clin Infect Dis 2000;30(Suppl 1):S5–14.

12. Detels R, Tarwater P, Phair JP, et al, Multicenter AIDS Cohort Study. Effectiveness of potent antiretroviral therapies on the incidence of opportunistic infections before and after AIDS diagnosis. AIDS 2001;15:347–55.

13. Mocroft A, Katlama C, Johnson AM, et al. AIDS across Europe, 1994-98: the EuroSIDA study. Lancet 2000;356:291–6.

14. Weverling GJ, Mocroft A, Ledergerber B, et al. Discontinuation of *Pneumocystis carinii* pneumonia prophylaxis after start of highly active antiretroviral therapy in HIV-1 infection. EuroSIDA Study Group. Lancet 1999;353:1293–8.

15. Buchacz K, Baker RK, Palella FJ, et al, HOPS Investigators. AIDS-defining opportunistic illnesses in US patients, 1994-2007: a cohort study. AIDS 2010;19(24):1549–59.

16. HIV in the United Kingdom: 2011 report. Available at: http://www.hpa.org.uk/webc/HPAwebFile/HPAweb_C/1317131685847. Accessed August 22, 2012.

17. Kaplan JE, Benson C, Holmes KH, et al; Centers for Disease Control and Prevention (CDC); National Institutes of Health; HIV Medicine Association of the Infectious Diseases Society of America. Guidelines for prevention and treatment of opportunistic infections in HIV-infected adults and adolescents: recommendations from CDC, the National Institutes of Health, and the HIV Medicine Association of the Infectious Diseases Society of America. MMWR Recomm Rep, in press.

18. Stansell JD, Osmond DH, Charlebois E, et al. Predictors of *Pneumocystis carinii* pneumonia in HIV-infected persons. Pulmonary complications of HIV infection study group. Am J Respir Crit Care Med 1997;155:60–6.

19. Walzer PD, Evans HE, Copas AJ, et al. Early predictors of mortality from *Pneumocystis jirovecii* pneumonia in HIV-infected patients: 1985-2006. Clin Infect Dis 2008;46:625–33.

20. Fisk DT, Meshnick S, Kazanjian PH. *Pneumocystis carinii* pneumonia in patients in the developing world who have acquired immunodeficiency syndrome. Clin Infect Dis 2003;36:70–8.

21. Wannamethee SG, Sirivichayakul S, Phillips AN, et al. Clinical and immunological features of human immunodeficiency virus infection in patients from Bangkok, Thailand. Int J Epidemiol 1998;27:289–95.

22. Weinberg A, Duarte MI. Respiratory complications in Brazilian patients infected with human immunodeficiency virus. Rev Inst Med Trop Sao Paulo 1993;35:129–39.

23. Mohar A, Romo J, Salido F, et al. The spectrum of clinical and pathological manifestations of AIDS in a consecutive series of autopsied patients in Mexico. AIDS 1992;6:467–73.

24. Morrow BM, Hsaio NY, Zampoli M, et al. *Pneumocystis* pneumonia in South African children with and without human immunodeficiency virus infection in the era of highly active antiretroviral therapy. Pediatr Infect Dis J 2010;29:535–9.

25. Worodria W, Okot-Nwang M, Yoo SD, et al. Causes of lower respiratory infection in HIV-infected Ugandan adults who are sputum AFB smear-negative. Int J Tuberc Lung Dis 2003;7:117–23.

26. Hartung TK, Chimbayo D, van Oosterhout JJ, et al. Etiology of suspected pneumonia in adults admitted to a high-dependency unit in Blantyre, Malawi. Am J Trop Med Hyg 2011;85:105–12.

27. Aderaye G, Bruchfeld J, Olsson M, et al. Occurrence of *Pneumocystis carinii* in HIV-positive patients with suspected pulmonary tuberculosis in Ethiopia. AIDS 2003;17:435–40.

28. Choukri F, Menotti J, Sarfati C, et al. Quantification and spread of *Pneumocystis jirovecii* in the surrounding air of patients with *Pneumocystis* pneumonia. Clin Infect Dis 2010;51:259–65.

29. Le Gal S, Damiani C, Rouillé A, et al. A cluster of *Pneumocystis* infections among renal transplant recipients: molecular evidence of colonized patients as potential infectious sources of *Pneumocystis jirovecii*. Clin Infect Dis 2012;54:e62–71.

30. Nevez G, Raccurt C, Jounieaux V, et al. Pneumocystosis versus pulmonary *Pneumocystis carinii* colonization in HIV-negative and HIV-positive patients. AIDS 1999;13:535–6.

31. Medrano FJ, Montes-Cano M, Conde M, et al. *Pneumocystis jirovecii* in general population. Emerg Infect Dis 2005;11:245–50.

32. Vargas SL, Ponce CA, Sanchez CA, et al. Pregnancy and asymptomatic carriage of *Pneumocystis jiroveci*. Emerg Infect Dis 2003;9:605–6.

33. Gutiérrez S, Respaldiza N, Campano E, et al. *Pneumocystis jirovecii* colonization in chronic pulmonary disease. Parasite 2011;18:121–6.

34. Morris A, Wei K, Afshar K, et al. Epidemiology and clinical significance of *Pneumocystis* colonization. J Infect Dis 2008;197:10–7.

35. Morris A, Norris KA. Colonization by *Pneumocystis jirovecii* and its role in disease. Clin Microbiol Rev 2012;25:297–317.

36. Calderón EJ, Rivero L, Respaldiza N, et al. Systemic inflammation in patients with chronic obstructive pulmonary disease who are colonized with *Pneumocystis jiroveci*. Clin Infect Dis 2007;45:e17–9.

37. Malin A, Miller R. *Pneumocystis carinii* pneumonia: presentation and diagnosis. Rev Med Microbiol 1992;3:80–7.

38. Miller RF, Millar AB, Weller IV, et al. Empirical treatment without bronchoscopy for *Pneumocystis carinii* pneumonia in the acquired immunodeficiency syndrome. Thorax 1989;44:559–64.

39. Kovacs JA, Hiemenz JW, Macher AM, et al. *Pneumocystis carinii* pneumonia: a comparison between patients with the acquired immunodeficiency syndrome and patients with other immunodeficiencies. Ann Intern Med 1984;100(5):663–71.

40. Zaman MK, White DA. Serum lactate dehydrogenase levels and *Pneumocystis* pneumonia. Diagnostic and prognostic significance. Am Rev Respir Dis 1988;137:796–800.

41. Watanabe T, Yasuoka A, Tanuma J, et al. Serum (1->3) beta-D-glucan as a noninvasive adjunct marker for the diagnosis of *Pneumocystis pneumonia* in patients with AIDS. Clin Infect Dis 2009; 49:1128–31.

42. Sax PE, Komarow L, Finkelman MA, et al. AIDS Clinical Trials Group Study A5164 Team. Blood (1->3)-beta-D-glucan as a diagnostic test for HIV-related *Pneumocystis jirovecii* pneumonia. Clin Infect Dis 2011;53:197–202.

43. Morris AM, Masur H. A serologic test to diagnose *Pneumocystis* pneumonia. Are we there yet? Clin Infect Dis 2011;53:2043–4.

44. Skelly MJ, Holzman RS, Merali S. S-adenosylmethionine levels in the diagnosis of *Pneumocystis carinii* pneumonia in patients with HIV infection. Clin Infect Dis 2008;46:467–71.

45. Wang P, Huang L, Davis JL, et al. A hydrophilic-interaction chromatography tandem mass spectroscopy method for quantitation of serum S-adenosylmethionine in patients infected with human immunodeficiency virus. Clin Chim Acta 2008;396:86–8.

46. Larsen HH, Huang L, Kovacs J, et al. A prospective, blinded study of quantitative touch-down polymerase chain reaction using oral-wash samples for diagnosis of *Pneumocystis* pneumonia in HIV-infected patients. J Infect Dis 2004;189:1679–83.

47. Alvarez-Martinez MJ, Miro JM, Valls ME, et al. Sensitivity and specificity of nested and real-time PCR for detection of *Pneumocystis jiroveci* in clinical specimens. Diagn Microbiol Infect Dis 2006;56:153–60.

48. Huggett JF, Taylor MS, Kocjan G, et al. Development and evaluation of a real-time PCR assay for detection of *Pneumocystis jirovecii* DNA in bronchoalveolar lavage fluid of HIV-infected patients. Thorax 2008;63:154–9.

49. Fisk M, Sage EK, Edwards SG, et al. Outcome from treatment of *Pneumocystis jirovecii* pneumonia with co-trimoxazole. Int J STD AIDS 2009;20:652–3.

50. Helweg-Larsen J, Benfield T, Atzori C, et al. Clinical efficacy of first- and second-line treatments for HIV-associated *Pneumocystis jirovecii* pneumonia: a tricentre cohort study. J Antimicrob Chemother 2009; 64:1282–90.

51. Benfield T, Atzori C, Miller RF, et al. Second-line salvage treatment of AIDS-associated *Pneumocystis jirovecii* pneumonia: a case series and systematic review. J Acquir Immune Defic Syndr 2008;48:63–7.

52. Miller RF, Allen E, Copas A, et al. Improved survival for HIV infected patients with severe *Pneumocystis jirovecii* pneumonia is independent of highly active antiretroviral therapy. Thorax 2006;61:716–21.

53. Davis JL, Morris A, Kallet RH, et al. Low tidal volume ventilation is associated with reduced mortality in HIV-infected patients with acute lung injury. Thorax 2008;63:988–93.

54. Radhi S, Alexander T, Ukwu M, et al. Outcome of HIV-associated *Pneumocystis pneumonia* in hospitalized patients from 2000 through 2003. BMC Infect Dis 2008;8:118.

55. Fei MW, Sant CA, Kim EJ, et al. Severity and outcomes of *Pneumocystis pneumonia* in patients newly diagnosed with HIV infection: an observational cohort study. Scand J Infect Dis 2009;41:672–8.

56. Arozullah AM, Yarnold PR, Weinstein RA, et al. A new pre-admission staging system for predicting inpatient mortality from HIV-associated *Pneumocystis carinii* pneumonia in the early highly active antiretroviral therapy (HAART) era. Am J Respir Crit Care Med 2000;161:1081–6.

57. Fei MW, Kim EJ, Sant CA, et al. Predicting mortality from HIV-associated *Pneumocystis pneumonia* at illness presentation: an observational cohort study. Thorax 2009;64:1070–6.

58. Armstrong-James D, Copas AJ, Walzer PD, et al. A prognostic scoring tool for identification of patients at high and low risk of death from HIV-associated *Pneumocystis jirovecii* pneumonia. Int J STD AIDS 2011;22:628–34.

59. Zolopa A, Andersen J, Powderly W, et al. Early antiretroviral therapy reduces AIDS progression/death in individuals with acute opportunistic infections: a multicenter randomized strategy trial. PLoS One 2009;4:e5575.

60. Grant PM, Komarow L, Andersen J, et al. Risk factor analyses for immune reconstitution inflammatory syndrome in a randomized study of early vs. deferred ART during an opportunistic infection. PLoS One 2010;5:e11416.

61. Jagannathan P, Davis E, Jacobson M, et al. Life-threatening immune reconstitution inflammatory syndrome after *Pneumocystis pneumonia*: a cautionary case series. AIDS 2009;23:1794–6.

62. D'Egidio GE, Kravcik S, Cooper CL, et al. *Pneumocystis jiroveci* pneumonia prophylaxis is not required with a CD4+ T-cell count <200 cells/microl when viral replication is suppressed. AIDS 2007;21:1711–5.

63. Cheng CY, Chen MY, Hsieh SM, et al. Risk of pneumocystosis after early discontinuation of prophylaxis among HIV-infected patients receiving highly active antiretroviral therapy. BMC Infect Dis 2010;10:126.

64. Opportunistic Infections Project Team of the Collaboration of Observational HIV Epidemiological Research in Europe (COHERE), Mocroft A, Reiss P, Kirk O, et al. Is it safe to discontinue primary *Pneumocystis jiroveci* pneumonia prophylaxis in patients with virologically suppressed HIV infection and a CD4 cell count <200 cells/microL? Clin Infect Dis 2010;51:611–9.

Other HIV-Associated Pneumonias

Jakrapun Pupaibool, MD[a], Andrew H. Limper, MD[b],*

KEYWORDS

- Nontuberculosis mycobacteria • Cytomegalovirus • Aspergillosis • Cryptococcosis
- Histoplasmosis • Coccidioidomycosis • Toxoplasmosis

KEY POINTS

- The lung is commonly involved with infectious complications in individuals infected with human immunodeficiency virus (HIV).
- In addition to *Pneumocystis* pneumonia discussed in another article in this issue, pulmonary infections in individuals infected with HIV can be related to nontuberculosis mycobacteria, cytomegalovirus, fungi, parasites, uncommon bacterial pneumonia, and other microorganisms.
- A high index of suspicion is needed, and awareness that the clinical presentation and treatment of pneumonia in patients with AIDS can be different from those in immunocompetent patients.
- Judicious use of invasive and noninvasive testing, as well as molecular biological techniques enhances the diagnosis and the prognosis of pulmonary infections in patients infected with HIV.

INTRODUCTION

The incidence and mortality of human immunodeficiency virus (HIV)-related opportunistic infections has decreased significantly from the era before antiretroviral therapy (ART).[1,2] However, HIV infection and its attendant risk for infectious complications remains one of the most important health care problems worldwide. Among infectious complications in patients with AIDS, the lung is the most frequently affected site.[3–5] Effective prophylaxis and antimicrobial therapy has made a significant impact on the incidence of common opportunistic infections such as *Pneumocystis jirovecii* pneumonia.[6] However, pulmonary infections from uncommon pathogens, and organisms not classically related to AIDS, as well as organisms without effective antimicrobial prophylaxis or those without established recommendations for primary prophylaxis have also been reported.

The differential diagnosis of pulmonary infections in patients with HIV is broad. The diagnostic approach should be individualized for each patient based on a detailed history of symptoms and environmental exposures, the physical examination, previous use of any antimicrobial prophylaxis, as well as the intensity and persistence of immune deficiency, which can be assessed by the CD4 cell count. These factors must be taken into account to determine the likelihood of any particular organism as the cause of pneumonia when developing the differential diagnosis for an individual patient.

The diagnosis and treatment of pneumonia in patients with AIDS can also be complicated by atypical presentation of the clinical manifestations of disease, unusual radiographic findings, the presence of multiple infections with different organisms,[7–12] noninfectious pulmonary complications,[13] immune reconstitution inflammatory

Disclosures: The authors have no financial, institutional, or other relevant relationships that would constitute a potential conflict of interest with this review.

Supported by: NIH-R01-HL-62150 to AHL, and funds from the Mayo Foundation.

[a] Division of Infectious Diseases, Mayo Clinic College of Medicine, Marian Hall 5-528, Rochester, MN 55905, USA; [b] Division of Pulmonary and Critical Care, Department of Internal Medicine, Mayo Clinic College of Medicine, Mayo Clinic, Gonda 18-South, Rochester, MN 55905, USA

* Corresponding author.

E-mail address: limper.andrew@mayo.edu

Clin Chest Med 34 (2013) 243–254

http://dx.doi.org/10.1016/j.ccm.2013.01.007

syndrome (IRIS), drug-drug interactions, and adverse drug reactions. Furthermore, the availability of definitive diagnostic tests, especially bronchoscopy, can be challenging in resource-poor areas.[14] Currently, there is no single comprehensive algorithm to serve as a guideline for determining the diagnosis of pneumonia in patients with HIV infection.

This review summarizes some of the major pulmonary infections from organisms other than *Pneumocystis jirovecii*, *Mycobacterium tuberculosis*, and *Streptococcus pneumoniae* in patients infected with HIV.

NONTUBERCULOUS MYCOBACTERIAL PNEUMONIA
The Organisms

Nontuberculous mycobacteria (NTM) can be isolated from water and soil. Unlike *M tuberculosis*, there are no known latent NTM infections. The mode of transmission of NTM is from recent acquisition through inhalation and ingestion. No isolation is required for patients hospitalized with pneumonia from NTM because there have been no documented cases of person-to-person transmission. Given that these organisms are ubiquitous in the environment, a positive respiratory sample culture must be interpreted with caution because a positive finding may represent either environmental contamination or transient airway colonization.[15] However, it is thought that colonization with NTM could precede disseminated infection.[16] Patients with advanced HIV infection with CD4 cell counts less than 50 cells/μL are at particular risk of developing infections from NTM.[17]

The diagnosis of pneumonia from NTM requires at least 2 positive expectorated sputum cultures or at least 1 positive bronchial wash/lavage sample. If granulomatous inflammation or acid-fast bacilli (AFB) are found on histopathology of a lung biopsy, only 1 positive culture from either sputum or lung biopsy or bronchial wash/lavage is required for a definitive diagnosis. However, in addition, appropriate pulmonary symptoms and radiographic abnormalities, as well as exclusion of other diagnoses, are required to fulfill the diagnostic criteria provided by the recommendations of the American Thoracic Society (ATS) and the Infectious Diseases Society of America (IDSA).[18]

Clinical Manifestations

The incidence of infections related to *Mycobacterium avium* complex (MAC), which consists of *M avium* and *M intracellulare*, has decreased substantially in the post-ART era.[19] However, MAC infections are still the most common NTM infection and the most common infection from NTM associated with IRIS in patients infected with HIV.[19,20] MAC rarely occurs as a cause of pneumonia in patients infected with HIV, especially as an isolated pulmonary infection without disseminated disease (**Fig. 1**).[21] *M kansasii* is the second most common NTM infection in patients infected with HIV.[22] Another NTM infection that exhibits clinical manifestations similar to those of MAC is *M simiae*.[8,23]

Most other NTM infections commonly manifest as disseminated infections with or without pulmonary involvement, except for *M kansasii* and *M xenopi*, which commonly present as localized pulmonary infection.[17,24,25] Disseminated disease and mycobacteremia from *M kansasii* is more common in patients infected with HIV compared with individuals without HIV.[26] Clinical manifestations of *M kansasii* infection are similar to those present during *M tuberculosis* infection except for the occurrence of meningitis, which is fairly uncommon in *M kansasii* infection.[27,28]

Constitutional symptoms, including fever, night sweats, decreased appetite, and weight loss are common among all NTM infections. Extrapulmonary manifestations should trigger clinicians to consider certain species of NTM more than the others. For instance, clinical features that may suggest infections from MAC and *M genavense*

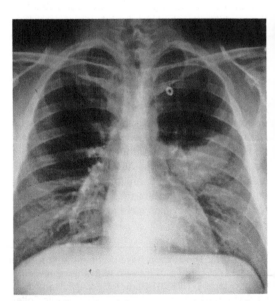

Fig. 1. Left upper lobe pneumonitis caused by *Mycobacterium avium* infection in a 32-year-old man infected with HIV presenting with cough, fever, sweats, and weight loss. Bronchoscopy with bronchoalveolar lavage established the infection; no other organisms were found.

include diarrhea, intra-abdominal adenopathy, and hepatosplenomegaly,[29–31] whereas skin, soft tissue, bone, and joint involvement suggest infections from rapid-growing mycobacteria (*M abscessus, M fortuitum, M chelonae*), and other NTMs such as *M malmoense, M szulgai,* and *M hemophilum*.[17,32,33]

Radiographic Findings

Typical radiographic findings of MAC pulmonary infection in immunocompetent hosts include upper lobe involvement with or without cavitation in men, and right middle lobe or lingular involvement in elderly women. In patients infected with HIV, no differences in radiographic findings by patient sex have been described. Multifocal bronchiectasis is the most common radiographic feature of MAC in HIV populations.[15]

In NTM infections other than MAC, pulmonary involvement as part of disseminated NTM disease presents more commonly compared with localized pulmonary infection in patients infected with HIV. Consequently, bilateral interstitial infiltrates are the most common radiographic features.[16,25] However, bilateral patchy infiltrates, cavitary lesions, pleural effusions, mediastinal adenopathy, or a normal chest radiograph can also be found. Although there are some differential radiographic features of pulmonary infection from *M kansasii* and *M tuberculosis*, they cannot be used to reliably distinguish one from another from the radiographic features alone.[34] Moreover, there are no specific radiographic features that can be used to distinguish among NTM pulmonary infections in patients infected with HIV.[16]

Treatment

Azithromycin or clarithromycin is recommended for primary prophylaxis in patients infected with HIV with CD4 cell counts less than 50 cells/μL.[35] No primary antimicrobial prophylaxis is currently recommended to prevent infections from NTM other than MAC.

The combination of clarithromycin or azithromycin, rifampin or rifabutin, and ethambutol, with or without the addition of amikacin or streptomycin is the usual antimicrobial regimen for effective treatment of MAC pulmonary disease. For pulmonary disease involving *M kansasii*, the regimen includes isoniazid, rifampin, and ethambutol. Besides MAC and *M kansasii*, there are no standard regimens to treat infections from infrequently encountered NTMs because of limited clinical evidence and published experience.[18]

In general, combinations of 3 or 4 antimicrobial agents to which the organism is susceptible are required. Four-drug regimens are used for patients with extensive pulmonary disease, disseminated infection, and mycobacteremia. Most NTMs are susceptible to the newer macrolides (clarithromycin or azithromycin) and fluoroquinolones (moxifloxacin, ciprofloxacin); these are the primary drugs used in most regimens to treat NTM infections. The third and fourth drugs can be chosen among isoniazid, rifampin, ethambutol, amikacin, doxycycline, and trimethoprim-sulfamethoxazole. Other antimicrobial agents to which the organism is susceptible can also be used. The regimen may also be guided by antibiograms reflecting organism sensitivities. However, the clinician must be aware of limitations because the exact correlation of in vitro susceptibility testing of certain drugs and clinical responses for MAC and uncommon NTMs are not always parallel or are still unknown. Consequently, in vitro susceptibility testing for infrequently encountered NTMs is not routinely recommended.[18]

Obtaining respiratory samples for cultures is essential in all patients (with or without HIV infection) suspected to have a pulmonary infection from NTM. It not only helps to guide antimicrobial therapy but also helps to determine the duration of treatment. At least 12 months of therapy after a negative respiratory sample culture is generally used as a guideline for treatment duration. In patients infected with HIV with AIDS, the treatment should also be continued until the CD4 cell count is more than 100 cells/μL for at least 6 months.[35]

FUNGAL PNEUMONIAS
Organisms

Medically important fungi that cause pulmonary infections in patients infected with HIV are categorized into 3 different groups in this review: *Aspergillus* species, *Cryptococcus neoformans*, and dimorphic fungi.

Aspergillus species are ubiquitous hyaline molds that can be isolated from air and soil. *A fumigatus* is the most common species that causes infections in patients infected with HIV.[36,37] Other common species include *A flavus, A niger, A terreus,* and *A nidulans.* The mode of pulmonary infection is usually from recent acquisition through inhalation. There is currently believed to be no latent state of infection. However, these fungi can colonize the respiratory tract in patients with preexisting pulmonary diseases and architectural distortion of the lung. In addition to neutropenia and corticosteroid use, which are the well-established major risk factors for infection, a CD4 cell count less than 50 cells/μL also represents a significant risk factor for invasive aspergillosis.[36–38]

Cryptococcus neoformans is a ubiquitous encapsulated yeast that is found worldwide. It can be isolated from aged pigeon droppings. *Cryptococcus gattii*, another *Cryptococcus* species that is found in tropical and subtropical climates, is not discussed in this review because it is typically a pathogen in individuals with an apparently healthy immune system. Infection with *Cryptococcus* is caused by inhaling spores or yeast cells.[39] The organism initially forms a primary pulmonary lymph node complex in a manner similar to tuberculosis.[40] Cryptococcal infection in patients infected with HIV is caused by either reactivation of latent infection or primary infection. Most cases of cryptococcal infection occur in patients with a CD4 cell count less than 200 cells/μL.[41]

The dimorphic fungi (*Histoplasma capsulatum*, *Blastomyces dermatitidis*, *Coccidioides* species, *Paracoccidioides braziliensis*, *Penicillium marneffei*) are endemic fungi that can be isolated from particular regions of the United States or certain parts of the world (**Table 1**). Thus, determining the patient's geographic and travel histories is helpful to exclude or suggest infections from certain organisms. The pathogenesis of infection is via inhalation of spores. These infections can be caused by either recent acquisition or reactivation of the latent state.

Clinical Manifestations

Invasive aspergillosis in patients infected with HIV most commonly presents as pneumonia, although disseminated infections involving multiple organs have also been reported.[36,38] The clinical symptoms are often nonspecific. Cough, dyspnea, and fever are the most common presenting symptoms; chest pain and hemoptysis present less commonly.[38,42] Tracheobronchial aspergillosis is another manifestation of invasive disease in patients infected with HIV.[36,38,42] Three forms of tracheobronchial aspergillosis have been described: the obstructive form, the ulcerative form, and the pseudomembranous form. Other well-known manifestations of *Aspergillus* pulmonary syndromes, such as aspergillomas, allergic bronchopulmonary aspergillosis, and chronic necrotizing pulmonary aspergillosis, are rarely reported in patients infected with HIV.[43–45] According to definitions from the European Organization for Research and Treatment of Cancer/ Invasive Fungal Infections Cooperative Group and the National Institute of Allergy and Infectious Diseases Mycoses Study Group (EORTC/MSG),[46] histopathologic evidence of tissue invasion by hyphal elements and culture isolation of *Aspergillus* are required to make a diagnosis of proven invasive aspergillosis. Galactomannan in serum and bronchoalveolar lavage (BAL) fluid can support a probable diagnosis of infection.

The most common manifestation of cryptococcal infection in patients infected with HIV is disseminated infection with meningitis.[47] Patients with localized pulmonary infection generally have a higher CD4 cell count than those with disseminated disease.[48] However, all patients infected with HIV with cryptococcal pneumonia should undergo a lumbar puncture examination to rule out central nervous system involvement.[49] Serum and cerebrospinal fluid cryptococcal antigen and fungal blood cultures should also be obtained to exclude disseminated disease. Serum cryptococcal antigen is an excellent screening test for disseminated disease in this population.[48]

Most patients infected with HIV with pneumonia from endemic fungi present with disseminated

Table 1
Endemic regional distribution of dimorphic fungi that cause pulmonary infections in individuals infected with HIV

Endemic Fungi	Endemic Areas
Histoplasma capsulatum	The Ohio, Missouri, and Mississippi River valleys in the United States; Mexico, Central America; certain areas in South American, Africa, and Asia
Blastomyces dermatitidis	Midwestern, southeastern, and south central United States; Canadian border around the Great Lakes and the St. Lawrence Seaway
Coccidioides imitis	Central and southern California (San Joaquin Valley, Mojave Desert), south central Arizona, southern New Mexico, and western Texas in the United States; Northern Mexico
Coccidioides posadasii	Southwest Mexico; Certain areas in Central American and South America
Paracoccidioides braziliensis	Certain areas in Mexico, Central America, and South American
Penicillium marneffei	Southeast Asia, Southern China, Taiwan, Hong Kong, and South Asia

disease. Molluscum-like skin lesions, hepatosplenomegaly, lymphadenopathy, and fungal isolation from blood and bone marrow cultures are present in disseminated histoplasmosis and penicilliosis.[50–55] Thus, skin scraping, lymph node aspiration, blood and bone marrow cultures can be used as alternatives to bronchoscopy to establish a definitive diagnosis. Cutaneous manifestations are relatively less common in disseminated blastomycosis, coccidioidomycosis, and paracoccidioidomycosis. Serology, serum antigen, and urine antigen are also useful in the diagnosis. However, definitive identification of organisms by smears and/or polymerase chain reaction (PCR) and isolation of organisms from respiratory samples are strongly encouraged because mixed infections can occur in the advanced stages of HIV infection.

Radiographic Findings

In a case series of pulmonary aspergillosis,[42] cavitary upper lobe lesions were the most common radiographic pattern, followed by bilateral alveolar or interstitial infiltrates, which were associated with disseminated infection, and focal alveolar infiltrates. The air crescent sign was not found. Respiratory sample cultures and tissue biopsy are necessary to confirm the diagnosis of invasive aspergillosis because there are no absolutely specific radiographic findings.

Radiographic findings in pulmonary cryptococcosis are varied. Bilateral diffuse interstitial infiltrates are the most common finding. Other findings include focal alveolar infiltrates, cavitary lesions, pleural effusions, and lymphadenopathy.[48,56–58] Ground-glass opacities similar to *Pneumocystis* pneumonia and miliary nodules similar to miliary tuberculosis have also been reported in patients infected with HIV.[59]

Bilateral nodular opacities or interstitial infiltrates are the most common radiographic findings in pneumonia from the endemic fungi.[50,60–65] Hilar adenopathy can be observed in histoplasmosis and coccidioidomycosis. However, the radiographic findings are varied and nonspecific in these infections.

Treatment

Primary antimicrobial prophylaxis regimens are not generally recommended for fungal infections in patients infected with HIV with a low CD4 cell count, with the exception of histoplasmosis, for which itraconazole is recommended when the CD4 cell count is less than 150 cells/μL for patients living in endemic areas where the incidence of histoplasmosis is more than 10 cases per 100 patient-years.[35,66] Fluconazole or itraconazole can also be considered for primary prophylaxis for patients living in endemic areas of coccidioidomycosis if the CD4 cell count is less than 250 cells/mL.[35]

The primary antifungal agent for invasive aspergillosis is voriconazole.[67] It has been shown to have more favorable outcomes compared with amphotericin B deoxycholate.[68] When required, the lipid formulations of amphotericin B are recommended over amphotericin B deoxycholate. Caspofungin, micafungin, and posaconazole are alternative agents for patients who are refractory to or intolerant of previous antifungal therapy.[67,69–71] Treatment can be discontinued when clinical symptoms resolve, there is evidence of resolution or stabilization of radiographic abnormalities, and the CD4 cell count is maintained at more than 200 cell/μL.[35]

The primary antifungal regimen for disseminated cryptococcosis is amphotericin B deoxycholate plus flucytosine for 2 weeks, followed by high-dose fluconazole (400 mg/d) for 8 weeks. For localized pulmonary cryptococcosis with asymptomatic or mild-to-moderate symptoms, fluconazole (400 mg/d) for 6 to 12 months is recommended. Secondary prophylaxis regimens are based on providing fluconazole (200 mg/d) until the CD4 cell count is greater than 100 cells/μL for at least 3 to 6 months.[35,49,71]

Regimens for treatment of endemic fungal pneumonias in patients infected with HIV should generally be designed to treat disseminated infection or at least aimed at treating moderately severe localized disease. The primary antifungal therapy for endemic fungal pulmonary infection with disseminated disease is initial therapy with lipid formulations of amphotericin B for 1 to 2 weeks or until clinical improvement, followed by itraconazole for 12 months, except for penicilliosis for which itraconazole should be provided for only 10 weeks.[35,66,71–73] Fluconazole can be used instead of itraconazole for coccidioidomycosis and paracoccidioidomycosis. Ketoconazole and sulfadiazine can be used for paracoccidioidomycosis after a favorable clinical response to initial therapy with amphotericin B.

Secondary prophylaxis is required until the CD4 cell count is more than 150 cells/μL for 6 months for histoplasmosis and blastomycosis, more than 250 cells/μL for 6 months for coccidioidomycosis, and more than 100 cells/μL for 6 months for penicilliosis. Secondary prophylaxis for paracoccidioidomycosis has not been well established and was not included in the latest guidelines.

VIRAL PNEUMONIA
Organisms

This review focuses only on cytomegalovirus (CMV) pneumonitis although other respiratory viruses such as influenza virus, parainfluenza virus, respiratory syncytial virus, adenovirus, and meta-pneumovius can also cause pneumonia in patients infected with HIV. CMV and herpes simplex virus (HSV) cause pneumonitis relatively rarely in patients infected with HIV.

Human CMV or Human herpesvirus 5 (HHV-5) is a double-stranded DNA virus that commonly infects most individuals early in life, and subsequently remains in a latent state in the individual throughout life. Most infections are caused by viral reactivation in patients with advanced immunocompromise. For patients infected with HIV, the infection typically occurs when the CD4 cell count decreases to less than 50 cells/μL.

Clinical Manifestations

The most common end-organ disease caused by CMV infection in patients infected with HIV is CMV retinitis. Other end-organ manifestations of CMV diseases include infections of the gastrointestinal tract (colitis, esophagitis) and central nervous system (ventriculitis, encephalitis, myelitis, radiculitis). Although CMV is one of the major pulmonary infections found in HIV-negative immunocompromised patients, such as solid organ and bone marrow transplant recipients, CMV pneumonitis occurs rarely in patients infected with HIV. However, it is not uncommon to detect CMV in BAL fluid in the presence of other infectious agents, particularly in coexistence with Pneumocystis jirovecii.

The significance of CMV in BAL fluid as a cause of pneumonia in patients infected with HIV remains controversial. The methods available to detect CMV in BAL fluid include cytologic examination, viral culture, and PCR. PCR detection of CMV in blood specimens does not help with the diagnosis of CMV pneumonitis. The diagnosis of CMV pneumonitis is more definitive when transbronchial or lung biopsy is performed and CMV cytopathic effects or inclusion bodies are identified within the tissue.[74]

Extrapulmonary manifestations of CMV are not associated with the detection of CMV in BAL fluid.[75,76] However, CMV pneumonitis should be suspected in patients infected with HIV who exhibit extrapulmonary CMV disease along with bilateral pulmonary infiltrates, and when other organisms responsible for pneumonia cannot be identified from BAL sampling.[74] The clinical manifestations of CMV pneumonitis are similar to those of Pneumocystis pneumonia except for the occasional presence of pleural effusions, which are only rarely found in Pneumocystis pneumonia.[76]

Radiographic Findings

Diffuse bilateral interstitial infiltrates or ground-grass opacities are characteristic radiographic features of pneumonia from many organisms in patients infected with HIV, including CMV pneumonitis and Pneumocystis pneumonia.[58,77]

Treatment

When CMV is identified in BAL fluid together with P jirovecii, this finding may simply represent viral shedding, reflecting the degree of low immunity in the HIV-infected host,[78] rather than coinfection with CMV. The coidentification of CMV along with P jirovecii is not significantly associated with increased mortality or severity of Pneumocystis pneumonia.[79–82]

For patients infected with HIV with bilateral interstitial pneumonia who have CMV in BAL fluid, anti-CMV treatment might be considered in the absence of other pathogens in the BAL fluid,[81] if CMV is found in BAL fluid in the presence of high levels of CMV viremia,[75] or if the patient has a poor response to anti-Pneumocystis therapy alone. There is also no strong evidence to support initiation of anti-CMV therapy for patients infected with HIV with positive CMV in BAL fluid who have Pneumocystis pneumonia requiring adjunctive corticosteroids.

If CMV is considered to be the cause of pulmonary infection, intravenous ganciclovir should be initiated. Alternative anti-CMV agents include foscarnet and cidofovir. Therapy can be switched to oral valganciclovir after at least 2 weeks of intravenous agents and clinic improvement, as well as stabilization of the observed radiologic findings. The treatment also should be continued until the CD4 cell count is greater than 100 cells/μL for 3 to 6 months.[35] ART should be instituted as soon as possible.

UNCOMMON BACTERIAL PNEUMONIA (NOCARDIOSIS, RHODOCOCCOSIS)
Organisms

Uncommon bacteria that can cause pulmonary infection in patients infected with HIV with a low CD4 cell count are discussed in this section, focusing on bacteria in the genera Nocardia and Rhodococcus. These organisms belong to the same family, Nocardiaceae. Bacteria in the genus Nocardia are gram-positive with partially acid-fast beading branching filaments, which can be isolated in soil worldwide. The most common species causing pulmonary infection is N asteroids, whereas N brasiliensis is the most common species causing lymphocutaneous infection.[83]

Rhodococcus equi is a gram-positive, weak acid-fast coccibacilli, which can be isolated from the stools of foals. Rhodococcosis is a rare zoonotic infection that occurs in immunocompromised patients, such as transplant recipients and individuals infected with HIV. Pulmonary nocardiosis and rhodococcosis are caused by recent acquisition of organisms through inhalation. Most patients have advanced AIDS with a CD4 cell count less than 50 cells/μL.[84,85]

Clinical Manifestations

Nonspecific symptoms including fever, cough, expectoration, and chest pain are common clinical symptoms in patients presenting with pulmonary nocardiosis or rhodococcosis. The lungs are usually the primary site of infection although direct inoculation through trauma and skin breakdown is possible. In immunocompromised patients, the infection progresses to disseminated disease with extrapulmonary involvement. Hematogenous spreading to the central nervous system and subcutaneous tissues causes brain and subcutaneous abscesses.

Although disseminated infection with extrapulmonary involvement is believed to be from hematogenous spread, isolation of *Nocardia* from blood is extremely uncommon in patients infected with HIV.[86,87] Nocardemia has been reported in patients with endovascular foreign bodies without HIV infection.[88–90] The prevalence of central nervous system involvement is 8.8%.[83] In contrast, *R equi* can be isolated from sputum and blood in approximately 50% of patients. The central nervous system is involved in 4.5% of infected individuals.[85] Extrapulmonary involvement in rhodococcosis is higher during relapse resulting from inadequate initial antimicrobial treatment.[91]

Radiographic Findings

Pulmonary consolidation with cavitation with or without mediastinal adenopathy are the most common radiographic findings of pulmonary nocardiosis[92,93] and rhodococcosis.[85,94–97]

Treatment

A 2-drug or 3-drug regimen is recommended for the initial treatment of nocardiosis. The regimen depends on in vitro susceptibility testing. Some species such as *N facinica*, *N nova*, and *N ottitidis-caviarum* can be resistant to trimethoprim-sulfamethoxazole.[98,99] Trimethoprim-sulfamethoxazole should be included in the regimen if the organism is susceptible to it and the patient is not allergic to sulfonamide antibiotics. The second and/or third agent(s) during the initial treatment can be chosen among amikacin, imipenem-cilastatin, and cephalosporins (ceftriaxone, cefotaxime, and cefepime).[99] Linezolid is also an alternative agent, but clinical data are limited. The therapy can be switched to oral trimethoprim-sulfamethoxazole with amoxicillin-clavulanate or minocycline or moxifloxacin after 3 to 6 weeks of intravenous therapy. The duration of treatment is usually in the range of 6 to 12 months, and should be based on radiographic response, clinical improvement, and host immune status.

There is no standard antimicrobial regimen for rhodococcosis. The most active antimicrobial agents include glycopeptides, carbapenems, aminoglycosides, fluoroquinolones, macrolides, trimethoprim-sulfamethoxazole, rifampin, tigecycline, and linezolid.[85,100,101] A combination of at least 2 intravenous antimicrobial agents based on in vitro susceptibility is recommended for the initial therapy, followed by a prolonged course of combined oral antimicrobial agents. The duration of treatment is also individualized for each patient depending on clinical and radiologic responses, as well as CD4 cell count measurements.[85,101]

PARASITIC PNEUMONIA
Organisms

Parasitic pneumonia is uncommon in patients infected with HIV. However, pulmonary infection from *Toxoplasma gondii* is more common compared with MAC, CMV, and HSV infections. Other parasites that have reportedly been implicated as causative agents for pneumonia in this population are cryptosporidia and microsporidia.[102–109] This review focuses on pulmonary toxoplasmosis.

Cats are the definitive hosts for *T gondii*. The routes of transmission to human are through ingestion of food contaminated with sporulated oocysts originating from cat feces or from the ingestion of undercooked meat of animals (pigs, sheep, birds, rodents) that harbor tissue cysts. Symptomatic infection in humans is generally from the reactivation of latent infection.

Clinical Manifestations

The most common manifestation of toxoplasmosis in patients infected with HIV is encephalitis. The incidence of pulmonary toxoplasmosis in patients infected with HIV has been reported in France,[110] but it is unknown in the United States. Many reported cases exhibit pneumonitis without encephalitis. The clinical presentation is nonspecific and includes fever, cough, and dyspnea.[111] The diagnosis is made by identification of toxoplasma tachyzoites in BAL fluid.[111,112]

Radiographic Findings

Diffuse bilateral interstitial or reticulonodular infiltrates are common radiographic findings of *Toxoplasma* pneumonitis.[111,113,114] No hilar or mediastinal adenopathy was observed in a small case series.[113] Because the clinical manifestations and radiographic findings are nonspecific, serology for *Toxoplasma* has a role in establishing the diagnosis of pulmonary toxoplasmosis. The diagnosis of pulmonary toxoplasmosis is much less likely when IgG antibodies are absent.

Treatment

The treatment of pulmonary toxoplasmosis is the same as for cerebral toxoplasmosis. The primary regimen is a combination of pyrimethamine-sulfadiazine. Folinic acid (leucovorin) is also provided to reduce hematologic toxicity from pyrimethamine. The combination of pyrimethamine-clindamycin or pyrimethamine-atovaquone are alternative regimens for patients with sulfa allergy.[35,115] Duration of therapy is at least 6 weeks if clinical and radiologic improvements are confirmed. Secondary prophylaxis is required to prevent recurrent disease until the CD4 cell count is greater than 200 cells/μL for 6 months.[35]

SUMMARY

The differential diagnosis of pneumonia in patients infected with HIV is broad. The clinical manifestations of pulmonary infections in this population are nonspecific. Radiographic findings are varied and nonpathognomonic for any particular organism and may overlap with noninfectious pulmonary diseases. Given the disseminated nature of many of these infections, the findings of diffuse bilateral interstitial infiltrates or ground-grass opacities are characteristic radiographic features of many of the organisms that cause pulmonary infections in this population, with the exception of pulmonary aspergillosis, nocardiosis, and rhodococcosis, which commonly present with cavitary pulmonary lesions. Bronchoscopy is required in most cases to establish a definitive diagnosis. It is essential that clinicians include testing for these uncommon HIV-associated pneumonias in the diagnostic evaluation of pulmonary disease in this population. The treatment duration for these infections is often prolonged because of low CD4 cell counts, and must be individualized to the clinical response and immune status of each patient. Primary and secondary prophylaxis depend on the CD4 cell count as well as other risk factors such as geographic location.

REFERENCES

1. Beck JM, Rosen MJ, Peavy HH. Pulmonary complications of HIV infection. Report of the Fourth NHLBI Workshop. Am J Respir Crit Care Med 2001;164: 2120–6.
2. Grubb JR, Moorman AC, Baker RK, et al. The changing spectrum of pulmonary disease in patients with HIV infection on antiretroviral therapy. AIDS 2006;20:1095–107.
3. Miller R. HIV-associated respiratory diseases. Lancet 1996;348:307–12.
4. Lazarous DG, O'Donnell AE. Pulmonary infections in the HIV-infected patient in the era of highly active antiretroviral therapy: an update. Curr Infect Dis Rep 2007;9:228–32.
5. Rosen MJ. Pulmonary complications of HIV infection. Respirology 2008;13:181–90.
6. Benito N, Rano A, Moreno A, et al. Pulmonary infiltrates in HIV-infected patients in the highly active antiretroviral therapy era in Spain. J Acquir Immune Defic Syndr 2001;27:35–43.
7. Schleicher GK, Feldman C. Dual infection with *Streptococcus pneumoniae* and *Mycobacterium tuberculosis* in HIV-seropositive patients with community acquired pneumonia. Int J Tuberc Lung Dis 2003;7:1207–8.
8. Huminer D, Dux S, Samra Z, et al. *Mycobacterium simiae* infection in Israeli patients with AIDS. Clin Infect Dis 1993;17:508–9.
9. Kitchen LW, Clark RA, Hoadley DJ, et al. Concurrent pulmonary *Blastomyces dermatitidis* and *Mycobacterium tuberculosis* infection in an HIV-1 seropositive man. J Infect Dis 1989;160:911–2.
10. Pistone T, Lacombe K, Poirot JL, et al. Imported concomitant coccidioidomycosis and histoplasmosis in an HIV-infected Colombian migrant in France. Trans R Soc Trop Med Hyg 2005;99:712–5.
11. Imai K, Koibuchi T, Kikuchi T, et al. Pulmonary nocardiosis caused by *Nocardia exalbida* complicating *Pneumocystis* pneumonia in an HIV-infected patient. J Infect Chemother 2011;17:547–51.
12. Inthraburan K, Wongsa A. Empyema thoracis due to nocardiosis and *Mycobacterium tuberculosis* mixed infections in an AIDS patient. Southeast Asian J Trop Med Public Health 2009;40:776–80.
13. Kanmogne GD. Noninfectious pulmonary complications of HIV/AIDS. Curr Opin Pulm Med 2005; 11:208–12.
14. Daley CL, Mugusi F, Chen LL, et al. Pulmonary complications of HIV infection in Dar es Salaam, Tanzania. Role of bronchoscopy and bronchoalveolar lavage. Am J Respir Crit Care Med 1996;154:105–10.
15. Shen MC, Lee SS, Huang TS, et al. Clinical significance of isolation of *Mycobacterium avium* complex from respiratory specimens. J Formos Med Assoc 2010;109:517–23.

16. El-Solh AA, Nopper J, Abdul-Khoudoud MR, et al. Clinical and radiographic manifestations of uncommon pulmonary nontuberculous mycobacterial disease in AIDS patients. Chest 1998;114:138–45.

17. Benator DA, Gordin FM. Nontuberculous mycobacteria in patients with human immunodeficiency virus infection. Semin Respir Infect 1996;11:285–300.

18. Griffith DE, Aksamit T, Brown-Elliott BA, et al. An official ATS/IDSA statement: diagnosis, treatment, and prevention of nontuberculous mycobacterial diseases. Am J Respir Crit Care Med 2007;175: 367–416.

19. Lawn SD, Bekker LG, Miller RF. Immune reconstitution disease associated with mycobacterial infections in HIV-infected individuals receiving antiretrovirals. Lancet Infect Dis 2005;5:361–73.

20. Phillips P, Bonner S, Gataric N, et al. Nontuberculous mycobacterial immune reconstitution syndrome in HIV-infected patients: spectrum of disease and long-term follow-up. Clin Infect Dis 2005;41:1483–97.

21. Hocqueloux L, Lesprit P, Herrmann JL, et al. Pulmonary Mycobacterium avium complex disease without dissemination in HIV-infected patients. Chest 1998;113:542–8.

22. Horsburgh CR Jr, Selik RM. The epidemiology of disseminated nontuberculous mycobacterial infection in the acquired immunodeficiency syndrome (AIDS). Am Rev Respir Dis 1989;139:4–7.

23. Al-Abdely HM, Revankar SG, Graybill JR. Disseminated Mycobacterium simiae infection in patients with AIDS. J Infect 2000;41:143–7.

24. Campo RE, Campo CE. Mycobacterium kansasii disease in patients infected with human immunodeficiency virus. Clin Infect Dis 1997;24:1233–8.

25. el-Helou P, Rachlis A, Fong I, et al. Mycobacterium xenopi infection in patients with human immunodeficiency virus infection. Clin Infect Dis 1997;25: 206–10.

26. Bloch KC, Zwerling L, Pletcher MJ, et al. Incidence and clinical implications of isolation of Mycobacterium kansasii: results of a 5-year, population-based study. Ann Intern Med 1998;129:698–704.

27. Flor A, Capdevila JA, Martin N, et al. Nontuberculous mycobacterial meningitis: report of two cases and review. Clin Infect Dis 1996;23:1266–73.

28. Canueto-Quintero J, Caballero-Granado FJ, Herrero-Romero M, et al. Epidemiological, clinical, and prognostic differences between the diseases caused by Mycobacterium kansasii and Mycobacterium tuberculosis in patients infected with human immunodeficiency virus: a multicenter study. Clin Infect Dis 2003;37:584–90.

29. Hsieh SM, Hung CC, Chen MY, et al. Clinical features and outcome in disseminated mycobacterial diseases in AIDS patients in Taiwan. AIDS 1998;12:1301–7.

30. Thomsen VO, Dragsted UB, Bauer J, et al. Disseminated infection with Mycobacterium genavense: a challenge to physicians and mycobacteriologists. J Clin Microbiol 1999;37:3901–5.

31. Monill JM, Franquet T, Sambeat MA, et al. Mycobacterium genavense infection in AIDS: imaging findings in eight patients. Eur Radiol 2001;11: 193–6.

32. Tappe D, Langmann P, Zilly M, et al. Osteomyelitis and skin ulcers caused by Mycobacterium szulgai in an AIDS patient. Scand J Infect Dis 2004;36: 883–5.

33. Hakawi AM, Alrajhi AA. Septic arthritis due to Mycobacterium szulgai in a patient with human immunodeficiency virus: case report. Scand J Infect Dis 2005;37:235–7.

34. Evans AJ, Crisp AJ, Hubbard RB, et al. Pulmonary Mycobacterium kansasii infection: comparison of radiological appearances with pulmonary tuberculosis. Thorax 1996;51:1243–7.

35. Kaplan JE, Benson C, Holmes KH, et al. Guidelines for prevention and treatment of opportunistic infections in HIV-infected adults and adolescents: recommendations from CDC, the National Institutes of Health, and the HIV Medicine Association of the Infectious Diseases Society of America. MMWR Recomm Rep 2009;58:1–207.

36. Mylonakis E, Barlam TF, Flanigan T, et al. Pulmonary aspergillosis and invasive disease in AIDS: review of 342 cases. Chest 1998;114:251–62.

37. Holding KJ, Dworkin MS, Wan PC, et al. Aspergillosis among people infected with human immunodeficiency virus: incidence and survival. Adult and Adolescent Spectrum of HIV Disease Project. Clin Infect Dis 2000;31:1253–7.

38. Denning DW, Follansbee SE, Scolaro M, et al. Pulmonary aspergillosis in the acquired immunodeficiency syndrome. N Engl J Med 1991;324:654–62.

39. Velagapudi R, Hsueh YP, Geunes-Boyer S, et al. Spores as infectious propagules of Cryptococcus neoformans. Infect Immun 2009;77:4345–55.

40. Baker RD. The primary pulmonary lymph node complex of crytptococcosis. Am J Clin Pathol 1976;65:83–92.

41. French N, Gray K, Watera C, et al. Cryptococcal infection in a cohort of HIV-1-infected Ugandan adults. AIDS 2002;16:1031–8.

42. Miller WT Jr, Sais GJ, Frank I, et al. Pulmonary aspergillosis in patients with AIDS. Clinical and radiographic correlations. Chest 1994;105:37–44.

43. Jain M. Allergic bronchopulmonary aspergillosis in an HIV-infected individual. Allergy Asthma Proc 2000;21:351–4.

44. Addrizzo-Harris DJ, Harkin TJ, McGuinness G, et al. Pulmonary aspergilloma and AIDS. A comparison of HIV-infected and HIV-negative individuals. Chest 1997;111:612–8.

45. Hasse B, Strebel B, Thurnheer R, et al. Chronic necrotizing pulmonary aspergillosis after tuberculosis in an HIV-positive woman: an unusual immune reconstitution phenomenon? AIDS 2005; 19:2179–81.

46. De Pauw B, Walsh TJ, Donnelly JP, et al. Revised definitions of invasive fungal disease from the European Organization for Research and Treatment of Cancer/Invasive Fungal Infections Cooperative Group and the National Institute of Allergy and Infectious Diseases Mycoses Study Group (EORTC/MSG) Consensus Group. Clin Infect Dis 2008;46:1813–21.

47. Clark RA, Greer D, Atkinson W, et al. Spectrum of *Cryptococcus neoformans* infection in 68 patients infected with human immunodeficiency virus. Rev Infect Dis 1990;12:768–77.

48. Meyohas MC, Roux P, Bollens D, et al. Pulmonary cryptococcosis: localized and disseminated infections in 27 patients with AIDS. Clin Infect Dis 1995;21:628–33.

49. Perfect JR, Dismukes WE, Dromer F, et al. Clinical practice guidelines for the management of cryptococcal disease: 2010 update by the Infectious Diseases Society of America. Clin Infect Dis 2010;50:291–322.

50. Ankobiah WA, Vaidya K, Powell S, et al. Disseminated histoplasmosis in AIDS. Clinicopathologic features in seven patients from a non-endemic area. N Y State J Med 1990;90:234–8.

51. Fredricks DN, Rojanasthien N, Jacobson MA. AIDS-related disseminated histoplasmosis in San Francisco, California. West J Med 1997;167:315–21.

52. Zhiyong Z, Mei K, Yanbin L. Disseminated *Penicillium marneffei* infection with fungemia and endobronchial disease in an AIDS patient in China. Med Princ Pract 2006;15:235–7.

53. Huber F, Nacher M, Aznar C, et al. AIDS-related *Histoplasma capsulatum* var. *capsulatum* infection: 25 years experience of French Guiana. AIDS 2008; 22:1047–53.

54. Lee N. Penicilliosis: an AIDS-defining disease in Asia. Hong Kong Med J 2008;14:88–9.

55. Cheng NC, Wong WW, Fung CP, et al. Unusual pulmonary manifestations of disseminated *Penicillium marneffei* infection in three AIDS patients. Med Mycol 1998;36:429–32.

56. Wasser L, Talavera W. Pulmonary cryptococcosis in AIDS. Chest 1987;92:692–5.

57. Clark RA, Greer DL, Valainis GT, et al. *Cryptococcus neoformans* pulmonary infection in HIV-1-infected patients. J Acquir Immune Defic Syndr 1990;3:480–4.

58. Cameron ML, Bartlett JA, Gallis HA, et al. Manifestations of pulmonary cryptococcosis in patients with acquired immunodeficiency syndrome. Rev Infect Dis 1991;13:64–7.

59. Friedman EP, Miller RF, Severn A, et al. Cryptococcal pneumonia in patients with the acquired immunodeficiency syndrome. Clin Radiol 1995;50: 756–60.

60. Herd AM, Greenfield SB, Thompson GW, et al. Miliary blastomycosis and HIV infection. CMAJ 1990;143:1329–30.

61. Srinath L, Ahkee S, Huang A, et al. Acute miliary blastomycosis in an AIDS patient. J Ky Med Assoc 1994;92:450–2.

62. Santos JW, Silveira ML, Santos FP, et al. Simultaneous chronic pulmonary paracoccidiodomycosis and disseminated cryptococcosis in a non-HIV patient. Mycopathologia 2005;159:373–6.

63. Marchiori E, Gasparetto EL, Escuissato DL, et al. Pulmonary paracoccidioidomycosis and AIDS: high-resolution CT findings in five patients. J Comput Assist Tomogr 2007;31:605–7.

64. Conces DJ Jr, Stockberger SM, Tarver RD, et al. Disseminated histoplasmosis in AIDS: findings on chest radiographs. AJR Am J Roentgenol 1993; 160:15–9.

65. Woods CW, McRill C, Plikaytis BD, et al. Coccidioidomycosis in human immunodeficiency virus-infected persons in Arizona, 1994-1997: incidence, risk factors, and prevention. J Infect Dis 2000;181: 1428–34.

66. Wheat LJ, Freifeld AG, Kleiman MB, et al. Clinical practice guidelines for the management of patients with histoplasmosis: 2007 update by the Infectious Diseases Society of America. Clin Infect Dis 2007; 45:807–25.

67. Walsh TJ, Anaissie EJ, Denning DW, et al. Treatment of aspergillosis: clinical practice guidelines of the Infectious Diseases Society of America. Clin Infect Dis 2008;46:327–60.

68. Herbrecht R, Denning DW, Patterson TF, et al. Voriconazole versus amphotericin B for primary therapy of invasive aspergillosis. N Engl J Med 2002;347:408–15.

69. Walsh TJ, Raad I, Patterson TF, et al. Treatment of invasive aspergillosis with posaconazole in patients who are refractory to or intolerant of conventional therapy: an externally controlled trial. Clin Infect Dis 2007;44:2–12.

70. Hiemenz JW, Raad II, Maertens JA, et al. Efficacy of caspofungin as salvage therapy for invasive aspergillosis compared to standard therapy in a historical cohort. Eur J Clin Microbiol Infect Dis 2010;29:1387–94.

71. Limper AH, Knox KS, Sarosi GA, et al. An official American Thoracic Society statement: treatment of fungal infections in adult pulmonary and critical care patients. Am J Respir Crit Care Med 2011; 183:96–128.

72. Galgiani JN, Ampel NM, Blair JE, et al. Coccidioidomycosis. Clin Infect Dis 2005;41:1217–23.

73. Chapman SW, Dismukes WE, Proia LA, et al. Clinical practice guidelines for the management of blastomycosis: 2008 update by the Infectious Diseases Society of America. Clin Infect Dis 2008;46:1801–12.

74. Rodriguez-Barradas MC, Stool E, Musher DM, et al. Diagnosing and treating cytomegalovirus pneumonia in patients with AIDS. Clin Infect Dis 1996;23:76–81.

75. Bower M, Barton SE, Nelson MR, et al. The significance of the detection of cytomegalovirus in the bronchoalveolar lavage fluid in AIDS patients with pneumonia. AIDS 1990;4:317–20.

76. Salomon N, Gomez T, Perlman DC, et al. Clinical features and outcomes of HIV-related cytomegalovirus pneumonia. AIDS 1997;11:319–24.

77. McGuinness G, Scholes JV, Garay SM, et al. Cytomegalovirus pneumonitis: spectrum of parenchymal CT findings with pathologic correlation in 21 AIDS patients. Radiology 1994;192:451–9.

78. Hyland M, Chan M, Hyland RH, et al. Associating poor outcome with the presence of cytomegalovirus in bronchoalveolar lavage from HIV patients with *Pneumocystis carinii* pneumonia. Chest 1995;107:595–7.

79. Miles PR, Baughman RP, Linnemann CC Jr. Cytomegalovirus in the bronchoalveolar lavage fluid of patients with AIDS. Chest 1990;97:1072–6.

80. Jacobson MA, Mills J, Rush J, et al. Morbidity and mortality of patients with AIDS and first-episode *Pneumocystis carinii* pneumonia unaffected by concomitant pulmonary cytomegalovirus infection. Am Rev Respir Dis 1991;144:6–9.

81. Hayner CE, Baughman RP, Linnemann CC Jr, et al. The relationship between cytomegalovirus retrieved by bronchoalveolar lavage and mortality in patients with HIV. Chest 1995;107:735–40.

82. Jensen AM, Lundgren JD, Benfield T, et al. Does cytomegalovirus predict a poor prognosis in *Pneumocystis carinii* pneumonia treated with corticosteroids? A note for caution. Chest 1995;108:411–4.

83. Beaman BL, Beaman L. *Nocardia* species: host-parasite relationships. Clin Microbiol Rev 1994;7:213–64.

84. Pintado V, Gomez-Mampaso E, Cobo J, et al. Nocardial infection in patients infected with the human immunodeficiency virus. Clin Microbiol Infect 2003;9:716–20.

85. Torres-Tortosa M, Arrizabalaga J, Villanueva JL, et al. Prognosis and clinical evaluation of infection caused by *Rhodococcus equi* in HIV-infected patients: a multicenter study of 67 cases. Chest 2003;123:1970–6.

86. Liu WL, Lai CC, Hsiao CH, et al. Bacteremic pneumonia caused by *Nocardia veterana* in an HIV-infected patient. Int J Infect Dis 2011;15:e430–2.

87. Minamoto GY, Sordillo EM. Disseminated nocardiosis in a patient with AIDS: diagnosis by blood and cerebrospinal fluid cultures. Clin Infect Dis 1998;26:242–3.

88. Kontoyiannis DP, Ruoff K, Hooper DC. *Nocardia* bacteremia. Report of 4 cases and review of the literature. Medicine (Baltimore) 1998;77:255–67.

89. Kontoyiannis DP, Jacobson KL, Whimbey EE, et al. Central venous catheter-associated *Nocardia* bacteremia: an unusual manifestation of nocardiosis. Clin Infect Dis 2000;31:617–8.

90. Al Akhrass F, Hachem R, Mohamed JA, et al. Central venous catheter-associated *Nocardia* bacteremia in cancer patients. Emerg Infect Dis 2011;17:1651–8.

91. Verville TD, Huycke MM, Greenfield RA, et al. *Rhodococcus equi* infections of humans. 12 cases and a review of the literature. Medicine (Baltimore) 1994;73:119–32.

92. Hwang JH, Koh WJ, Suh GY, et al. Pulmonary nocardiosis with multiple cavitary nodules in a HIV-negative immunocompromised patient. Intern Med 2004;43:852–4.

93. Kramer MR, Uttamchandani RB. The radiographic appearance of pulmonary nocardiosis associated with AIDS. Chest 1990;98:382–5.

94. Arlotti M, Zoboli G, Moscatelli GL, et al. *Rhodococcus equi* infection in HIV-positive subjects: a retrospective analysis of 24 cases. Scand J Infect Dis 1996;28:463–7.

95. Wicky S, Cartei F, Mayor B, et al. Radiological findings in nine AIDS patients with *Rhodococcus equi* pneumonia. Eur Radiol 1996;6:826–30.

96. Muntaner L, Leyes M, Payeras A, et al. Radiologic features of *Rhodococcus equi* pneumonia in AIDS. Eur J Radiol 1997;24:66–70.

97. Li HJ, Cheng JL. Imaging and pathological findings of AIDS complicated by pulmonary *Rhodococcus equi* infection. Chin Med J (Engl) 2011;124:968–72.

98. Brown-Elliott BA, Biehle J, Conville PS, et al. Sulfonamide resistance in isolates of *Nocardia* spp. from a US multicenter survey. J Clin Microbiol 2012;50:670–2.

99. Uhde KB, Pathak S, McCullum I Jr, et al. Antimicrobial-resistant *Nocardia* isolates, United States, 1995-2004. Clin Infect Dis 2010;51:1445–8.

100. Topino S, Galati V, Grilli E, et al. *Rhodococcus equi* infection in HIV-infected individuals: case reports and review of the literature. AIDS Patient Care STDS 2010;24:211–22.

101. Ferretti F, Boschini A, Iabichino C, et al. Disseminated *Rhodococcus equi* infection in HIV infection despite highly active antiretroviral therapy. BMC Infect Dis 2011;11:343.

102. Forgacs P, Tarshis A, Ma P, et al. Intestinal and bronchial cryptosporidiosis in an immunodeficient homosexual man. Ann Intern Med 1983;99:793–4.

103. Weber R, Kuster H, Visvesvara GS, et al. Disseminated microsporidiosis due to *Encephalitozoon hellem*: pulmonary colonization, microhematuria, and mild conjunctivitis in a patient with AIDS. Clin Infect Dis 1993;17:415–9.

104. Dupont C, Bougnoux ME, Turner L, et al. Microbiological findings about pulmonary cryptosporidiosis in two AIDS patients. J Clin Microbiol 1996; 34:227–9.

105. Poirot JL, Deluol AM, Antoine M, et al. Bronchopulmonary cryptosporidiosis in four HIV-infected patients. J Eukaryot Microbiol 1996;43:78S–9S.

106. Scaglia M, Sacchi L, Croppo GP, et al. Pulmonary microsporidiosis due to *Encephalitozoon hellem* in a patient with AIDS. J Infect 1997;34:119–26.

107. Matos O, Lobo ML, Antunes F. Methodology of the diagnosis of microsporidiosis in urine and pulmonary specimens from AIDS patients. J Eukaryot Microbiol 2001;(Suppl):69S–70S.

108. Sodqi M, Brazille P, Gonzalez-Canali G, et al. Unusual pulmonary *Enterocytozoon bieneusi* microsporidiosis in an AIDS patient: case report and review. Scand J Infect Dis 2004;36:230–1.

109. Palmieri F, Cicalini S, Froio N, et al. Pulmonary cryptosporidiosis in an AIDS patient: successful treatment with paromomycin plus azithromycin. Int J STD AIDS 2005;16:515–7.

110. Belanger F, Derouin F, Grangeot-Keros L, et al. Incidence and risk factors of toxoplasmosis in a cohort of human immunodeficiency virus-infected patients: 1988-1995. HEMOCO and SEROCO Study Groups. Clin Infect Dis 1999;28:575–81.

111. Rabaud C, May T, Lucet JC, et al. Pulmonary toxoplasmosis in patients infected with human immunodeficiency virus: a French National Survey. Clin Infect Dis 1996;23:1249–54.

112. Bonilla CA, Rosa UW. *Toxoplasma gondii* pneumonia in patients with the acquired immunodeficiency syndrome: diagnosis by bronchoalveolar lavage. South Med J 1994;87:659–63.

113. Goodman PC, Schnapp LM. Pulmonary toxoplasmosis in AIDS. Radiology 1992;184:791–3.

114. Mariuz P, Bosler EM, Luft BJ. Toxoplasma pneumonia. Semin Respir Infect 1997;12:40–3.

115. Dannemann B, McCutchan JA, Israelski D, et al. Treatment of toxoplasmic encephalitis in patients with AIDS. A randomized trial comparing pyrimethamine plus clindamycin to pyrimethamine plus sulfadiazine. The California Collaborative Treatment Group. Ann Intern Med 1992;116:33–43.

Human Immunodeficiency Virus–Associated Lung Malignancies

Allison A. Lambert, MD[a,b], Christian A. Merlo, MD, MPH[a,b],
Gregory D. Kirk, MD, MPH, PhD[a,b],*

KEYWORDS

- HIV/AIDS • Lung cancer • Kaposi sarcoma • Non-Hodgkin lymphoma • Antiretroviral therapy
- Cigarette smoking

KEY POINTS

- Rates of Kaposi sarcoma (KS) and non-Hodgkin lymphoma (NHL) have reduced substantially following the widespread uptake of highly active antiretroviral therapy (HAART), but still represent a substantial disease burden with significant mortality.
- Immune reconstitution inflammatory syndrome infrequently occurs in KS and NHL following HAART initiation, but may have serious clinical consequences, especially in pulmonary KS. However, HAART remains the best strategy to lower the risk for KS or NHL.
- Lung cancer represents the most common non-AIDS–defining cancer, presenting at advanced stages with substantial mortality.
- HIV appears to increase the risk of lung cancer independent of smoking, although the underlying mechanisms remain to be elucidated.
- The prevalence of smoking among HIV-infected persons is extremely high; smoking cessation needs to assume greater priority in HIV primary care.

INTRODUCTION

With the improved survival attributable to highly active antiretroviral therapy (HAART),[1–3] human immunodeficiency virus (HIV) has been transformed into a chronic disease. Growing numbers of HIV-infected persons in the United States are surviving to older ages; however, a changing spectrum of diseases with reduced AIDS-defining conditions but increased non-AIDS disease is being observed.[4–6] Life expectancy for a newly diagnosed HIV-infected person is now approaching that of the general population.[7] HIV-infected persons are well recognized to have a high burden of cigarette smoking. With reductions in HIV-infected persons experiencing profound immunodeficiency but with prolonged survival of persons with extensive tobacco use, monitoring of the changing patterns of morbidity and mortality is needed. Temporal patterns of lung malignancies in HIV exemplify these dramatic shifts in incidence and etiology, and raise concerns regarding the future burden of disease. Understanding the epidemiology and pathogenesis of lung malignancies among HIV-infected patients can help inform approaches for improving the diagnosis, management, and prevention of these malignancies in this evolving patient population.

Before the introduction of HAART, mortality among HIV-infected patients was defined largely by opportunistic infections and by AIDS-defining malignancies, particularly Kaposi sarcoma (KS)

a Department of Medicine, Johns Hopkins School of Medicine, 1830 Monument Street, Baltimore, MD, USA;
b Department of Epidemiology, Johns Hopkins Bloomberg School of Public Health, Baltimore, MD 21205, USA
* Corresponding author. Department of Epidemiology, Johns Hopkins University, 615 N. Wolfe Street, E-6533, Baltimore, MD 21205.
E-mail address: gkirk@jhsph.edu

Clin Chest Med 34 (2013) 255–272
http://dx.doi.org/10.1016/j.ccm.2013.01.008
0272-5231/13/$ – see front matter © 2013 Elsevier Inc. All rights reserved.

and non-Hodgkin lymphoma (NHL).[8] However, with the introduction of HAART, morbidity and mortality attributable to opportunistic infections and AIDS-defining malignancies has declined. One recent study found that 39% of Department of Defense patients with HIV who died in the post-HAART era had a CD4 count greater than 200 cells/mL, illustrating the lack of immunosuppression at the time of death and highlighting the changing morbidity and mortality affecting HIV-infected patients.[8] As the incidence of KS and NHL declines, non–AIDS-defining cancers (NADC) comprise an increasing proportion of malignancies among HIV-infected patients.[10] Furthermore, the incidence of NADC is increased among HIV-infected patients when compared with the general population.[10,11] Engels and colleagues[12] reported that in the pre-HAART era, NADC comprised 31.4% of cancer diagnoses; however, the proportion of NADC increased to 58% of cancer diagnoses during post-HAART years. Primary lung cancer is the second most commonly diagnosed malignancy in the United States, with more people dying of lung cancer than any other type of cancer each year.[13] First recognized in the HIV setting in early 1984,[14] lung cancer remains the most common NADC.[9,12,15–18] In light of the increasing risk of NADC, and more specifically lung cancer, clinicians need to better recognize, diagnose, treat and ideally, prevent lung cancer in this population. This review of lung malignancies in HIV briefly highlights key epidemiologic and clinical features in the pulmonary involvement of AIDS-defining malignancies of KS and NHL. Focusing on lung cancer, the authors sequentially discuss the epidemiology and mechanisms, clinical presentation, pathology, treatment and outcomes, and prevention. Finally, the important knowledge gaps and future directions for research related to HIV-associated lung malignancies are highlighted.

AIDS-DEFINING MALIGNANCIES OF THE LUNG: KAPOSI SARCOMA AND NON-HODGKIN LYMPHOMA

KS and NHL are AIDS-defining cancers (ADC) and represent the most common malignancies that occur following the development of AIDS.[10] A U.S. study linking AIDS and cancer registries from 1980–2002 reported 6.7% of patients were diagnosed with KS and 2.3% with NHL within 1 year of AIDS diagnosis. Overall, rates of both KS and NHL significantly declined in the mid-1990s around the time of the introduction of HAART (**Fig. 1**A, B); these rates have plateaued during the HAART era.[10] Although the lungs are not typically the primary site of disease, pulmonary involvement for both KS and NHL is relatively common.

Kaposi Sarcoma

HIV/AIDS-associated KS most commonly occurs in homosexual or bisexual men infected with the human herpes virus-8 (HHV-8), also known as the KS-associated herpes virus (KSHV). In a review of AIDS and cancer registries from 1980 to 2002, 89% of KS cases occurred among men who have sex with men (MSM).[10] The higher burden of KS among MSM has been attributed to differences in the seroprevalence of KSHV between HIV risk groups.[19] HIV/AIDS-associated KS occurs at advanced stages of immunosuppression (ie, lower CD4 cell counts),[20–24] and displays a more rapid course in comparison with classic or endemic KS.[25,26] Although disease is rarely isolated to the lungs, pulmonary involvement occurs frequently in HIV-infected patients with extensive mucocutaneous disease. Pulmonary KS is present in approximately 30% of patients; however, the rates of clinical diagnosis before autopsy are highly disparate.[27] HIV-infected patients with pulmonary KS have significantly lower CD4 counts and shorter survival times than those without pulmonary manifestations of KS.[26]

Patients generally present with vague respiratory symptoms, most commonly dyspnea and cough, and can have nonspecific imaging findings, making the workup of these symptoms in this at-risk patient population challenging.[24,28] In the HAART era, the current CD4 count is the patient characteristic most predictive of risk for KS.[29] Imaging findings of peribronchovascular nodularity and thickening, interlobular septal thickening, and fissural nodularity consistent with KS often parallel bronchoscopic findings; however, patients can present with parenchymal findings noted on computed tomography (CT) without evidence of endobronchial lesions.[30,31] Diagnosis can be made via bronchoscopic visualization of typical KS-appearing endobronchial lesions, if present. The utility and yield of bronchoscopic evaluation is variable because of the nature of KS lesions, with intermittent presence of endobronchial lesions, unpredictable proximity to airway, irregular extension into the submucosal space, and, sometimes, microscopic size.[24] Pleural effusions, if present, are often related to a secondary infection; thoracentesis with pleural fluid analysis is rarely diagnostic. Gallium-thallium radionuclide imaging is helpful in distinguishing pulmonary KS from pulmonary infection because KS is thallium avid and does not take up gallium, in contrast to infected lung.[32]

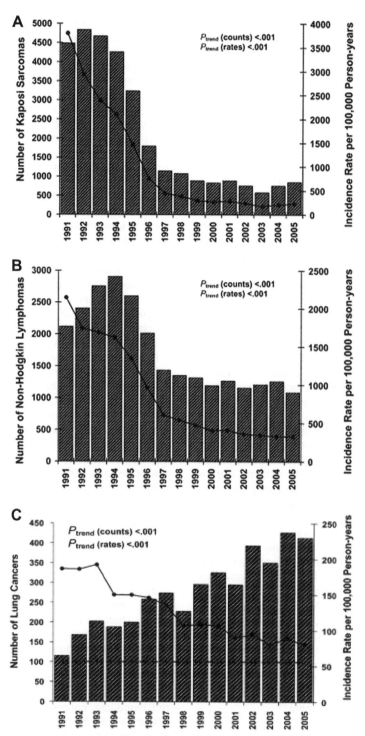

Fig. 1. Trends in cancer incidence among people living with AIDS in the United States during 1991 to 2005. Estimated counts (ie, number of cancers) and standardized incidence rates of Kaposi sarcoma (*A*), non-Hodgkin lymphoma (*B*), and lung cancer (*C*). Bars depict the estimated counts and points connected by lines depict the incidence rates standardized to the 2000 US AIDS population by age group, race, and sex. Trends in cancer counts and rates were estimated with linear regression. Two-sided *P* values were calculated using the χ^2 test. (*Adapted from* Shiels MS, Pfeiffer RM, Gail MH, et al. Cancer burden in the HIV-infected population in the United States. J Natl Cancer Inst 2011;103(9):759–60; with permission.)

Despite a dramatic decrease in the prevalence of KS with the introduction of HAART, KS is associated with significant mortality burden. However, it remains difficult to determine whether KS represents the proximate cause of death or if KS is simply strongly associated with AIDS. A review of causes of death among HIV-infected patients from 1990 to 2003 found that 11% of patients with HIV died of KS in the pre-HAART era compared to 12.8% in the post-HAART era.[8] Although the proportionate mortality due to KS has been relatively constant, survival following a KS diagnoses has improved. Two-year survival of HIV/AIDS KS patients has increased from 30% in the pre-HAART era to as high as 85% since HAART availability.[29,33] These changes in survival are largely attributable to HAART. Higher CD4 count and isolated KS as the AIDS-defining illness are associated with improved outcomes when compared with poorly controlled HIV with concomitant opportunistic infections.[34] The primary treatment for HIV/AIDS KS is reversal of immunodeficiency through use of effective antiretroviral therapy (ART); regression of lesions is generally observed with restoration of immune function.

Paradoxically, an immune reconstitution inflammatory syndrome (IRIS) may occasionally occur in patients with KS following ART initiation.[35–37] In contrast to many other opportunistic infections present at ART initiation, IRIS appears to occur more commonly in patients with KS. IRIS complications are more severe in KS patients and can result in death; these complications are more pronounced among patients with pulmonary KS or other visceral involvement.[38,39] Tumor-directed therapy involves combination myelosuppressive chemotherapy, with radiation therapy used in selected cases; both of these treatments can be challenging to tolerate in the setting of advanced AIDS.[40,41] Cytotoxic chemotherapy also may play a role in management of KS-associated IRIS.[35,37] For unclear reasons, pulmonary KS portends a substantially worse prognosis, whether in the setting of simply having a KS diagnosis or if IRIS occurs. A single-institution study in the HAART era reported 5-year survival of 49% in pulmonary KS compared with 82% in HIV/AIDS KS patients without pulmonary involvement.[26]

Non-Hodgkin Lymphoma

Severe immunosuppression is the hallmark of HIV/AIDS-associated NHL, which most commonly manifests with central nervous system (CNS) involvement in the setting of advanced HIV/AIDS disease. NHL is an ADC with the risk strongly related to the degree of immunosuppression, often occurring at CD4 cell counts of fewer than 50 cells/mL. Subsequently, NHL has also demonstrated declining rates since the introduction of HAART (see **Fig. 1**).[42]

Epstein-Barr virus (EBV) has been associated with the majority of HIV-associated NHL cases, although the degree of involvement varies in relation to the subtype of lymphoma.[43,44] Around 60% of AIDS-related lymphomas are diffuse large-cell lymphomas, typically presenting in the setting of advanced AIDS and at extranodal sites. Burkitt or Burkitt-like lymphoma comprises around 40% of AIDS-related NHL, uniformly expresses characteristic translocations of the c-myc gene, and may occur at a lesser degree of immunodeficiency than large-cell lymphomas.[43,45] Primary pulmonary lymphoma (PPL) is an infrequent cause of AIDS-related lymphoma, and is of the large-cell type with uniform EBV expression.[46] Rarely, immune-compromised HIV-infected patients may manifest lymphoma of the pleura or other body cavities (primary effusion lymphoma [PEL]), which are strongly associated with KSHV infection, in addition to EBV.[47]

Relative to CNS involvement, pulmonary NHL occurs infrequently in HIV-infected patients. In a retrospective review of AIDS patients undergoing autopsy at 2 San Francisco hospitals from 1982 to 1991,[48] 5.8% of NHL patients experienced isolated pulmonary localization without other systemic manifestations, and the lung was the most common organ involved in those with an extranodal site of disease (70%). HIV-infected patients with pulmonary NHL often present with pneumonic or pleural disease; the most common symptoms are constitutional (95%), cough (71%), and dyspnea (63%). The majority of patients have an abnormal examination, manifest most commonly by tachypnea (74%). Ninety-seven percent of patients have abnormal radiographic findings, with lobar consolidation (40%), nodules (40%), reticular infiltrates (24%), and masses (24%) seen on chest radiography. Thoracic lymphadenopathy may be present[49,50] but is thought to be uncommon. Pleural and serum lactate dehydrogenase levels are often substantially elevated, but this represent sensitive but not specific markers of NHL. Pleural fluid analysis is typically exudative, with elevated white and red blood cell counts and a low glucose level. Transbronchial biopsy specimens were diagnostic in 58% of cases in a retrospective series of patients, whereas pleural cytologic evaluation, closed needle pleural biopsy, and open lung biopsy were diagnostic in 75%, 100%, and 75% of cases, respectively.[48]

Persons with HIV/AIDS-associated NHL demonstrate persistently elevated mortality despite HAART availability, likely related to NHL occurrence primarily at extremely advanced stages of HIV disease.[51] During the pre-HAART era, 80% of patients with HIV-associated NHL had advanced NHL (stage IV) at the time of diagnosis.[48] In the pre-HAART era, less than 20% of persons with AIDS and non-CNS NHL survived 2 years; however, since the introduction of HAART in 1996, 2-year survival has increased to 43% in these patients. Simultaneous diagnosis of non-CNS NHL and HIV appears to be associated with even better survival, likely due to the added benefit of HAART initiation.[33] Although NHL rates have declined during the HAART era (along with overall mortality rates), the proportionate mortality caused by NHL in the setting of HIV has not changed substantially.[8,12,52] Treatment of NHL in HIV-infected patients has involved HAART along with administration of first-line chemotherapy. In recent years, salvage high-dose chemotherapy and autologous peripheral-blood stem cell transplantation have become available to HIV-infected patients who were previously excluded from these therapies because of concern for toxicity and severe immunodeficiency.[53]

Similar to KS, the occurrence of NHL in the period following HAART initiation has been described, although IRIS clearly is more common in relation to KS. The use of highly potent, newer HAART regimens in persons with profound immunosuppression may increase the likelihood of IRIS and NHL diagnosis.[54] Despite the risk for IRIS, HAART remains the most effective tool for reversing immune suppression and minimizing the likelihood of development of KS or NHL.

PRIMARY LUNG CANCER IN HIV
Epidemiology and Mechanisms

This section summarizes the current literature on HIV-associated lung cancer, highlighting how the epidemiologic data can inform and complement mechanistic studies. As illustrated in **Fig. 2**, as ADC have declined with the advent of HAART, rates of NADC, of which lung cancer is the most common, have increased. In contrast to these data using all HIV-infected patients as the denominator, data from AIDS registries have demonstrated a substantially increasing burden of lung cancer among AIDS patients, although incidence rates appear to have stabilized or declined among this subset with an existing AIDS diagnosis (see **Fig. 2C**).[55]

HIV as an Independent Risk Factor

The epidemiologic data regarding the association of HIV with lung cancer has been recently reviewed.[9] Most epidemiologic studies report standardized incidence ratios (SIR) to compare the ratio of the observed incidence of lung cancer in clinic-based HIV-infected populations with the expected incidence in the general population.[56] Depending on the population characteristics, SIRs for HIV range from 0.7 to 6.59 in the post-HAART

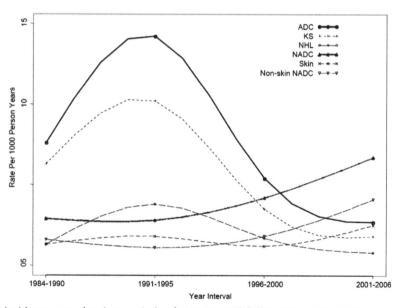

Fig. 2. Cancer incidence rates by time periods of HAART availability. ADC, AIDS-defining cancer; KS, Kaposi sarcoma; NADC, non-AIDS–defining cancer; NHL, non-Hodgkin lymphoma. (*From* Crum-Cianflone N, Hullsiek KH, Marconi V, et al. Trends in the incidence of cancers among HIV-infected persons and the impact of antiretroviral therapy: a 20-year cohort study. AIDS 2009;23:41–50; with permission.)

Table 1
Studies of the risk of lung cancer associated with HIV infection

Authors,[Ref.] Year	Study Population	Years of Study	No. of HIV+ in Follow-Up	No. of HIV+ LC Cases	SIR (95% CI)
HIV/AIDS Registry Linkage Studies					
Parker et al,[100,a] 1998	Texas	1990–1995	26181	36	6.5 (4.9–8.9)
Grulich et al,[101,a] 1999	NSW, Australia	1980–1993	3616	6	3.8 (1.4–8.3)
Cooksley et al,[102] 1999	Harris County, Texas	1975–1994	14986	18	0.7 (0.4–1.1)
Frisch et al,[11,a] 2001	USA	1978–1996	302834	808	4.5 (4.2–4.8)
Grulich et al,[103] 2002	Australia	1980–1999	13067	17	1.4 (0.8–2.3)
Allardice et al,[104] 2003	Scotland	1981–1996	2574	5	4.1 (1.3–9.5)
Dal Maso et al,[105,a] 2003	Italy	1985–1998	12104	22	2.4 (1.5–3.7)
Newnham et al,[106] 2005	England	1985–2001	33190	38	2.2 (1.6–3.1)
Engels et al,[10,a] 2006	USA	1980–2002	375933	393	2.6 (2.1–3.1)
Mbulaiteye et al,[107] 2006	Uganda	1989–2002	12607	4	5.0 (1.0–15)
Galceran et al,[108,a] 2007	Catalonia, Spain	1981–1999	1659	4	9.4 (2.4–24)
Dal Maso et al,[109,a] 2009	Italy	1986–2005	21951	42	4.1 (2.9–5.5)
Polesel et al,[110,a] 2010	Italy	1986–2004	21951	59	1.8 (1.0–3.2)
Cohort/Database Studies					
Serraino et al,[111] 2000	France; Italy	1982–1998	5281	4	2.9 (0.7–7.4)
Phelps et al,[112] 2001	Multisite USA	1993–2000	1310	4	6.4 (3.7–11)
Herida et al,[113] 2003	France	1992–1999	77025	99	2.1 (1.7–2.7)
Bower et al,[61] 2003	London HIV clinic	1986–2001	8400	11	8.9 (4.9–20)
Clifford et al,[114] 2005	Switzerland	1985–2003	7304	14	3.2 (1.7–5.4)
Engels et al,[57] 2006	Baltimore HIV clinic	1989–2003	5238	33	2.5 (1.6–3.5)
Serraino et al,[115] 2007	France; Italy	1985–2005	8074	14	1.7 (0.9–2.8)
Patel et al,[116] 2008	Multisite USA	1992–2003	54780	140	3.3 (2.8–3.9)
Levine et al,[117] 2010	Multisite USA	1994–2004	2651	12	3.3 (1.7–5.7)
Meta-Analyses					
Grulich et al,[62] 2007	Multisite	Varied	444172	1016	2.7 (1.9–3.9)
Shiels et al,[18] 2009	Multisite	Varied	625716	847	2.6 (2.1–3.1)

Studies are listed chronologically by publication date and grouped by study design of an HIV/AIDS and cancer registry linkage, a cohort or an administrative database design. Estimates of risk for lung cancer associated with HIV are presented and compared with the lung cancer cases that would have been expected in the general population with similar age and demographic characteristics. Adjustment for individual tobacco use was not possible in these studies.

Abbreviations: CI, confidence interval; LC, lung cancer; NSW, New South Wales; SIR, standardized incidence ratio.

[a] Studies included only persons with AIDS diagnoses.

Data from Kirk GD, Merlo CA. HIV infection in the etiology of lung cancer: confounding, causality, and consequences. Proc Am Thorac Soc 2011;8:327.

era.[12,18,56–58] In a summary of these studies (**Table 1**), only 1 of 22 reported a nonsignificantly decreased risk of lung cancer among HIV-infected patients compared with the general population (SIR 0.7). The remaining 21 studies all reported an increased risk of lung cancer associated with HIV infection; 17 studies found a statistically significant association of HIV with lung cancer. Despite lung cancer being the most common NADC, individual studies were usually limited by small numbers of cases, and the precision of the estimates was limited.

Whether HIV infection independently increases the risk of lung cancer has been debated extensively, largely because tobacco remains an important potential confounder of the association between HIV and lung cancer. HIV-infected patients have substantially higher smoking prevalence, with estimates ranging from 30% to 85% compared with the estimated 20% to 25% of the general population who are smokers.[9] Studies of HIV and lung cancer have therefore been challenged by the requirements of having large numbers of HIV-infected persons with data available on individual smoking behavior, following for prolonged periods to identify adequate outcomes of lung cancer, and then comparing to an epidemiologically appropriate comparison group (in contrast to simply comparing with the general population).

Several studies have had a design adequate to address the potential confounding of smoking (**Table 2**). Sigel and colleagues[15] evaluated a cohort of demographically similar HIV-infected and uninfected patients from the Veterans Aging Cohort Study Virtual Cohort and Veterans Affairs Central Cancer Registry during the post-HAART era. HIV-infected patients were more likely to be current smokers with a baseline history of drug abuse, alcohol abuse, hepatitis C virus infection, and a history of bacterial pneumonia. After adjusting for age, gender, race/ethnicity, baseline chronic obstructive pulmonary disease, bacterial pneumonia and smoking, they found HIV to be independently associated with lung cancer. Among HIV-infected and uninfected injection drug users (IDUs) enrolled in the AIDS Link to the Intravenous Experience (ALIVE) Study in Baltimore, studies of death from lung cancer and of incident lung cancer were performed. ALIVE has individual smoking behavior collected systematically rather than through medical records, in identical fashion among HIV-positive and HIV-negative IDUs. After adjusting for individual smoking behavior and other risk factors, both studies demonstrated an independent association between HIV and lung cancer, with an estimated 2- to 4-fold increased risk.[16,58] By contrast, Silverberg and colleagues[9] reported a nonsignificantly increased risk of lung cancer among managed care patients with HIV in comparison with those without HIV, after adjusting for current smoking status obtained through medical record review. Differences in these findings could represent variability in the HIV risk groups (eg, IDU, MSM), sociodemographic characteristics, HIV clinical status, or smoking behavior of the study populations, or heterogeneity in the methods used for ascertaining smoking exposure. However, when considering all of the studies, these data support the hypothesis that HIV infection plays an independent role in the increased risk of lung cancer, even after accounting for tobacco use.

The Role of Immunosuppression

One proposed mechanism for the increased risk of lung cancer in this population is that persistent HIV-associated immunosuppression results in reduced immune surveillance and a subsequent increased risk of malignancy. Epidemiologic data in support of the role of immune suppression should demonstrate a higher risk in persons with AIDS or advanced immunodeficiency as measured by current or nadir CD4 cell count. In data from the AIDS/Cancer Match study, a national linkage of HIV/AIDS and cancer registries, Engels and colleagues[12] report SIRs of 4.7 (95% confidence interval [CI] 3.0–6.9) during the post-AIDS diagnosis period, compared with 2.3 (95% CI 1.8–2.8) during the pre-AIDS diagnosis period. The SIRs during the pre-HAART and post-HAART time periods

Table 2
Studies of risk of lung cancer associated with HIV infection compared with an HIV-uninfected control group, with adjustment for individual smoking exposure

Authors,[Ref.] Year	Population	Years of Study	No. of HIV+ in Follow-Up	No. of HIV+ LC Cases	No. of HIV− in Follow-Up	No. of HIV− LC Cases	IRR (95% CI)
Phelps et al,[112] 2001	Multisite USA	1993–2000	871	4	439	1	3.3
Kirk et al,[16] 2007	Baltimore IDUs	1988–2005	1192	14	894	13	3.8 (1.6–7.9)
Shiels et al,[58] 2010	Baltimore IDUs	1988–2006	1072	13	1423	16	2.3 (1.1–5.1)
Silverberg et al,[60] 2011	California HMO patients	1996–2008	20775	56	215158	380	1.2 (0.9–1.6)
Sigel et al,[15] 2012	US Veterans	1997–2008	37294	457	75750	614	1.7 (1.5–1.9)

Abbreviations: CI, confidence interval; HMO, health maintenance organization; IDU, intravenous drug user; IRR, incidence rate ratio; LC, lung cancer.

Data from Kirk GD, Merlo CA. HIV infection in the etiology of lung cancer: confounding, causality, and consequences. Proc Am Thorac Soc 2011;8:329.

included in the study were equal, at 2.6 (both statistically significant). In further analysis from the AIDS/Cancer Match study, Frisch and colleagues[11] found lung cancer to be one of several non-AIDS–defining malignancies meeting all 3 of their criteria for potential association with immunosuppression. Although the investigators raised concerns that potential methodological limitations and confounding by tobacco use could have influenced the findings, these data illustrate an increase in the relative risk of lung cancer with the progression of HIV to AIDS. In a meta-analysis of NADC, Shiels and colleagues[18] also reported increased lung cancer among persons with AIDS.

At the time of diagnosis of lung cancer, most HIV-infected patients have a CD4 count of greater than 200 cells/μL. Analysis of Parisian hospital records noted a median CD4 count of 364/mm^3, whereas a prospective study by Shiels and colleagues[58] found a median of 267 cells/mm^3.[59] By contrast, several studies have failed to demonstrate a strong association between the incidence of lung cancer in HIV-infected patients and CD4 count.[16,17,58] In the post-HAART era, while a significantly elevated risk of lung cancer was observed as compared with the general population, incidence did not vary greatly by CD4 count.[17] Engels and colleagues[57] noted an inverse relationship between the incidence of lung cancer and HIV viral load; however, no relationship was observed between the incidence of lung cancer and current or nadir CD4 count. The ALIVE Study similarly uncovered no association between CD4 count or HIV RNA load with mortality due to lung cancer. The median CD4 count among HIV-infected patients with lung cancer was 260 cells/μL.[16]

By contrast, several studies have found an association between the incidence of lung cancer and immunosuppression. In the Kaiser-Permanente managed care population database, the risk for lung cancer among HIV-infected patients was significant among HIV patients with CD4 counts of fewer than 200 cells/μL, with a relative risk of 2.2 (95% CI 1.3–3.6) compared with their non-HIV counterparts.[60] A small British study revealed no substantial change in the degree of immunosuppression between HIV-infected patients diagnosed with lung cancer in the pre- and post-HAART eras.[61] In a meta-analysis including patients who were immunosuppressed either from HIV infection or solid organ transplantation, rates of lung cancers were increased among both populations. Furthermore, among those with kidney failure, the risk of lung cancer was much greater after transplantation than during dialysis, suggesting that immune suppression was distinctly associated with increased risk.[62] A strong dose-response

relationship was observed between increasing risk of lung cancer and lower current CD4 cell counts in an analysis of a large French hospital database.[63]

Impact of HAART

Besides contributing to prolonged survival and the increased risk of lung cancer associated with aging, HAART itself has been suggested to be directly oncogenic and to potentially contribute to the development of lung cancer in HIV-infected patients.[64] On the cellular level, zidovudine and didanosine have been shown to elicit mutagenic responses in vitro. Furthermore, zidovudine-didanosine coexposure potentiated zidovudine-DNA incorporation and mutagenic responses, but at concentrations 3 to 30 times the peak plasma levels seen in patients. With the development of potent, less toxic antiretrovirals, exposure to these older medications is now relatively rare, except in resource-limited settings. It remains unclear whether newer regimens have any direct mutagenic effects.

Genomic instability has been hypothesized to increase the risk of lung cancer in HIV. Microsatellite alterations, but not the loss of heterozygosity, were significantly increased in lung cancer tissue samples from HIV-infected patients when compared with samples from HIV-indeterminant patients.[65] While genomic instability has been suggested as a potential mechanism in lung carcinogenesis, little is known about the putative molecular effects of these alterations.

Infections and Chronic Inflammation

Prior pulmonary infections have been associated with an increased risk of lung cancer in the general population, likely related to a chronic inflammatory process.[66–68] Similarly, pulmonary infections have been theorized to increase the risk of lung cancer among HIV-infected patients.[16,69] HIV-infected persons are at substantially higher risk for bacterial pneumonia as well as *Pneumocystis*, mycobacterial, and viral respiratory infections. Risk for these infections appears to be further increased with immunodeficiency and smoking. Repeated bacterial pneumonias have been associated with an increased risk of lung cancer among HIV-infected persons with AIDS.[70]

Cancers known to be associated with human papillomavirus (HPV) (anal, vaginal, penile, nasopharyngeal, laryngeal, and oral) are increased in HIV-infected patients.[18] Although HPV has been hypothesized to contribute to the increased incidence of lung cancer among HIV-infected patients, the data remain inconclusive. HPV detection in bronchial carcinoma is variable. Despite this, bronchial carcinoma induced by asbestos and radiation exposure can be modeled using an HPV-18 immortalized bronchial cell line.[71]

CLINICAL PRESENTATION

The age at diagnosis of lung cancer has been consistently reported to be lower among HIV-infected patients than in HIV-uninfected patients. In a review of lung cancer diagnoses at Johns Hopkins Hospital from 1986 to 2004, HIV-infected patients were generally diagnosed between 40 and 60 years of age, rather than between 50 and 80 years of age in the HIV-indeterminate cohort. Demopoulos and colleagues[72] similarly found a younger age of presentation of lung cancer in HIV-infected patients when reviewing the Cancer Registry files at Bellevue Hospital in New York. In this cohort, HIV-infected patients diagnosed with lung cancer presented at the age of 50, rather than 60 years. In France from 1993 to 2002, the median age at diagnosis of lung cancer among HIV-infected patients was 45 years compared with 63 years in the general population.[59] Lastly, in a review of HIV-infected patients with lung cancer followed in a Baltimore clinic from 1989 to 2002, the incidence of lung cancer increased with age, whereas the SIR decreased with age, indicating that excess risk was greatest at younger ages.[57]

However, several studies have noted that there are substantial differences in the age distribution of the HIV population compared with the general population.[72,73] Shiels and colleagues[74] adjusted for the underlying population structures (Fig. 3A) and reevaluated differences in the observed age at cancer diagnosis for a variety of cancers among HIV-infected patients. For most cancers, the younger age distribution of the AIDS population compared with the general population accounted for the observed difference in age at diagnosis. For lung cancer (see Fig. 3B), the younger age of cancer diagnosis among HIV-infected patients persisted, albeit of a substantially smaller magnitude of 3 to 4 years rather than the previously described presentation at an age 10 to 20 years younger than the general population.

PATHOLOGY

Adenocarcinoma appears to be the most common pathologic type of lung cancer among HIV-infected patients, similar to the general population.[15,17,57,73] In contrast to these data, Hakimian and colleagues[75] focused on the post-HAART era in a single-center retrospective analysis of 34 patients with lung cancer and HIV, of whom 30 (88%) were diagnosed with non–small cell lung cancer (NSCLC) and 4 (12%) with small cell lung cancer; no adenocarcinoma cases were identified. In the general population, most nonsmokers who develop lung cancer are diagnosed with adenocarcinoma as opposed to squamous cell carcinoma, which is more commonly diagnosed among smokers. Thus, the consistently observed preponderance of adenocarcinoma among HIV-infected patients with lung cancer has led researchers to question the relationship between tobacco use and lung cancer in these patients. However, it should be recognized that HIV-associated lung cancer has been reported almost exclusively among current or former smokers.

UNIQUE TREATMENT OUTCOMES AND CONCERNS IN HIV-ASSOCIATED LUNG CANCER
Disease Stage at Diagnosis and Survival

HIV-infected patients often present with an advanced stage of lung cancer (Table 3), although it remains unclear whether the disease stage is increased in comparison with HIV-uninfected patients with lung cancer. In analysis of cases of lung cancer in the Veterans Affairs system where similar access to care and screening patterns would be expected by HIV status, Sigel and colleagues[15] found that stage at diagnosis did not differ between HIV-infected and HIV-uninfected patients in the post-HAART era. However, substantial data indicate that HIV-infected cases of lung cancer present at more advanced disease stage. An analysis of post-HAART era data by Chaturvedi and colleagues[17] indicated that more than 50% of HIV-infected patients diagnosed with lung cancer had distant disease at initial presentation, arguing against a strong contribution of increased surveillance in HIV-positive patients to explain their higher cancer risk. A French retrospective review found that more than 70% of patients presented with stage IIIB or stage IV disease.[59] Hakimian and colleagues[75] reported that 80% of NSCLC patients were diagnosed with stage IIIB/IV disease. In the ALIVE study, the stage of lung cancer at presentation was more advanced among HIV-infected than HIV-uninfected IDUs, both groups having limited access to care.[58] Similarly, in a large HIV–cancer registry match study from Texas, 337 HIV-infected patients with lung cancer displayed more distant stage disease at presentation compared with the more than 156,000 HIV-uninfected patients with lung cancer.[76]

Following a diagnosis of lung cancer, mortality appears to be higher in HIV-infected than in

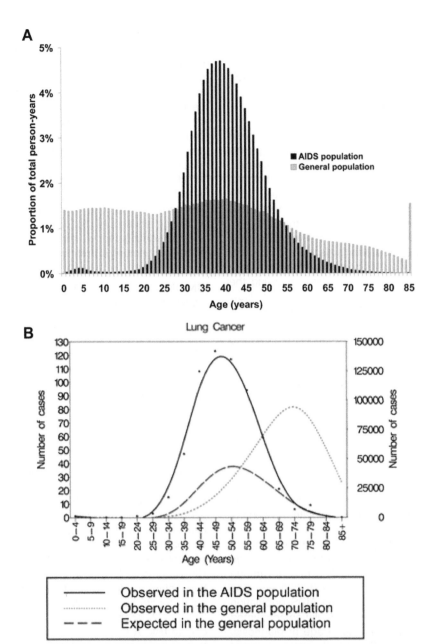

Fig. 3. Age at cancer diagnosis among persons with AIDS and the general population in the United States, 1996 to 2007. (*A*) The younger, more restricted age distribution of the AIDS population compared with the general population. These differences in population structure contribute to the observed younger ages of cancer diagnosis reported among persons with AIDS. To illustrate this with lung cancer, (*B*) displays the younger observed age distribution of cases of lung cancer in persons with AIDS (*solid line*) compared with the general population (*dotted line*). However, after standardizing the age of the general population to that of the AIDS population, the expected age distribution in the general population (*dashed line*) is more similar to the AIDS population. (*Adapted from* Shiels MS, Pfeiffer RM, Engels EA. Age at cancer diagnosis among persons with AIDS in the United States. Ann Intern Med 2010;153(7):455–7; with permission.)

HIV-uninfected patients. Conflicting evidence exists as to whether this simply represents a more advanced disease stage at diagnosis or if there truly is lower survival with HIV. Reduced

uptake, greater toxicity, and more limited responses to cancer treatment have been proposed as potential mechanisms to explain poor survival in HIV-associated lung cancer. In several studies

Table 3
Overview of selected studies describing clinical outcomes in HIV-associated lung cancer patients

Study	Bower[61]	Brock[73]	D'Jaen [PMID 21062730]	Hakimian[75]	Shiels[58]	Sigel[15]
Number of cases	11	92	75	34	13	457
Type of cohort	Hospital database (UK)	Hospital database (USA)	International database	2 Hospital databases (USA)	IDU cohort linked to cancer registry (USA)	Veterans cohort linked to cancer registry (USA)
Years of study	1986–2001	1986–2004	1996–2008	1996–2003	1988–2006	1997–2008
Age at cancer diagnosis	45[a]	46 (42–53)	50 (32–75)[c]	44 (34–77)[c]	46 (40–49)	51 (34–83)[c]
Stage at diagnosis	54% IV	68.5% IV	77% IIIB/IV	53% IV	64% Distant	68% III/IV
CD4 count at cancer diagnosis	160	305 (82–428)	340 (0–1456)	>200	267 (199–437)[b]	286 (139–448)
Histology	Adeno 45% Squamous 36%	Adeno 48% Squamous 17% Small cell 8%	Adeno 46% Squamous 35% Small & Large-cell 19%	NSCLC 88% Small cell 12%	Adeno 8% Squamous 42%	Adeno 36% Squamous 30% Small cell 8%
Survival (months)	4–5 (range 2–15+)	6.3 (2.3–11.4)	9	8.2 (no IQR)	4.7 (2.5–9.2)	—

Data presented represent the median values (IQR: Interquartile range), unless otherwise indicated.
Abbreviations: Adeno, adenocarcinoma; IDU, injection drug user; NSCLC, non-small cell lung cancer; squamous, squamous cell cancer.
[a] Mean.
[b] Measured at study entry.
[c] Range of values.

that reported clinical outcomes for patients with HIV-associated lung cancer, presentation was generally advanced and survival times were dismal (see **Table 3**). In a retrospective review of diagnoses of lung cancer among HIV-infected patients at Johns Hopkins Hospital from 1986 to 2004, lung cancer survival was shorter among HIV-infected patients (median survival: 6.3 months vs 9.4 months; $P = 0.002$). However, after accounting for stage of cancer (HIV-infected patients: 87% stage IIIB/IV; 69% distant metastases compared with 68% and 47% in HIV-indeterminate patients, respectively), the differences in survival were attenuated.[73] In a retrospective review of patients with HIV and lung cancer, the median survival of patients with stage IIIB or stage IV NSCLC was 5.2 months, and 7.2 months for the few patients with small cell lung cancer, all of whom had extensive disease.[75] In the large study from Texas, HIV infection was associated with significantly higher lung cancer–specific mortality (hazard ratio 1.34, 95% CI 1.15–1.56).[76] Among NSCLC patients in this study, HIV-infected patients were notably around 60% less likely to receive cancer treatment. By contrast, another large, population-based registry match study that linked cancer registry with Medicare data to ascertain HIV status among older NSCLC patients (median age of 75 years for both HIV-uninfected and HIV-uninfected cases), no significant differences in survival were observed by HIV status.[77]

Irrespective of how much HIV infection contributes to excess mortality in lung cancer compared with HIV-uninfected persons, mortality of persons with HIV and lung cancer appears to be primarily driven by lung cancer.[33,78] A French retrospective review of records at 2 hospitals from 1993 to 2002 found that 64% of patients did not respond to treatment, with 86% of the patients dying from progressive lung cancer rather than HIV-related complications or opportunistic infections. In this cohort, the median survival of patients with a CD4 count of less than 300/mm^3 was 3 months, compared with 11 months among patients with a CD4 count of at least 300/mm^3.[59] ALIVE also found a high rate of mortality due to lung cancer, with no deaths due to AIDS and shorter survival time, approximately 0.39 years (interquartile range [IQR] 0.21–0.77), compared with HIV-uninfected cases of lung cancer (0.72 years, IQR 0.36–1.7).[58]

Treatment of any type or stage of lung cancer among HIV-infected patients is generally the same as for HIV-uninfected patients, although several unique considerations should be evaluated before initiation of treatment. It is important to recognize that in the era of HAART, HIV status should not be a primary factor in the treatment decisions for lung cancer.[77,79] At present, there are no HIV-specific guidelines for the treatment of lung cancer or for dose adjustments of concurrently used anticancer and antiretroviral drugs.[80] Improved access to evidence-based, state-of-the-art cancer therapies for HIV-infected patients with lung cancer should be a clinical priority.[81]

Before initiation of cancer treatment, functional status should be evaluated to help guide the timing and enhance tolerability of the therapy to be administered. In patients with HIV, assessment of functional status may assume even greater priority. If possible, based on the clinical context, many clinicians would advocate for initiation of HAART to improve performance status before undergoing chemotherapy. In a retrospective review of a tumor registry at 2 Maryland hospitals, 20% of patients with HIV and lung cancer received these diagnoses concurrently.[75] Although no guidelines currently exist for this scenario, HAART was usually started first.

Monitoring for venous thromboembolism (VTE) among HIV-associated patients with lung cancer presents an equally unclear area. The increased incidence of VTE among patients with lung cancer is well established, particularly related to chemotherapy, extensive cancer disease, and indwelling catheters.[82] Substantial data also suggest that HIV-infected patients have a heightened risk for VTE.[83,84] Mechanisms remain unclear, but proposed VTE risk factors in the setting of HIV infection include advanced HIV disease (eg, elevated viral load, lower CD4 counts, history of opportunistic infections), injection drug use and direct effects of antiretrovirals.[85–89] Diagnosis and risk stratification of VTE is further complicated by the presence of known biomarkers of VTE (eg, elevated von Willebrand factor and auto-antibodies to phospholipids; depressed anticoagulant protein C and S and antithrombin III) in the blood of HIV patients, caused either directly or indirectly by HIV infection.[83,88] VTE prophylaxis is not currently recommended as part of routine care for HIV-infected patients with lung cancer; further data are needed to clarify VTE risk and inform appropriate management in the setting of comorbid HIV and lung cancer.

PREVENTION
Smoking Cessation

In the current primary care guidelines for the management of HIV-infected persons by the HIV Medicine Association of the Infectious Diseases Society of America, screening for tobacco use is not explicitly recommended.[90] Smoking prevalence varies between different racial, socioeconomic, and

HIV risk groups, but appears to range from 30% to 85%.[9] In a cross-sectional survey of nearly 350 HIV-infected patients, 47% were current smokers and 63% were ever smokers; male gender, older age, lower educational attainment, and heavy alcohol or injection drug use were associated with being a smoker.[91] In an urban IDU population smoking was nearly ubiquitous, although only moderate levels of nicotine dependence were observed; there were no substantial differences in smoking behavior (eg, age at first smoking, pack-years, nicotine addiction) between HIV-infected and HIV-uninfected IDUs.[92] Among nearly 900 HIV-infected Veterans Administration patients, 63% were current smokers and 22% were former smokers. Current smokers complained of increased respiratory symptoms and reported decreased quality of life.[93] Among New York Medicaid patients with HIV, two-thirds were current smokers, smoking an average of 16 cigarettes per day for a mean of 23 years' duration. More than 80% of the smokers with HIV were in the precontemplative or contemplative stages of quitting; however, nearly half of the patients (46%) expressed interest in accessing a free or low-cost smoking-cessation program.[94]

Several other studies have indicated that smoking cessation is of substantial interest to HIV-infected patients; however, significant provider, insurance, financial, and other barriers to using evidence-based approaches to smoking cessation in HIV care persist. Furthermore, it remains unclear whether smoking-cessation programs need to be tailored to the specific needs of HIV-infected patients. Tobacco cessation should be promoted in any patient who is a smoker, although cessation is of critical importance among HIV-infected patients. In addition to tobacco-related complications common to all smokers (eg, lung cancer, obstructive lung disease, atherosclerosis), tobacco use among HIV-infected patients is associated with increased risk for less common complications such as oral candidiasis, hairy leukoplakia, and bacterial pneumonia.[93,95,96] These complications, along with the risk of lung cancer, should motivate both the patient and the primary care provider to address tobacco cessation as a priority. Smoking-cessation behaviors and interventions are reviewed in further detail in the article by Browning and colleagues elsewhere in this issue.

Screening for Lung Cancer

Infectious Diseases Society of America guidelines for primary care do not recommend any routine screening for lung cancer. However, they do recommend obtaining a baseline chest radiograph (CXR) in any patient with a history of positive tuberculosis screening test or with preexisting lung disease, in case future abnormalities on imaging arise.[90] Findings from the National Lung Screening Trial (NLST) showed that low-dose CT scanning reduced mortality from lung cancer by 20% when compared with CXR screening among older, high-risk smokers.[97] Although there is still much debate regarding the risk of lung cancer posed by HIV infection, NLST recommendations for screening among older smokers may apply to HIV-infected patients as well, although the benefits and harms of screening may be different in HIV-infected patients. Given the high burden of tobacco use and the concern for earlier onset of lung cancer among HIV-infected patients, growing discussions have focused on whether CT screening should be performed on HIV-infected smokers, although there exist no data in support of this approach. When considering CT imaging of the chest as part of malignancy screening in HIV-infected patients, clinicians will likely be faced with the need for interpretation of an even greater number of ambiguous radiographic abnormalities. In a retrospective evaluation of 42 HIV-infected patients with abnormal CXRs and an absence of pulmonary symptoms admitted to 2 Seattle hospitals between 1996 and 1998, Gold and colleagues[98] found that the most frequent thoracic radiographic abnormalities were nodular disease (52%), followed by adenopathy (17%) and infiltrate (12%). The final diagnosis in these patients was most commonly tuberculosis (26%), nontuberculosis mycobacteria (24%), KS (12%), lymphoproliferative disorder (7%) and other neoplasia (6%). Nearly 40% of these diagnoses were obtained via bronchoscopy, suggesting that aggressive evaluation of radiographic abnormalities in HIV-infected patients was justified. However, the role for invasive testing in the setting of CT screening is unknown. Besides pulmonary nodules, lymphadenopathy is also commonly found on thoracic imaging of HIV-infected patients. The differential diagnosis of lymphadenopathy is broad, and the diagnostic approach (reviewed by Lichtenberger and colleagues[99]) may involve characterizing lymphadenopathy as low-attenuation (eg, mycobacterial or fungal infection), or enhancing (eg, multicentric Castleman disease, KS, or bacillary angiomatosis).[99]

SUMMARY

HIV-associated lung malignancies contribute to substantial morbidity and mortality in the HIV-infected population. Immunosuppression is the primary risk factor for HIV/AIDS-associated KS and NHL. Following widespread uptake of HAART, rates of KS and NHL have declined substantially. After HAART initiation, IRIS, especially in pulmonary KS, has been associated with serious clinical consequences and death. However, effective HAART remains the best strategy to lower the risk for KS or NHL. Concurrent with declines in KS and NHL, NADC, of which lung cancer is the most common, have increased in incidence and importance. HIV-associated lung cancer occurs almost exclusively among smokers and generally among those with significant immune deficiency. Compared with HIV-uninfected populations, the onset of lung cancer in HIV-infected individuals occurs 3 to 4 years earlier, generally with advanced cancer stage at diagnosis, and worse survival. Adenocarcinoma is the most frequent histologic type. Despite the high smoking prevalence in HIV populations, HIV appears to increase the risk of lung cancer independent of smoking, although the underlying mechanisms remain unclear. Smoking cessation needs to assume greater priority in HIV primary care.

REFERENCES

1. Palella FJ Jr, Delaney KM, Moorman AC, et al. Declining morbidity and mortality among patients with advanced human immunodeficiency virus infection. HIV Outpatient Study Investigators. N Engl J Med 1998;338(13):853–60.
2. Sterne JA, Hernan MA, Ledergerber B, et al. Long-term effectiveness of potent antiretroviral therapy in preventing AIDS and death: a prospective cohort study. Lancet 2005;366(9483):378–84.
3. Detels R, Munoz A, McFarlane G, et al. Effectiveness of potent antiretroviral therapy on time to AIDS and death in men with known HIV infection duration. Multicenter AIDS Cohort Study Investigators. JAMA 1998;280(17):1497–503.
4. Survival after introduction of HAART in people with known duration of HIV-1 infection. The CASCADE Collaboration. Concerted Action on SeroConversion to AIDS and Death in Europe. Lancet 2000; 355(9210):1158–9.
5. High KP, Brennan-Ing M, Clifford DB, et al. HIV and aging: state of knowledge and areas of critical need for research. A report to the NIH Office of AIDS Research by the HIV and Aging Working Group. J Acquir Immune Defic Syndr 2012; 60(Suppl 1):S1–18.
6. Hasse B, Ledergerber B, Furrer H, et al. Morbidity and aging in HIV-infected persons: the Swiss HIV cohort study. Clin Infect Dis 2011;53(11):1130–9.
7. van Sighem AI, Gras LA, Reiss P, et al. Life expectancy of recently diagnosed asymptomatic HIV-infected patients approaches that of uninfected individuals. AIDS 2010;24(10):1527–35.
8. Crum NF, Riffenburgh RH, Wegner S, et al. Comparisons of causes of death and mortality rates among HIV-infected persons: analysis of the pre-, early, and late HAART (highly active antiretroviral therapy) eras. J Acquir Immune Defic Syndr 2006;41(2):194–200.
9. Kirk GD, Merlo CA. HIV infection in the etiology of lung cancer: confounding, causality, and consequences. Proc Am Thorac Soc 2011;8(3): 326–32.
10. Engels EA, Pfeiffer RM, Goedert JJ, et al. Trends in cancer risk among people with AIDS in the United States 1980-2002. AIDS 2006;20(12): 1645–54.
11. Frisch M, Biggar RJ, Engels EA, et al. Association of cancer with AIDS-related immunosuppression in adults. JAMA 2001;285(13):1736–45.
12. Engels EA, Biggar RJ, Hall HI, et al. Cancer risk in people infected with human immunodeficiency virus in the United States. Int J Cancer 2008; 123(1):187–94.
13. Cancer facts & figures 2011. Atlanta, GA: American Cancer Society; 2011.
14. Irwin LE, Begandy MK, Moore TM. Adenosquamous carcinoma of the lung and the acquired immunodeficiency syndrome. Ann Intern Med 1984;100(1):158.
15. Sigel K, Wisnivesky J, Gordon K, et al. HIV as an independent risk factor for incident lung cancer. AIDS 2012;26(8):1017–25.
16. Kirk GD, Merlo C, O' Driscoll P, et al. HIV infection is associated with an increased risk for lung cancer, independent of smoking. Clin Infect Dis 2007; 45(1):103–10.
17. Chaturvedi AK, Pfeiffer RM, Chang L, et al. Elevated risk of lung cancer among people with AIDS. AIDS 2007;21(2):207–13.
18. Shiels MS, Cole SR, Kirk GD, et al. A meta-analysis of the incidence of non-AIDS cancers in HIV-infected individuals. J Acquir Immune Defic Syndr 2009;52(5):611–22.
19. Gambus G, Bourboulia D, Esteve A, et al. Prevalence and distribution of HHV-8 in different subpopulations, with and without HIV infection, in Spain. AIDS 2001;15(9):1167–74.
20. Renwick N, Halaby T, Weverling GJ, et al. Seroconversion for human herpesvirus 8 during HIV infection is highly predictive of Kaposi's sarcoma. AIDS 1998;12(18):2481–8.
21. Kramer A, Biggar RJ, Hampl H, et al. Immunologic markers of progression to acquired immunodeficiency syndrome are time-dependent and illness-specific. Am J Epidemiol 1992;136(1):71–80.
22. Gallafent JH, Buskin SE, De Turk PB, et al. Profile of patients with Kaposi's sarcoma in the era of highly active antiretroviral therapy. J Clin Oncol 2005; 23(6):1253–60.

23. Huang L, Schnapp LM, Gruden JF, et al. Presentation of AIDS-related pulmonary Kaposi's sarcoma diagnosed by bronchoscopy. Am J Respir Crit Care Med 1996;153(4 Pt 1):1385–90.

24. Aboulafia DM. The epidemiologic, pathologic, and clinical features of AIDS-associated pulmonary Kaposi's sarcoma. Chest 2000;117(4):1128–45.

25. Angeletti PC, Zhang L, Wood C. The viral etiology of AIDS-associated malignancies. Adv Pharmacol 2008;56:509–57.

26. Palmieri C, Dhillon T, Thirlwell C, et al. Pulmonary Kaposi sarcoma in the era of highly active antiretroviral therapy. HIV Med 2006;7(5):291–3.

27. Murray JF, Mason RJ. Murray and Nadel's textbook of respiratory medicine. ScienceDirect (Online service). 5th edition. Philadelphia: Saunders/Elsevier; 2010. Available at: http://www.mdconsult.com/public/book/view?title=Mason:+Murray+&+Nadel's+Textbook+of+Respiratory+Medicine. Accessed December 20, 2012.

28. Ognibene FP, Steis RG, Macher AM, et al. Kaposi's sarcoma causing pulmonary infiltrates and respiratory failure in the acquired immunodeficiency syndrome. Ann Intern Med 1985;102(4):471–5.

29. Lodi S, Guiguet M, Costagliola D, et al. Kaposi sarcoma incidence and survival among HIV-infected homosexual men after HIV seroconversion. J Natl Cancer Inst 2010;102(11):784–92.

30. Gruden JF, Huang L, Webb WR, et al. AIDS-related Kaposi sarcoma of the lung: radiographic findings and staging system with bronchoscopic correlation. Radiology 1995;195(2):545–52.

31. Gasparetto TD, Marchiori E, Lourenco S, et al. Pulmonary involvement in Kaposi sarcoma: correlation between imaging and pathology. Orphanet J Rare Dis 2009;4:18.

32. Lee VW, Fuller JD, O'Brien MJ, et al. Pulmonary Kaposi sarcoma in patients with AIDS: scintigraphic diagnosis with sequential thallium and gallium scanning. Radiology 1991;180(2):409–12.

33. Biggar RJ, Engels EA, Ly S, et al. Survival after cancer diagnosis in persons with AIDS. J Acquir Immune Defic Syndr 2005;39(3):293–9.

34. Stebbing J, Sanitt A, Nelson M, et al. A prognostic index for AIDS-associated Kaposi's sarcoma in the era of highly active antiretroviral therapy. Lancet 2006;367(9521):1495–502.

35. Feller L, Anagnostopoulos C, Wood NH, et al. Human immunodeficiency virus-associated Kaposi sarcoma as an immune reconstitution inflammatory syndrome: a literature review and case report. J Periodontol 2008;79(2):362–8.

36. Bower M, Nelson M, Young AM, et al. Immune reconstitution inflammatory syndrome associated with Kaposi's sarcoma. J Clin Oncol 2005;23(22):5224–8.

37. Leidner RS, Aboulafia DM. Recrudescent Kaposi's sarcoma after initiation of HAART: a manifestation of immune reconstitution syndrome. AIDS Patient Care STDS 2005;19(10):635–44.

38. Achenbach CJ, Harrington RD, Dhanireddy S, et al. Paradoxical immune reconstitution inflammatory syndrome in HIV-infected patients treated with combination antiretroviral therapy after AIDS-defining opportunistic infection. Clin Infect Dis 2012;54(3):424–33.

39. Stover KR, Molitorisz S, Swiatlo E, et al. A fatal case of Kaposi sarcoma due to immune reconstitution inflammatory syndrome. Am J Med Sci 2012;343(5):421–5.

40. Cadranel JL, Kammoun S, Chevret S, et al. Results of chemotherapy in 30 AIDS patients with symptomatic pulmonary Kaposi's sarcoma. Thorax 1994;49(10):958–60.

41. Kirova YM, Belembaogo E, Frikha H, et al. Radiotherapy in the management of epidemic Kaposi's sarcoma: a retrospective study of 643 cases. Radiother Oncol 1998;46(1):19–22.

42. Simard EP, Pfeiffer RM, Engels EA. Cumulative incidence of cancer among individuals with acquired immunodeficiency syndrome in the United States. Cancer 2011;117(5):1089–96.

43. Cadranel J, Naccache J, Wislez M, et al. Pulmonary malignancies in the immunocompromised patient. Respiration 1999;66(4):289–309.

44. Restrepo CS, Chen MM, Martinez-Jimenez S, et al. Chest neoplasms with infectious etiologies. World J Radiol 2011;3(12):279–88.

45. Knowles DM. Biologic aspects of AIDS-associated non-Hodgkin's lymphoma. Curr Opin Oncol 1993;5(5):845–51.

46. Ray P, Antoine M, Mary-Krause M, et al. AIDS-related primary pulmonary lymphoma. Am J Respir Crit Care Med 1998;158(4):1221–9.

47. Cesarman E, Chang Y, Moore PS, et al. Kaposi's sarcoma-associated herpesvirus-like DNA sequences in AIDS-related body-cavity-based lymphomas. N Engl J Med 1995;332(18):1186–91.

48. Eisner MD, Kaplan LD, Herndier B, et al. The pulmonary manifestations of AIDS-related non-Hodgkin's lymphoma. Chest 1996;110(3):729–36.

49. Miller RF, Jones EL, Duddy MJ, et al. Progressive intrathoracic lymphadenopathy: EBV associated non-Hodgkin's lymphoma. Sex Transm Infect 2002;78(1):13–7.

50. Allen CM, Al-Jahdali HH, Irion KL, et al. Imaging lung manifestations of HIV/AIDS. Ann Thorac Med 2010;5(4):201–16.

51. Gerard L, Galicier L, Maillard A, et al. Systemic non-Hodgkin lymphoma in HIV-infected patients with effective suppression of HIV replication: persistent occurrence but improved survival. J Acquir Immune Defic Syndr 2002;30(5):478–84.

52. Kirk O, Pedersen C, Cozzi-Lepri A, et al. Non-Hodgkin lymphoma in HIV-infected patients in the era of highly active antiretroviral therapy. Blood 2001;98(12):3406–12.

53. Re A, Michieli M, Casari S, et al. High-dose therapy and autologous peripheral blood stem cell transplantation as salvage treatment for AIDS-related lymphoma: long-term results of the Italian Cooperative Group on AIDS and Tumors (GICAT) study with analysis of prognostic factors. Blood 2009; 114(7):1306–13.

54. Huhn GD, Badri S, Vibhakar S, et al. Early development of non-Hodgkin lymphoma following initiation of newer class antiretroviral therapy among HIV-infected patients—implications for immune reconstitution. AIDS Res Ther 2010;7:44.

55. Shiels MS, Pfeiffer RM, Gail MH, et al. Cancer burden in the HIV-infected population in the United States. J Natl Cancer Inst 2011;103(9):753–62.

56. Cadranel J, Garfield D, Lavole A, et al. Lung cancer in HIV infected patients: facts, questions and challenges. Thorax 2006;61(11):1000–8.

57. Engels EA, Brock MV, Chen J, et al. Elevated incidence of lung cancer among HIV-infected individuals. J Clin Oncol 2006;24(9):1383–8.

58. Shiels MS, Cole SR, Mehta SH, et al. Lung cancer incidence and mortality among HIV-infected and HIV-uninfected injection drug users. J Acquir Immune Defic Syndr 2010;55(4):510–5.

59. Spano JP, Massiani MA, Bentata M, et al. Lung cancer in patients with HIV Infection and review of the literature. Med Oncol 2004;21(2):109–15.

60. Silverberg MJ, Chao C, Leyden WA, et al. HIV infection, immunodeficiency, viral replication, and the risk of cancer. Cancer Epidemiol Biomarkers Prev 2011;20(12):2551–9.

61. Bower M, Powles T, Nelson M, et al. HIV-related lung cancer in the era of highly active antiretroviral therapy. AIDS 2003;17(3):371–5.

62. Grulich AE, van Leeuwen MT, Falster MO, et al. Incidence of cancers in people with HIV/AIDS compared with immunosuppressed transplant recipients: a meta-analysis. Lancet 2007;370(9581):59–67.

63. Guiguet M, Boue F, Cadranel J, et al. Effect of immunodeficiency, HIV viral load, and antiretroviral therapy on the risk of individual malignancies (FHDH-ANRS CO4): a prospective cohort study. Lancet Oncol 2009;10(12):1152–9.

64. Meng Q, Walker DM, Olivero OA, et al. Zidovudine-didanosine coexposure potentiates DNA incorporation of zidovudine and mutagenesis in human cells. Proc Natl Acad Sci U S A 2000;97(23): 12667–71.

65. Wistuba II, Behrens C, Milchgrub S, et al. Comparison of molecular changes in lung cancers in HIV-positive and HIV-indeterminate subjects. JAMA 1998;279(19):1554–9.

66. Chaturvedi AK, Gaydos CA, Agreda P, et al. Chlamydia pneumoniae infection and risk for lung cancer. Cancer Epidemiol Biomarkers Prev 2010; 19(6):1498–505.

67. Alavanja MC, Brownson RC, Boice JD Jr, et al. Pre-existing lung disease and lung cancer among nonsmoking women. Am J Epidemiol 1992;136(6): 623–32.

68. Brownson RC, Alavanja MC. Previous lung disease and lung cancer risk among women (United States). Cancer Causes Control 2000;11(9):853–8.

69. Engels EA. Inflammation in the development of lung cancer: epidemiological evidence. Expert Rev Anticancer Ther 2008;8(4):605–15.

70. Shebl FM, Engels EA, Goedert JJ, et al. Pulmonary infections and risk of lung cancer among persons with AIDS. J Acquir Immune Defic Syndr 2010; 55(3):375–9.

71. Syrjanen KJ. HPV infections and lung cancer. J Clin Pathol 2002;55(12):885–91.

72. Demopoulos BP, Vamvakas E, Ehrlich JE, et al. Non-acquired immunodeficiency syndrome-defining malignancies in patients infected with human immunodeficiency virus. Arch Pathol Lab Med 2003;127(5):589–92.

73. Brock MV, Hooker CM, Engels EA, et al. Delayed diagnosis and elevated mortality in an urban population with HIV and lung cancer: implications for patient care. J Acquir Immune Defic Syndr 2006; 43(1):47–55.

74. Shiels MS, Pfeiffer RM, Engels EA. Age at cancer diagnosis among persons with AIDS in the United States. Ann Intern Med 2010;153(7):452–60.

75. Hakimian R, Fang H, Thomas L, et al. Lung cancer in HIV-infected patients in the era of highly active antiretroviral therapy. J Thorac Oncol 2007;2(4): 268–72.

76. Suneja G, Shiels MS, Melville SK, et al. Disparities in the treatment and outcomes of lung cancer among HIV-infected people in Texas. AIDS 2013; 27(3):459–68.

77. Rengan R, Mitra N, Liao K, et al. Effect of HIV on survival in patients with non-small-cell lung cancer in the era of highly active antiretroviral therapy: a population-based study. Lancet Oncol 2012; 13(12):1203–9.

78. Riedel DJ, Mwangi EI, Fantry LE, et al. High cancer-related mortality in an Urban, predominantly African-American, HIV-infected population. AIDS 2012. [Epub ahead of print].

79. Aboulafia DM. Decision making in non-AIDS-defining malignancies. Lancet Oncol 2012;13(12): 1172–3.

80. Rudek MA, Flexner C, Ambinder RF. Use of antineoplastic agents in patients with cancer who have HIV/AIDS. Lancet Oncol 2011;12(9): 905–12.

81. Persad GC, Little RF, Grady C. Including persons with HIV infection in cancer clinical trials. J Clin Oncol 2008;26(7):1027–32.

82. Lee AY, Levine MN. Venous thromboembolism and cancer: risks and outcomes. Circulation 2003; 107(23 Suppl 1):I17–21.

83. Auerbach E, Aboulafia DM. Venous and arterial thromboembolic complications associated with HIV infection and highly active antiretroviral therapy. Semin Thromb Hemost 2012;38(8):830–8.

84. Klein SK, Slim EJ, de Kruif MD, et al. Is chronic HIV infection associated with venous thrombotic disease? A systematic review. Neth J Med 2005; 63(4):129–36.

85. Rasmussen LD, Dybdal M, Gerstoft J, et al. HIV and risk of venous thromboembolism: a Danish nationwide population-based cohort study. HIV Med 2011;12(4):202–10.

86. Fultz SL, McGinnis KA, Skanderson M, et al. Association of venous thromboembolism with human immunodeficiency virus and mortality in veterans. Am J Med 2004;116(6):420–3.

87. Ahonkhai AA, Gebo KA, Streiff MB, et al. Venous thromboembolism in patients with HIV/AIDS: a case-control study. J Acquir Immune Defic Syndr 2008;48(3):310–4.

88. Jacobson MC, Dezube BJ, Aboulafia DM. Thrombotic complications in patients infected with HIV in the era of highly active antiretroviral therapy: a case series. Clin Infect Dis 2004;39(8):1214–22.

89. George SL, Swindells S, Knudson R, et al. Unexplained thrombosis in HIV-infected patients receiving protease inhibitors: report of seven cases. Am J Med 1999;107(6):624–30.

90. Aberg JA, Kaplan JE, Libman H, et al. Primary care guidelines for the management of persons infected with human immunodeficiency virus: 2009 update by the HIV medicine Association of the Infectious Diseases Society of America. Clin Infect Dis 2009;49(5):651–81.

91. Gritz ER, Vidrine DJ, Lazev AB, et al. Smoking behavior in a low-income multiethnic HIV/AIDS population. Nicotine Tob Res 2004;6(1):71–7.

92. Marshall MM, Kirk GD, Caporaso NE, et al. Tobacco use and nicotine dependence among HIV-infected and uninfected injection drug users. Addict Behav 2011;36(1–2):61–7.

93. Crothers K, Griffith TA, McGinnis KA, et al. The impact of cigarette smoking on mortality, quality of life, and comorbid illness among HIV-positive veterans. J Gen Intern Med 2005;20(12):1142–5.

94. Burkhalter JE, Springer CM, Chhabra R, et al. Tobacco use and readiness to quit smoking in low-income HIV-infected persons. Nicotine Tob Res 2005;7(4):511–22.

95. Burns DN, Kramer A, Yellin F, et al. Cigarette smoking: a modifier of human immunodeficiency virus type 1 infection? J Acquir Immune Defic Syndr 1991;4(1):76–83.

96. Conley LJ, Bush TJ, Buchbinder SP, et al. The association between cigarette smoking and selected HIV-related medical conditions. AIDS 1996;10(10):1121–6.

97. Aberle DR, Adams AM, Berg CD, et al. Reduced lung-cancer mortality with low-dose computed tomographic screening. N Engl J Med 2011; 365(5):395–409.

98. Gold JA, Rom WN, Harkin TJ. Significance of abnormal chest radiograph findings in patients with HIV-1 infection without respiratory symptoms. Chest 2002;121(5):1472–7.

99. Lichtenberger JP, Sharma A, Zachary KC, et al. What a differential a virus makes: a practical approach to thoracic imaging findings in the context of HIV infection—part 2, extrapulmonary findings, chronic lung disease, and immune reconstitution syndrome. Am J Roentgenol 2012;198(6):1305–12.

100. Parker MS, Leveno DM, Campbell TJ, et al. AIDS-related bronchogenic carcinoma: fact or fiction? Chest 1998;113(1):154–61.

101. Grulich AE, Wan X, Law MG, et al. Risk of cancer in people with AIDS. AIDS 1999;13(7):839–43.

102. Cooksley CD, Hwang LY, Waller DK, et al. HIV-related malignancies: community-based study using linkage of cancer registry and HIV registry data. Int J STD AIDS 1999;10(12):795–802.

103. Grulich AE, Li Y, McDonald A, et al. Rates of non-AIDS-defining cancers in people with HIV infection before and after AIDS diagnosis. AIDS 2002;16(8): 1155–61.

104. Allardice GM, Hole DJ, Brewster DH, et al. Incidence of malignant neoplasms among HIV-infected persons in Scotland. Br J Cancer 2003; 89(3):505–7.

105. Dal Maso L, Franceschi S, Polesel J, et al. Risk of cancer in persons with AIDS in Italy, 1985-1998. Br J Cancer 2003;89(1):94–100.

106. Newnham A, Harris J, Evans HS, et al. The risk of cancer in HIV-infected people in southeast England: a cohort study. Br J Cancer 2005;92(1): 194–200.

107. Mbulaiteye SM, Katabira ET, Wabinga H, et al. Spectrum of cancers among HIV-infected persons in Africa: the Uganda AIDS-Cancer Registry Match Study. Int J Cancer 2006;118(4):985–90.

108. Galceran J, Marcos-Gragera R, Soler M, et al. Cancer incidence in AIDS patients in Catalonia, Spain. Eur J Cancer 2007;43(6):1085–91.

109. Dal Maso L, Polesel J, Serraino D, et al. Pattern of cancer risk in persons with AIDS in Italy in the HAART era. Br J Cancer 2009;100(5):840–7.

110. Polesel J, Franceschi S, Suligoi B, et al. Cancer incidence in people with AIDS in Italy. Int J Cancer 2010;127(6):1437–45.

111. Serraino D, Boschini A, Carrieri P, et al. Cancer risk among men with, or at risk of, HIV infection in southern Europe. AIDS 2000;14(5):553–9.

112. Phelps RM, Smith DK, Heilig CM, et al. Cancer incidence in women with or at risk for HIV. Int J Cancer 2001;94(5):753–7.

113. Herida M, Mary-Krause M, Kaphan R, et al. Incidence of non-AIDS-defining cancers before and during the highly active antiretroviral therapy era in a cohort of human immunodeficiency virus-infected patients. J Clin Oncol 2003;21(18): 3447–53.

114. Clifford GM, Polesel J, Rickenbach M, et al. Cancer risk in the Swiss HIV Cohort Study: associations with immunodeficiency, smoking, and highly active antiretroviral therapy. J Natl Cancer Inst 2005; 97(6):425–32.

115. Serraino D, Piselli P, Busnach G, et al. Risk of cancer following immunosuppression in organ transplant recipients and in HIV-positive individuals in southern Europe. Eur J Cancer 2007;43(14):2117–23.

116. Patel P, Hanson DL, Sullivan PS, et al. Incidence of types of cancer among HIV-infected persons compared with the general population in the United States, 1992-2003. Ann Intern Med 2008;148(10): 728–36.

117. Levine AM, Seaberg EC, Hessol NA, et al. HIV as a risk factor for lung cancer in women: data from the Women's Interagency HIV Study. J Clin Oncol 2010;28(9):1514–9.

Human Immunodeficiency Virus–Associated Obstructive Lung Diseases

Matthew R. Gingo, MD, MS[a], Alison Morris, MD, MS[a],
Kristina Crothers, MD[b],*

KEYWORDS

- Chronic obstructive pulmonary disease • Emphysema • Asthma • HIV • AIDS
- Smoking-related lung disease

KEY POINTS

- Obstructive lung disease is common among persons infected by human immunodeficiency virus (HIV), and HIV infection appears to be an independent risk factor for the diagnosis of chronic obstructive pulmonary disease (COPD).
- Early and progressive emphysema and COPD likely contribute to significant morbidity in HIV-infected persons.
- In addition to smoking, other likely contributors to the pathogenesis of COPD in HIV infection include microbial colonization, elevated HIV viral levels, and possible immune reconstitution with antiretrovirals.
- Asthma is a phenotype of obstructive lung disease that is commonly diagnosed in HIV-infected persons, and may have unique mechanisms related to metabolic disease in HIV and inflammation related to chronic HIV infection.
- Smoking cessation, monitoring for infectious complications of inhaled corticosteroids, and pulmonary rehabilitation are aspects of the treatment of obstructive lung disease that are important considerations in HIV-infected persons.

INTRODUCTION

Obstructive lung disease includes the most common lung conditions in the general population, asthma and chronic obstructive pulmonary disease (COPD). Although they are described as two separate disorders, there is much overlap in their pathology, physiology, and clinical manifestations.[1] Both conditions are becoming more common in the developing world: asthma likely from multiple factors,[2,3] and COPD from smoking.[4] Obstructive lung disease is increasingly recognized as a common comorbidity in individuals infected by human immunodeficiency virus (HIV). Beyond the typical risk factors, HIV infection may itself be an independent risk factor for obstructive lung disease.

This article reviews the evidence for HIV infection as a risk factor for obstructive lung diseases, namely COPD and asthma. Studies identifying

Funding: National Institutes of Health/National Heart, Lung, and Blood Institute K23 HL108697 (M.R.G.); R01 HL083461, R01 HL 090339, and HL083461S (A.M.); R01 HL 090342 (K.C.).
a Division of Pulmonary, Allergy, and Critical Care Medicine, Department of Medicine, University of Pittsburgh School of Medicine, 628 NW MUH, 3459 Fifth Avenue, Pittsburgh, PA 15213, USA; b Division of Pulmonary and Critical Care Medicine, Department of Medicine, Harborview Medical Center, University of Washington School of Medicine, 325 Ninth Avenue, Box 359762, Seattle, WA 98104, USA
* Corresponding author.
E-mail address: kcrothers@medicine.washington.edu

Clin Chest Med 34 (2013) 273–282
http://dx.doi.org/10.1016/j.ccm.2013.02.002
0272-5231/13/$ – see front matter © 2013 Elsevier Inc. All rights reserved.

chestmed.theclinics.com

potential mechanisms leading to airways disease (airflow obstruction and airway hyperreactivity) are discussed. Finally, the treatment of HIV-related obstructive lung disease is considered.

INCREASED RISK OF COPD/EMPHYSEMA

The Global Initiative on Obstructive Lung Disease (GOLD) group defines COPD as "persistent airflow limitation that is usually progressive" and "associated with an enhanced chronic inflammatory response in the airways and the lung."[5] COPD results from emphysema, inflammation of small airways, bronchoconstriction, excess mucus in the airways, or a combination of these factors. Fixed airflow obstruction is required to diagnose COPD, and is defined by GOLD criteria as a ratio of the forced expiratory volume in 1 second (FEV$_1$) over the forced vital capacity (FVC) of less than 70%. COPD can also be diagnosed based on a ratio of the FEV$_1$/FVC that is below the lower limit of normal (less than the fifth percentile). Impaired diffusing capacity of the lung for carbon monoxide (DLco) can be a manifestation of significant emphysema.[6,7]

Cigarette smoking is the major risk factor for development of COPD. However, as not all smokers develop COPD, other factors appear to be involved,[8] including genetic factors such as α1-antitrypsin deficiency, and factors such as race and gender. Occupational and environmental factors can also play a significant role.[9–12] HIV-infected individuals may represent another population with an increased susceptibility to COPD.

Before the advent of effective antiretroviral therapy (ART), abnormalities of pulmonary function associated with HIV were first noted by the Pulmonary Complications of HIV Infection Study (PCHIS). In a longitudinal evaluation of pulmonary function in 1300 participants, HIV-infected persons had more dyspnea in comparison with HIV-uninfected persons, and injection drug users (IDU) reported more cough and sputum production.[13] Lower diffusing capacity for carbon monoxide (DLco) was more common in those with respiratory symptoms, smokers, and IDU, and HIV-infected persons had a lower DLco percent predicted. These findings need to be interpreted with caution because the prevalence of African Americans was different in the groups, and the DLco prediction equations did not account for race. Also, DLco tended to be lower in those persons with CD4$^+$ cell counts less than 200 cells/μL.

Early in the HIV epidemic, it was thought DLco impairment was primarily due to HIV-related inflammation or infection, and that DLco was worse with more severe HIV disease.[14–17] However, data from Diaz and colleagues[18] demonstrated that emphysema was an important determinant of a decreased DLco. HIV-infected smokers without a history of pulmonary infections had emphysema by either pulmonary function testing (PFT) or computed tomography (CT) scans,[19] and emphysema also occurred in HIV-infected persons who were nonsmokers. Twenty-three percent of HIV-infected smokers without a history of pulmonary infections had emphysema by either PFT or CT scan compared with only 2% of HIV-uninfected controls matched for age and smoking, and 37% of HIV-infected persons with a smoking history of more than 12 pack-years had emphysema compared with none of the HIV-uninfected controls. Diaz and colleagues[18] reported a series of 4 HIV-infected nonsmokers who had air-trapping, decreased DLco, and emphysema on CT scan. These observations suggest that before ART became available, HIV was a risk factor for COPD or interacted with other risk factor(s) in the development of COPD, particularly of the emphysema subtype.[18]

Since the advent of effective combination ART, several studies have sought to determine the prevalence and risk factors for COPD, and for abnormal pulmonary function associated with HIV infection. Two studies from the Veterans Aging Cohort Study (VACS) suggest that HIV infection is an independent risk factor for COPD.[20,21] The first assessed 1014 HIV-infected and 713 HIV-uninfected men enrolled at 5 VACS sites for diagnoses of COPD determined by International Classification of Diseases (ICD)-9 diagnostic codes and patient self-report on questionnaire. Unadjusted prevalence of COPD in HIV-infected versus HIV-uninfected subjects by ICD-9 codes was 10% versus 9% ($P = .4$) and by participant self-report 15% versus 12% ($P = .04$). After adjusting for differences in age, smoking, race/ethnicity, and other potential confounders such as IDU and alcohol abuse, HIV-infected subjects were approximately 50% to 60% more likely to have COPD than HIV-uninfected subjects by either ICD-9 codes or patient self-report. The second VACS study tracked the incidence of lung disease by ICD-9 diagnosis in 33,420 HIV-infected veterans and 66,840 HIV-uninfected veterans matched by age, sex, race and ethnicity, and site.[21] The incidence of new COPD diagnosis was 20.3 per 1000 person-years, and incident COPD was 8% greater in HIV-infected persons 50 years and older and 17% greater in HIV-infected persons younger than 50 years, compared with HIV-uninfected persons controlling for age, race and ethnicity, sex, alcohol disorders, drug abuse, and hepatitis C infection. In a subgroup with data to control for smoking history, HIV-infected participants had an even greater incidence rate compared with HIV-uninfected persons: 11% greater in persons 50 years and older and 25% greater in persons younger than 50 years. The difference in rates between HIV-infected and uninfected persons was greater at younger ages, suggesting a potential earlier onset of lung disease in HIV-infected persons; a competing risk for mortality could also account for a lower relative difference in older HIV-infected compared with uninfected individuals.

Pulmonary function has recently been measured in several cohorts that include HIV-infected persons (**Table 1**).[22–28] In HIV-infected persons, airflow obstruction is common, possibly more common than would be expected. Spirometry from 234 HIV-infected individuals found 8.6% had an FEV_1/FVC below the 5% lower limit of age, race, and gender predicted normal,[22] and lower FEV_1/FVC was associated with older age, smoking, history of bacterial pneumonia, and ART use. In a separate cohort of 167 HIV-infected outpatients, an FEV_1/FVC of less than 0.7 was found in 21.0%, and airflow obstruction was associated with smoking, IDU, and ART use.[23] Another cohort of 98 individuals had a 16.3% prevalence of obstructive lung disease (FEV_1/FVC <0.70 and FEV_1 <80% predicted), which was associated with age, smoking, intravenous drug use, and history of *Pneumocystis* pneumonia.[25] Compared with data from the National Health and Nutrition Evaluation Survey III, this HIV cohort appeared to have greater prevalence of obstructive lung disease even with a similar prevalence of smoking. In a cohort of intravenous drug abusers, airflow obstruction (FEV_1/FVC <0.70) was present in 16.8% of HIV-infected participants,[26] and HIV-infected participants with a viral load greater than 200,000 copies/mL were approximately 3.4 times more likely than HIV-uninfected participants to have obstructive lung disease. HIV-infected participants with controlled viral loads had rates of obstruction similar to those of HIV-uninfected participants.

Diffusion impairment (a common manifestation of emphysema) remains a frequent abnormality in the current HIV era. In one recent study, 64% of HIV-infected individuals had a DL_{CO} of less than 80% predicted,[23] and in another, 43% had a DL_{CO} less than 1.645 residual standard deviations below predicted values.[27] Diffusion impairment, worse in smokers, is also common in never smokers. In these 2 studies, 48% and 9% of never smokers, respectively, had impaired diffusing capacity. Reduced diffusing capacity was also associated with use of pneumonia prophylaxis.[23] In longitudinal follow-up, DL_{CO}

declined significantly and to a greater degree than other lung function parameters.[27] In addition, a comparison of lung function between 229 HIV-infected and 213 HIV-uninfected participants from the Multicenter AIDS Cohort and VACS studies found that HIV infection was independently associated with impaired diffusing capacity.[29]

The decrease in DL_{CO} likely has significant clinical relevance. In the authors' experience, lower DL_{CO} is a significant predictor of mortality.[30] In a cohort of 237 HIV-infected participants followed for 3 years on average, individuals who died had a significantly lower DL_{CO} (51.3% predicted vs 66.0% predicted, $P = .004$). The odds of death if the DL_{CO} was below 60% predicted were significantly greater independent of age, smoking history, ART use, and CD4 cell count (adjusted odds ratio 6.31, 95% confidence interval 1.21–32.9, $P = .029$). These findings suggest that lung diseases in HIV-infected individuals are an important health concern and either directly contribute to mortality or are a marker of an underlying systemic process.

MECHANISTIC FACTORS ASSOCIATED WITH COPD

In addition to smoking, HIV-related factors appear to contribute to COPD/emphysema as the disease appears to be accelerated in HIV-infected smokers and is also seen in nonsmokers. Poorly controlled HIV has been associated with worse pulmonary function[21,26] and a greater decline in lung function.[28] In the VACS study, lung diseases such as asthma and COPD were less likely in those with lower HIV RNA levels and use of ART at baseline. The AIDS Linked to Intravenous Experience study directly measured pulmonary function and also found that individuals with HIV viral levels higher than 200,000 copies/mL had worse airway obstruction.[26] In a follow-up longitudinal study of this cohort, high viral loads (>75,000 copies/mL) or low CD4 counts (<100 cells/μL) were associated with a greater decline in FEV_1 and FVC over time.[28] These studies suggest that the pathogenesis of COPD in HIV is related to worse HIV control (either a direct viral effect or effects of HIV sequelae such as infections). However, 2 studies have found that use of ART is also associated with worse lung function.[22,23] Biological mechanisms to explain this paradox could be related to differences in timing of ART initiation between populations; those in whom ART is initiated at a lower CD4 cell count could experience worsening in lung function on ART, potentially from increases in autoimmunity or renewed immunologic response to low-level lung pathogens.[31,32]

Table 1
Studies of pulmonary function in HIV-infected individuals during the combination ART era

Authors,[Ref.] Year	Design and Population	Important Findings
George et al,[22] 2009	Cross-sectional analysis of spirometry data from 234 HIV-infected individuals recruited from an HIV clinic in Los Angeles, California	31% of participants had at least 1 respiratory symptom Prevalence of an FEV_1/FVC below the age-adjusted lower limit of normal was 8.6% and <0.7 was 6.8% Worse airflow obstruction was associated with older age, more pack-years of smoking, history of bacterial pneumonia, and use of ART
Gingo et al,[23] 2010	Cross-sectional analysis of pre- and post-bronchodilator spirometry and DLco data from 167 HIV-infected participants recruited from an HIV clinic at the University of Pittsburgh, Pennsylvania	47% of participants had at least 1 respiratory symptom; 21% had irreversible airflow obstruction (post-bronchodilator FEV_1/FVC <0.7) High prevalence of diffusing impairment (64% had a DLco <80% predicted), including never smokers (47%) Only 15% had pulmonary function testing in the past Airflow obstruction was associated with increased pack-years of smoking, intravenous drug use, and use of antiretroviral medication
Cui et al,[24] 2010	Cross-sectional analysis of spirometry from 119 HIV-infected participants from an HIV clinic	20% had abnormal spirometry 53% had at least 1 respiratory symptom FEV_1 was lower with more pack-years of smoking, nonwhite race, male sex, and restrictive lung disease Symptoms were more common with current smoking and antiretroviral use
Hirani et al,[25] 2011	Cross-sectional analysis of spirometry and St George's Respiratory Questionnaire data from 98 consecutive HIV-infected patients seen for routine care at Thomas Jefferson University in Philadelphia, Pennsylvania	16% had obstructive lung disease (FEV_1/FVC <0.7 and FEV_1 <80% predicted). SGRQ mean was 7, 17 in smokers, and 28 in those with airflow obstruction Airflow obstruction associated with greater age, smoking, and history of PCP Cohort was compared with the NHANES III dataset, which had similar rates of smoking; HIV cohort was found to have greater prevalence of COPD
Drummond et al,[26] 2012	Spirometry obtained in 1077 participants from the AIDS Linked to Intravenous Experience study cohort in Baltimore, Maryland	16.8% of HIV-infected participants had airflow obstruction (FEV_1/FVC <0.7) Higher viral loads (>200,000 copies/mL) were associated with airflow obstruction No association between HIV status or CD4 counts and airflow obstruction
Kristoffersen et al,[27] 2012	Prospective cohort of 88 HIV-infected participants, with repeat spirometry in 63 participants with a mean follow-up of 4.4 y; Denmark	10% prevalence of airflow obstruction (FEV_1/FVC <0.7) at baseline that increased to 19% at follow-up 4.4 y later Reduced DLco (below the 90% CI of predicted) was common at baseline (40%) and remained constant over 4.4 y

(continued on next page)

Table 1
(continued)

Authors,[Ref.] Year	Design and Population	Important Findings
Drummond et al,[28] 2013	Serial spirometry on 1064 participants in AIDS Linked to Intravenous Experience	HIV-infected persons with a viral load >75,000 copies/mL or a CD4 count <100 cells/μL had significantly greater decline in FEV_1 and FVC over time No significant difference in FEV_1/FVC by HIV status HIV-infected participants with controlled disease had no difference in lung-function change compared with HIV-uninfected participants

Abbreviations: ART, antiretroviral therapy; CI, confidence interval; COPD, chronic obstructive pulmonary disease; DL_{CO}, diffusing capacity of the lung; FEV_1, forced expiratory volume in 1 second; FVC, forced vital capacity; HIV, human immunodeficiency virus; NHANES, National Health and Nutrition Evaluation Survey; PCP, *Pneumocystis* pneumonia; SGRQ, St George's Respiratory Questionnaire.

Microbial colonization may play a role in the pathogenesis of COPD in HIV. Several studies have implicated colonization with *Pneumocystis jirovecii*, a common HIV-associated infection, in the pathogenesis of obstructive lung disease in HIV. In a cohort of 42 HIV-infected individuals, those with *P jirovecii*, detectable only by nested polymerase chain reaction of the mitochondrial large subunit rRNA in oral washes or induced sputum, had worse airflow and more obstructive lung disease by pulmonary function studies.[33] In macaque models of HIV infection, monkeys that become colonized with *Pneumocystis* (detection of *Pneumocystis* DNA in lung or airway samples) develop worse airflow obstruction and emphysema.[34,35] A non-immunosuppressed rodent model has also shown development of COPD-like changes in mice exposed to both cigarette smoke and *Pneumocystis*.[36] HIV infection is associated with a greater probability of colonization with *Pneumocystis*, which may explain in part the increased prevalence of obstructive lung disease in HIV-infected persons.[37] Several studies have identified the lung microbiome community as unique in HIV-infected persons.[38–40] One study found an increase in *Tropheryma whipplei* in HIV-infected persons, but a relationship between *T whipplei* and lung function is not known.[41]

ASTHMA IN HIV INFECTION

Asthma is characterized by airway inflammation and inducible or reversible airway obstruction (airway hyperreactivity). Asthma is associated with morbidity related to episodes of dyspnea and functional impairment, and increased mortality in some populations.[2,42] Before the advent of ART,

not all studies showed a significant association, but HIV-infected persons were more likely to have airway hyperreactivity.[43,44] Airway hyperreactivity in the pre-ART era was associated with smoking and atopy. Data are limited in the ART era regarding the association between HIV and asthma. In the VACS cohort, which was predominantly older male smokers, asthma diagnosis was not more common in HIV-infected individuals.[21] However, 2 studies in children have shown that asthma symptoms and inhaler use are more common in HIV-infected children in the ART era and in those children taking ART medications.[45–47]

Self-reported asthma diagnosis is commonly used in epidemiologic studies. Two recent studies found that 11% and 21% of HIV-infected persons had an asthma diagnosis by history (doctor-diagnosed asthma),[24,48] in contrast to a prevalence of approximately 9% in the general population.[49,50] There was also a 4% and 9% prevalence, respectively, of bronchodilator reversibility by American Thoracic Society/European Respiratory Society criteria with PFT in these studies, which is potentially higher than is expected in the general population.[50] In the general population, most adults with asthma are diagnosed in childhood.[51] By contrast, 55% of the HIV-infected individuals reported onset of asthma as an adult, often after diagnosis of HIV.[48]

Asthma in HIV infection is common, and there may be distinct phenotypes of asthma associated with HIV. Airway inflammation in HIV could have unique mechanisms related to allergy/atopy, metabolic disease, and chronic inflammation, possibly stimulated by underlying infections.[50] In the study by Gingo and colleagues,[48] doctor-diagnosed asthma was associated with female sex, being obese, not being on ART, and a history of bacterial or *Pneumocystis* pneumonia, and there was a strong association between doctor-diagnosed asthma and high sputum eosinophil counts. In addition, approximately 10% of the cohort had high sputum eosinophil counts, suggesting an increase in T-helper 2 type inflammation in the airways of HIV-infected persons. Doctor-diagnosed asthma and bronchodilator reversibility were also associated with cytokines that can be elevated in chronic HIV infection, namely RANTES and macrophage inflammatory proteins 1α and 1β.[52]

TREATMENT CONSIDERATIONS FOR OBSTRUCTIVE LUNG DISEASE IN HIV

Although there are a few studies of smoking cessation therapy in HIV-infected persons, there are no studies of therapy specific to obstructive lung disease in HIV. In the absence of other data, the general treatment guidelines from various respiratory societies should be followed as for other patient populations. However, several factors are important to keep in mind when approaching HIV-infected patients with obstructive lung disease. The first is the high prevalence of smoking and the significant impact that smoking has on mortality in the HIV population. Rates of current smoking are nearly 2-fold higher in most HIV-infected than in HIV-uninfected populations.[53] However, health care providers of HIV-infected patients may be less aware of current smoking and less confident in their ability to counsel their patients regarding smoking cessation.[54] Current smoking is associated with increased respiratory symptoms, COPD, bacterial pneumonia, and decreased quality of life among HIV-infected patients.[55] In addition, the population-attributable

risk of death associated with smoking is twice as high in HIV-infected individuals than in HIV-uninfected persons, and HIV-infected smokers lose more life years to smoking than to HIV infection.[56] These findings highlight the need to increase efforts at smoking cessation among patients with HIV. Smoking-cessation interventions can be effectively applied in HIV-infected populations, and are reviewed in detail in the article by Browning and colleagues elsewhere in this issue.[57–60]

Respiratory medications commonly recommended for obstructive lung diseases warrant careful consideration in HIV-infected populations. Inhaled corticosteroids (ICS), in particular, may pose increased risk of complications in HIV-infected individuals. ICS are associated with oral candidiasis, bacterial pneumonia,[61] and tuberculosis in the HIV-uninfected population.[62] These complications of ICS could be augmented by HIV infection, particularly as bacterial pneumonia continues to be a major comorbidity in HIV, even with ART and relatively controlled CD4 counts.[63,64] In addition, there are certain ICS (fluticasone in particular) whose metabolism is slowed by the presence of certain antiretroviral medications (ritonavir). This interaction leads to increased levels of systemic steroids, and side effects of chronic steroid therapy such as osteoporosis and Cushing disease.[65–67] Further studies are needed to assess the safety and/or effectiveness of ICS in this population.

Pulmonary rehabilitation programs may be of increased importance in HIV patients with COPD. Obstructive lung disease (COPD and/or asthma) was independently associated with self-reported increased physical disability among HIV-infected veterans,[68] and the combination of HIV infection and COPD had a significant impact on physical functioning.[69] Pulmonary rehabilitation

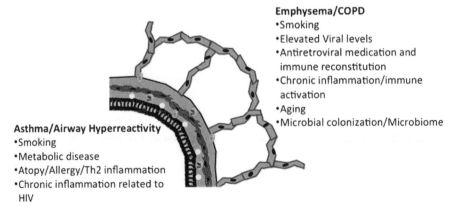

Emphysema/COPD
• Smoking
• Elevated Viral levels
• Antiretroviral medication and
  immune reconstitution
• Chronic inflammation/immune
  activation
• Aging
• Microbial colonization/Microbiome

Asthma/Airway Hyperreactivity
• Smoking
• Metabolic disease
• Atopy/Allergy/Th2 inflammation
• Chronic inflammation related to
  HIV

Fig. 1. Mechanisms related to obstructive lung disease in human immunodeficiency virus (HIV)-infected persons grouped by association with chronic obstructive pulmonary disease (COPD)/emphysema and association with asthma/airway hyperreactivity.

significantly improves physical functioning in HIV-uninfected patients with COPD.[70] HIV may exaggerate the systemic and skeletal manifestations associated with decrements in physical capacity encountered in HIV-uninfected COPD. There are skeletal muscle dysfunctions and mitochondrial abnormalities related to HIV infection and its treatment.[71] Peak aerobic capacity was decreased by 41% in HIV-infected patients,[72] and respiratory muscle function was decreased in otherwise healthy HIV-infected patients in comparison with HIV-uninfected patients.[73] In HIV-infected patients, exercise training is safe and has potential benefits,[74,75] but studies to determine the role and optimal type of exercise training in HIV-infected patients, particularly those with COPD, are needed.

SUMMARY

HIV-infected individuals appear to have an increased risk for obstructive lung diseases, although whether this represents increased emphysema, chronic bronchitis, asthma, or a combination of these disorders has not been fully evaluated. Although part of the increased risk of obstructive lung disease, particularly COPD, may be related to smoking and drug abuse, the apparent risk for COPD remains elevated in HIV-infected persons even after controlling for these and other potential confounders.[19–21] Recent studies of pulmonary function in HIV-infected persons have elucidated some factors that may be important in the pathogenesis of obstructive lung disease in HIV: poor HIV control contributing to COPD and decline in lung function, and metabolic disease and inflammation associated with asthma and airway hyperreactivity (**Fig. 1**). Further possible mechanisms are currently being elucidated, such as chronic immune activation and immune senescence leading to early aging in HIV patients, as described in the article by Fitzpatrick and colleagues elsewhere in this issue.

Given the increasing age of HIV-infected individuals and the high prevalence of smoking, health care providers are likely to encounter a substantial number of HIV-infected patients with obstructive lung diseases. Undiagnosed airway obstruction is associated with impaired health and functional status, thus making identification of COPD and asthma important.[76] Studies are needed to determine whether the pharmacologic and nonpharmacologic management strategies for obstructive lung diseases should differ among HIV-infected and HIV-uninfected patients. A better understanding of treatments to appropriately manage obstructive lung disease in HIV-infected patients is essential to optimize health benefits such as decreased symptoms and exacerbations of disease, to improve exercise capacity and quality of life, and to increase smoking cessation.[77,78]

REFERENCES

1. Gibson PG, Simpson JL. The overlap syndrome of asthma and COPD: what are its features and how important is it? Thorax 2009;64(8):728–35.
2. Akinbami LJ, Moorman JE, Bailey C, et al. Trends in asthma prevalence, health care use, and mortality in the United States, 2001-2010. NCHS Data Brief 2012;(94):1–8.
3. Kazani S, Israel E. Update in asthma 2011. Am J Respir Crit Care Med 2012;186(1):35–40.
4. Thun MJ, Carter BD, Feskanich D, et al. 50-year trends in smoking-related mortality in the United States. N Engl J Med 2013;368(4):351–64.
5. Vestbo J, Hurd SS, Agusti AG, et al. Global strategy for the diagnosis, management and prevention of chronic obstructive pulmonary disease, GOLD executive summary. Am J Respir Crit Care Med 2013;187(4):347–65.
6. Haraguchi M, Shimura S, Hida W, et al. Pulmonary function and regional distribution of emphysema as determined by high-resolution computed tomography. Respiration 1998;65(2):125–9.
7. Park KJ, Bergin CJ, Clausen JL. Quantitation of emphysema with three-dimensional CT densitometry: comparison with two-dimensional analysis, visual emphysema scores, and pulmonary function test results. Radiology 1999;211(2):541–7.
8. Mannino DM. COPD: epidemiology, prevalence, morbidity and mortality, and disease heterogeneity. Chest 2002;121(Suppl 5):121S–6S.
9. Sandford AJ, Silverman EK. Chronic obstructive pulmonary disease. 1: susceptibility factors for COPD the genotype-environment interaction. Thorax 2002;57(8):736–41.
10. Chapman KR. Chronic obstructive pulmonary disease: are women more susceptible than men? Clin Chest Med 2004;25(2):331–41.
11. Silverman EK, Weiss ST, Drazen JM, et al. Gender-related differences in severe, early-onset chronic obstructive pulmonary disease. Am J Respir Crit Care Med 2000;162(6):2152–8.
12. Petty TL, Weinmann GG. Building a national strategy for the prevention and management of and research in chronic obstructive pulmonary disease. National Heart, Lung, and Blood Institute Workshop Summary. Bethesda, Maryland, August 29-31, 1995. JAMA 1997;277(3):246–53.
13. Rosen MJ, Lou Y, Kvale PA, et al. Pulmonary function tests in HIV-infected patients without AIDS. Pulmonary Complications of HIV Infection Study Group. Am J Respir Crit Care Med 1995;152(2):738–45.

14. Diaz PT, King MA, Pacht ER, et al. The pathophysiology of pulmonary diffusion impairment in human immunodeficiency virus infection. Am J Respir Crit Care Med 1999;160(1):272–7.

15. Mitchell DM, Fleming J, Pinching AJ, et al. Pulmonary function in human immunodeficiency virus infection. A prospective 18-month study of serial lung function in 474 patients. Am Rev Respir Dis 1992;146(3):745–51.

16. Nieman RB, Fleming J, Coker RJ, et al. Reduced carbon monoxide transfer factor (TLCO) in human immunodeficiency virus type I (HIV-I) infection as a predictor for faster progression to AIDS. Thorax 1993;48(5):481–5.

17. Shaw RJ, Roussak C, Forster SM, et al. Lung function abnormalities in patients infected with the human immunodeficiency virus with and without overt pneumonitis. Thorax 1988;43(6):436–40.

18. Diaz PT, Clanton TL, Pacht ER. Emphysema-like pulmonary disease associated with human immunodeficiency virus infection. Ann Intern Med 1992;116(2):124–8.

19. Diaz PT, King MA, Pacht ER, et al. Increased susceptibility to pulmonary emphysema among HIV-seropositive smokers. Ann Intern Med 2000;132(5):369–72.

20. Crothers K, Butt AA, Gibert CL, et al. Increased COPD among HIV-positive compared to HIV-negative veterans. Chest 2006;130(5):1326–33.

21. Crothers K, Huang L, Goulet JL, et al. HIV infection and risk for incident pulmonary diseases in the combination antiretroviral therapy era. Am J Respir Crit Care Med 2011;183(3):388–95.

22. George MP, Kannass M, Huang L, et al. Respiratory symptoms and airway obstruction in HIV-infected subjects in the HAART era. PLoS One 2009;4(7):e6328.

23. Gingo MR, George MP, Kessinger CJ, et al. Pulmonary function abnormalities in HIV-infected patients during the current antiretroviral therapy era. Am J Respir Crit Care Med 2010;182(6):790–6.

24. Cui Q, Carruthers S, McIvor A, et al. Effect of smoking on lung function, respiratory symptoms and respiratory diseases amongst HIV-positive subjects: a cross-sectional study. AIDS Res Ther 2010;7:6.

25. Hirani A, Cavallazzi R, Vasu T, et al. Prevalence of obstructive lung disease in HIV population: a cross sectional study. Respir Med 2011;105(11):1655–61.

26. Drummond MB, Kirk GD, Astemborski J, et al. Association between obstructive lung disease and markers of HIV infection in a high-risk cohort. Thorax 2012;67(4):309–14.

27. Kristoffersen US, Lebech AM, Mortensen J, et al. Changes in lung function of HIV-infected patients: a 4.5-year follow-up study. Clin Physiol Funct Imaging 2012;32(4):288–95.

28. Drummond MB, Merlo CA, Astemborski J, et al. The effect of HIV infection on longitudinal lung function decline among injection drug users: a prospective cohort. AIDS 2013. [Epub ahead of print].

29. Crothers K, Kleerup EC, Wongtrakool C, et al. HIV infection is associated with impaired pulmonary diffusing capacity. CROI 2012. Seattle, Mar 7, 2012 (Meeting Abstracts).

30. Gingo MR, Morris A. Pathogenesis of HIV and the lung. Curr HIV/AIDS Rep 2013;10(1):42–50.

31. Crothers K, Huang L. Pulmonary complications of immune reconstitution inflammatory syndromes in HIV-infected patients. Respirology 2009;14(4):486–94.

32. Mori S, Levin P. A brief review of potential mechanisms of immune reconstitution inflammatory syndrome in HIV following antiretroviral therapy. Int J STD AIDS 2009;20(7):447–52.

33. Morris A, Alexander T, Radhi S, et al. Airway obstruction is increased in pneumocystis-colonized human immunodeficiency virus-infected outpatients. J Clin Microbiol 2009;47(11):3773–6.

34. Kling HM, Shipley TW, Patil SP, et al. Relationship of Pneumocystis jirovecii humoral immunity to prevention of colonization and chronic obstructive pulmonary disease in a primate model of HIV infection. Infect Immun 2010;78(10):4320–30.

35. Shipley TW, Kling HM, Morris A, et al. Persistent Pneumocystis colonization leads to the development of chronic obstructive pulmonary disease in a nonhuman primate model of AIDS. J Infect Dis 2010;202(2):302–12.

36. Christensen PJ, Preston AM, Ling T, et al. Pneumocystis murina infection and cigarette smoke exposure interact to cause increased organism burden, development of airspace enlargement, and pulmonary inflammation in mice. Infect Immun 2008;76(8):3481–90.

37. Morris A, George MP, Crothers K, et al. HIV and chronic obstructive pulmonary disease: is it worse and why? Proc Am Thorac Soc 2011;8(3):320–5.

38. Ireland AW, Ghedin E, Pop M, et al. Comparison of the respiratory microbiome in HIV-infected and HIV-uninfected individuals. Am J Respir Crit Care Med 2012;185(Meeting Abstracts):A4045.

39. Twigg HL, Nelson D, Dong Q, et al. Analysis of the respiratory microbiome using bronchoalveolar lavage from HIV-infected and uninfected subjects. Am J Respir Crit Care Med 2010;181(Meeting Abstracts):A5629.

40. Twigg HL, Nelson D, Dong Q, et al. Analysis of the respiratory microbiome using bronchoalveolar lavage from HIV-infected and uninfected subjects. Am J Respir Crit Care Med 2011;183(Meeting Abstracts):A6257.

41. Lozupone C, Cota-Gomez A, Palmer BE, et al. Widespread colonization of the lung by tropheryma whipplei in HIV infection. Am J Respir Crit Care Med 2013. [Epub ahead of print].

42. Pac A, Tobiasz-Adamczyk B, Brzyska M, et al. The role of different predictors in 20-year mortality among Krakow older citizens. Arch Gerontol Geriatr 2013;56(3):524–30.

43. Poirier CD, Inhaber N, Lalonde RG, et al. Prevalence of bronchial hyperresponsiveness among HIV-infected men. Am J Respir Crit Care Med 2001; 164(4):542–5.

44. Wallace JM, Stone GS, Browdy BL, et al. Nonspecific airway hyperresponsiveness in HIV disease. Pulmonary Complications of HIV Infection Study Group. Chest 1997;111(1):121–7.

45. Foster SB, Paul ME, Kozinetz CA, et al. Prevalence of asthma in children and young adults with HIV infection. J Allergy Clin Immunol 2007;119(3):750–2.

46. Foster SB, McIntosh K, Thompson B, et al. Increased incidence of asthma in HIV-infected children treated with highly active antiretroviral therapy in the National Institutes of Health Women and Infants Transmission Study. J Allergy Clin Immunol 2008;122(1):159–65.

47. Gutin F, Butt A, Alame W, et al. Asthma in immunecompetent children with human immunodeficiency virus. Ann Allergy Asthma Immunol 2009;102(5):438.

48. Gingo MR, Wenzel SE, Steele C, et al. Asthma diagnosis and airway bronchodilator response in HIV-infected patients. J Allergy Clin Immunol 2012; 129(3):708–714.e8.

49. Bridevaux PO, Probst-Hensch NM, Schindler C, et al. Prevalence of airflow obstruction in smokers and never-smokers in Switzerland. Eur Respir J 2010;36(6):1259–69.

50. Appleton SL, Adams RJ, Wilson DH, et al. Spirometric criteria for asthma: adding further evidence to the debate. J Allergy Clin Immunol 2005;116(5): 976–82.

51. Miranda C, Busacker A, Balzar S, et al. Distinguishing severe asthma phenotypes: role of age at onset and eosinophilic inflammation. J Allergy Clin Immunol 2004;113(1):101–8.

52. Cocchi F, DeVico AL, Garzino-Demo A, et al. Identification of RANTES, MIP-1 alpha, and MIP-1 beta as the major HIV-suppressive factors produced by CD8+ T cells. Science 1995;270(5243):1811–5.

53. Centers for Disease Control and Prevention (CDC). Cigarette smoking among adults—United States, 2004. MMWR Morb Mortal Wkly Rep 2005;54(44): 1121–4.

54. Crothers K, Goulet JL, Rodriguez-Barradas MC, et al. Decreased awareness of current smoking among health care providers of HIV-positive compared to HIV-negative veterans. J Gen Intern Med 2007;22(6):749–54.

55. Crothers K, Griffith TA, McGinnis KA, et al. The impact of cigarette smoking on mortality, quality of life, and comorbid illness among HIV-positive veterans. J Gen Intern Med 2005;20(12):1142–5.

56. Helleberg M, Afzal S, Kronborg G, et al. Mortality attributable to smoking among HIV-1-Infected Individuals: a nationwide, population-based cohort study. Clin Infect Dis 2013;56(5):727–34.

57. Cummins D, Trotter G, Moussa M, et al. Smoking cessation for clients who are HIV-positive. Nurs Stand 2005;20(12):41–7.

58. Vidrine DJ, Arduino RC, Lazev AB, et al. A randomized trial of a proactive cellular telephone intervention for smokers living with HIV/AIDS. AIDS 2006;20(2):253–60.

59. Wewers ME, Neidig JL, Kihm KE. The feasibility of a nurse-managed, peer-led tobacco cessation intervention among HIV-positive smokers. J Assoc Nurses AIDS Care 2000;11(6):37–44.

60. Ferketich AK, Diaz P, Browning KK, et al. Safety of varenicline among smokers enrolled in the Lung HIV Study. Nicotine Tob Res 2013;15(1):247–54.

61. Calverley PM, Anderson JA, Celli B, et al. Salmeterol and fluticasone propionate and survival in chronic obstructive pulmonary disease. N Engl J Med 2007;356(8):775–89.

62. Brassard P, Suissa S, Kezouh A, et al. Inhaled corticosteroids and risk of tuberculosis in patients with respiratory diseases. Am J Respir Crit Care Med 2011;183(5):675–8.

63. Hirschtick RE, Glassroth J, Jordan MC, et al. Bacterial pneumonia in persons infected with the human immunodeficiency virus. Pulmonary Complications of HIV Infection Study Group. N Engl J Med 1995; 333(13):845–51.

64. Segal LN, Methe BA, Nolan A, et al. HIV-1 and bacterial pneumonia in the era of antiretroviral therapy. Proc Am Thorac Soc 2011;8(3):282–7.

65. Foisy MM, Yakiwchuk EM, Chiu I, et al. Adrenal suppression and Cushing's syndrome secondary to an interaction between ritonavir and fluticasone: a review of the literature. HIV Med 2008;9(6):389–96.

66. Kaviani N, Bukberg P, Manessis A, et al. Iatrogenic osteoporosis, bilateral hip osteonecrosis, and secondary adrenal suppression in an HIV-infected patient receiving inhaled corticosteroids and ritonavir-boosted HAART. Endocr Pract 2011;17(1): 74–8.

67. Kedem E, Shahar E, Hassoun G, et al. Iatrogenic Cushing's syndrome due to coadministration of ritonavir and inhaled budesonide in an asthmatic human immunodeficiency virus infected patient. J Asthma 2010;47(7):830–1.

68. Oursler KK, Goulet JL, Leaf DA, et al. Association of comorbidity with physical disability in older HIV-infected adults. AIDS Patient Care STDS 2006; 20(11):782–91.

69. Oursler KK, Goulet JL, Crystal S, et al. Association of age and comorbidity with physical function in HIV-infected and uninfected patients: results from the Veterans Aging Cohort Study. AIDS Patient Care STDS 2011;25(1):13–20.

70. Nici L, Donner C, Wouters E, et al. American Thoracic Society/European Respiratory Society statement on pulmonary rehabilitation. Am J Respir Crit Care Med 2006;173(12):1390–413.

71. Authier FJ, Chariot P, Gherardi RK. Skeletal muscle involvement in human immunodeficiency virus (HIV)-infected patients in the era of highly active antiretroviral therapy (HAART). Muscle Nerve 2005; 32(3):247–60.

72. Oursler KK, Sorkin JD, Smith BA, et al. Reduced aerobic capacity and physical functioning in older HIV-infected men. AIDS Res Hum Retroviruses 2006;22(11):1113–21.

73. Schulz L, Nagaraja HN, Rague N, et al. Respiratory muscle dysfunction associated with human immunodeficiency virus infection. Am J Respir Crit Care Med 1997;155(3):1080–4.

74. Nixon S, O'Brien K, Glazier RH, et al. Aerobic exercise interventions for adults living with HIV/AIDS. Cochrane Database Syst Rev 2010;(8):CD001796.

75. O'Brien K, Nixon S, Glazier RH, et al. Progressive resistive exercise interventions for adults living with HIV/AIDS. Cochrane Database Syst Rev 2004;(4):CD004248.

76. Coultas DB, Mapel D, Gagnon R, et al. The health impact of undiagnosed airflow obstruction in a national sample of United States adults. Am J Respir Crit Care Med 2001;164(3):372–7.

77. Sin DD, McAlister FA, Man SF, et al. Contemporary management of chronic obstructive pulmonary disease: scientific review. JAMA 2003;290(17): 2301–12.

78. Tomas LH, Varkey B. Improving health-related quality of life in chronic obstructive pulmonary disease. Curr Opin Pulm Med 2004;10(2):120–7.

Human Immunodeficiency Virus–Associated Pulmonary Arterial Hypertension

Christopher F. Barnett, MD, MPH, Priscilla Y. Hsue, MD*

KEYWORDS

- Pulmonary arterial hypertension • HIV • AIDS • Antiretroviral therapy

KEY POINTS

- As patients with human immunodeficiency virus (HIV) infection worldwide survive longer, the prevalence of HIV-associated pulmonary arterial hypertension (HIV-PAH) is likely to increase.
- The development of PAH in HIV-infected individuals is associated with worse functional capacity and survival.
- The underlying mechanism leading to HIV-PAH remains unclear and is an area of active investigation.
- The optimal approach to therapy for individuals with HIV-PAH is uncertain, but should include aggressive management of HIV infection and careful use of PAH-specific therapies given possible significant drug interactions.

INTRODUCTION

Modern treatment with antiretroviral therapy (ART) has improved survival for patients with human immunodeficiency virus (HIV) infection. Cardiovascular disease and other non-AIDS conditions are increasingly becoming key health concerns as this patient population continues to age.[1–3] HIV-infected patients are more likely than the general population to develop cardiovascular disease, probably because of a combination of traditional risk factors, HIV-related inflammation, and effects of antiretroviral drugs.[4] Among the cardiovascular complications of HIV infection, HIV-associated pulmonary arterial hypertension (PAH) is especially severe and is associated with significant mortality.[5]

Pulmonary hypertension (PH) is a disease process associated with an increase in the mean pulmonary artery pressure (mPAP). PAH defines an increase in the mPAP specifically related to arteriopathy of the pulmonary vasculature. PAH can be idiopathic, familial, or secondary to a variety of conditions such as connective tissue disease, congenital systemic-to-pulmonary shunts, drugs and toxins, liver cirrhosis, or HIV infection.[6] PAH leads to a progressive increase in mPAP and pulmonary vascular resistance (PVR), and a decrease in cardiac output (CO). Pulmonary artery pressure may normalize or decrease as progressive right heart failure occurs and CO decreases, ultimately leading to exercise limitation and death.

HIV could represent a major cause of PAH (HIV-PAH). There are 34 million individuals worldwide with HIV infection.[7] Given that PAH occurs in 0.5% of patients with HIV, there may be as many as 200,000 patients with HIV infections affected by PAH worldwide.[8] If the natural history of PAH is as ominous in HIV infection as it is in other

Conflicts of Interest: Dr Barnett has no conflicts of interest to declare. Dr Hsue has received honorarium from Gilead.

Grant Support: Dr Hsue is supported by grants from the NIH (R01HL095130, R01HL91526, and R01HL090480).

Division of Cardiology, San Francisco General Hospital, University of California, San Francisco, 1001 Potrero Avenue, Room 5G1, San Francisco, CA 94110, USA

* Corresponding author.

E-mail address: phsue@medsfgh.ucsf.edu

patient populations, PAH could become a major health care concern in the future.

EPIDEMIOLOGY

Since the first case was identified in 1987,[9] PAH has become a well-recognized complication of HIV infection. The initial prevalence estimate of 0.5% was derived from a large Swiss cohort of 1200 largely untreated HIV-infected individuals who used injection drugs.[10] Prevalence estimates have varied considerably over time.[8] The most recent estimates come from a prospective cohort study of 7648 HIV-infected individuals in France. Participants were screened for unexplained dyspnea using a questionnaire followed by echocardiography and pulmonary artery catheterization (PAC), yielding a prevalence of HIV-PAH of 0.46% (95% confidence interval 0.32–0.64),[11] similar to that determined in the original Swiss cohort.

Prevalence estimates have varied depending on the population being studied, as seen in several echocardiographic studies that have evaluated the prevalence of elevated pulmonary artery systolic pressures (PASP) in the setting of HIV infection. In a study performed at San Francisco General Hospital, tricuspid regurgitant jet velocity (TRV) and right atrial pressure were used to estimate PASP in 196 HIV-infected individuals and 52 age-matched uninfected controls.[12] HIV-infected individuals had a higher PASP compared with controls (median 27.5 mm Hg, interquartile range 22–33 mm Hg, compared with 22 mm Hg, interquartile range 18–25 mm Hg; $P<.001$). A PASP of greater than 30 or 40 mm Hg was found in 35.2% of HIV patients compared with 6.6% of controls ($P<.001$), and 7.7% of HIV patients compared with 1.9% of controls ($P = .005$), respectively. After adjustment for age, gender, smoking, stimulant use, and intravenous drug use, HIV-infected individuals had a 5 mm Hg higher mean PASP and a 7-fold greater odds of having a pulmonary artery systolic pressure greater than 30 mm Hg ($P<.001$). A study of 656 HIV-infected individuals demonstrated that among individuals with a detectable tricuspid regurgitant (TR) jet, 57% had evidence of PH defined as right ventricular (RV) pressure greater than 30 mm Hg.[13] Finally, a study of HIV-infected individuals in Spain reported that 9.9% of individuals had a TRV greater than 2.8 m/s.[14] A retrospective study in patients attending the National Institutes of Health HIV clinic showed that 9.3% of patients had a TRV of 2.5 m/s or greater (PASP 30 mm Hg) and 0.4% had a TRV of at least 3.0 m/s (PASP 41 mm Hg).[5]

The cohorts included in these studies varied greatly, and the reason for significant differences seen in the prevalence could be related to demographics, intravenous drug use, or mode of transmission. Also notable is the large number of individuals who had echocardiographic abnormalities, but who did not meet criteria for a diagnosis of PAH. This finding raises the possibility that many more patients could have early or mild forms of PAH.[5,13]

PATHOGENESIS

Patients with HIV and PAH have plexogenic lesions, similar to patients with other diseases associated with PAH (**Fig. 1**), but whether the pathogenesis of disease is similar to PAH in these HIV-uninfected populations is unknown.[15] Possible mechanisms that may be important in HIV-PAH include effects of HIV viral proteins, immune activation induced by HIV, or risk factors that are common in the HIV-infected population. Diastolic dysfunction, which is common in HIV, might also contribute to findings of elevated right-sided heart pressures.[16]

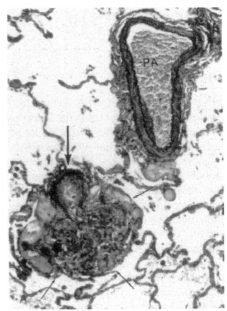

Fig. 1. Elastic stain of lung reveals a predominantly unremarkable pulmonary artery (PA) with only a focal area of intimal sclerosis; immediately adjacent, there is a small muscular pulmonary artery (*thick arrow*) with severe intimal thickening and elastic tissue destruction that leads into an irregular mass of proliferating and focally dilated vascular channels (*outlined by thin arrows*), consistent with a plexiform lesion (Elastica van Gieson stain; original magnification 150×). (*From* Kim KK, Factor SM. Membranoproliferative glomerulonephritis and plexogenic pulmonary arteriopathy in a homosexual man with acquired immunodeficiency syndrome. Human Pathol 1987;18: 1295; with permission.)

HIV has never been shown to directly infect pulmonary vascular endothelial cells,[17,18] but HIV viral antigens are present in pulmonary endothelium and may directly stimulate abnormal apoptosis, growth, and proliferation.[19] Gp120, a viral protein necessary for the binding and entry of HIV into macrophages, has been shown to target human lung endothelial cells, increase markers of apoptosis, and stimulate the secretion of endothelin-1, a protein that is a potent vasoconstrictor.[17] The negative factor (nef) antigen, critical for the maintenance of viral loads and for host-cell signaling interactions, has been localized to multiple pulmonary and vascular cells types.[20] Primates infected with a simian immunodeficiency virus (SIV) expressing HIV nef protein develop lesions resembling plexiform lesions, and colocalization of HIV-1 nef has been demonstrated in pulmonary artery endothelial cells of HIV-infected individuals with PAH, but not in uninfected individuals or in individuals with idiopathic PAH.[20,21] Specific nef signature sequences have been associated with PAH in 2 different HIV cohorts.[22] Bone morphogenic protein receptor 2 (BMPR-2) mutations are associated with familial PAH and result in decreased signaling through BMPR-2.[23] The HIV-1 tat (transcriptional transactivator) protein represses BMPR-2 gene expression in human macrophages in vitro, interfering with BMP–BMPR-2 transcriptional regulation.[23] Exogenous tat protein has also been shown to activate endothelial cells, resulting in the release of growth factors,[23] supporting the hypothesis that HIV viral proteins could induce aberrant endothelial function, leading to PAH.

There are other mechanisms by which HIV could cause PAH. HIV infection induces a chronic inflammatory state characterized by persistent immune activation and dysregulation,[24] which could indirectly induce the release of proinflammatory cytokines and growth factors that could produce PAH.[25] Even in the setting of effectively treated HIV infection, chronic inflammation persists and is independently associated with increased cardiovascular risk.[26] Sputum inflammatory markers and activated CD8+ T cells are associated with elevated TRV and elevated PASP,[27] demonstrating that HIV-associated inflammation may play a role in HIV-PAH. Increased expression of platelet-derived growth factor, a potent stimulus of smooth muscle cell and fibroblast growth and migration, has also been noted in lung tissue from patients with HIV-PAH.[18] Similarly, vascular endothelial growth factor A induces vascular permeability and endothelial cell proliferation, and is produced by T cells infected by HIV in vivo.[28]

Coinfections associated with HIV have also been postulated to play a role. Human herpesvirus (HHV)-8 has been reported to be associated with PAH histologically.[29] HHV-8 is associated with Kaposi sarcoma,[30] and homosexual HIV-infected individuals have a high prevalence of HHV-8 infection ranging from 30% to 60%.[31] However, HHV-8 infection has not been consistently associated with HIV and PAH in several studies.[12,32,33]

Other risk behaviors associated with HIV infection might also play a role in HIV-PAH. Stimulant drug use is common in HIV-infected populations, and HIV-infected individuals who use stimulant drugs are more likely to develop HIV-PAH.[12] Injection drug use may act as a "second hit" in HIV and contribute to development of HIV-PAH.[34] This hypothesis is supported by a recent study of rhesus macaques infected with SIV and treated with intramuscular morphine for 31 weeks. Animals developed significant pulmonary vascular remodeling including plexiform lesions, whereas animals either infected with SIV alone or treated with morphine alone did not.[35]

SURVIVAL

Survival reported for patients with HIV-PAH has consistently been worse than for either HIV infection or idiopathic PAH.[36,37] In patients with HIV-PAH, mortality is most often secondary to PAH leading to right heart failure. Survival estimates for HIV-PAH come from a few large cohort studies and have varied over time, probably in part because of the availability of therapies for HIV and PAH.

The first series to evaluate survival was a prospective cohort study of 19 HIV-PAH patients in a comparison with 19 HIV-infected controls performed before the wide availability of ART or PAH-specific therapy.[36] Survival in HIV-PAH was 58%, 32%, and 21% at 1, 2, and 3 years, markedly worse than controls (**Fig. 2**). A lower CD4+ T-lymphocyte count and the diagnosis of PAH were associated with worse survival.

The most recent data on survival of patients with HIV-PAH come from the French cohort. This series includes 77 patients with HIV-PAH evaluated between 2000 and 2008 and managed with modern therapy for HIV and PAH.[38] In univariate analysis, a history of right-sided heart failure, baseline New York Heart Association Functional Class (NYHA FC) IV, cardiac index less than 2.8 L/min/m^2, detectable HIV viral load, and CD4 count less than 200 cells/μL were associated with poor survival. In multivariate analysis, a low cardiac index and a low CD4 count remained associated with worse survival. Overall survival was 88%, 72%, and 63% at 1, 3, and 5 years, significantly better than prior series. In patients who

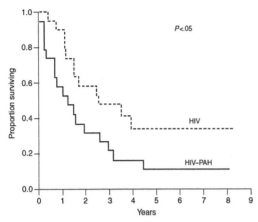

Fig. 2. Kaplan-Meier plot demonstrating the probability of survival in patients with HIV infection and PAH compared with matched HIV-infected controls without PAH before the modern era of antiretroviral and PAH-specific therapy. (*Reprinted* with permission of the American Thoracic Society. Copyright (c) 2013 American Thoracic Society. *From* Opravil M, Pechere M, Speich R, et al. HIV-associated primary pulmonary hypertension. A case control study. Swiss HIV Cohort Study. Am J Respir Crit Care Med 1997;155:992. Official journal of the American Thoracic Society.)

received PAH-specific therapy, survival was 66% compared with 72% in those who did not.

CLINICAL PRESENTATION AND DIAGNOSIS

Presenting complaints of HIV-PAH are the same as those for patients with idiopathic PAH. Symptoms are often nonspecific and insidious, so they are attributed to other complications of HIV or HIV itself. The time from presentation to the diagnosis is often long, from 6 months to 2 years. In a series of patients diagnosed with HIV-PAH before the year 2000, the most common presenting symptom was progressive shortness of breath (85%) followed by pedal edema (30%), nonproductive cough (19%), fatigue (13%), presyncope or syncope (12%), and chest pain (7%).[15]

Physical examination may be unremarkable, but often demonstrates typical findings of right-sided heart failure and volume overload. Auscultation may reveal a right-sided heave or S3, jugular veins may be distended, and there may be peripheral edema. The lung examination is frequently normal in patients with PAH, and abnormal lung findings may suggest an alternative diagnosis. The electrocardiogram may show signs of RV hypertrophy with right axis deviation and right atrial enlargement. A chest radiograph may reveal right heart enlargement and enlargement of the pulmonary arteries without lung findings.[15] For most patients with HIV who have symptoms suggestive of PAH on initial evaluation, the next diagnostic test will usually be an echocardiogram, but routine screening with echocardiography for PAH in HIV-infected patients without a clinical suspicion of PAH may not be a useful or cost-effective approach.[39]

Echocardiography may not be sufficient to rule out PAH in individuals with a compatible clinical picture. Spectral Doppler is used to determine the peak velocity of the TR jet, which can be entered into modified Bernoulli equation to estimate the PASP (**Fig. 3**). This estimate may be unreliable if the peak TRV cannot be determined because there is minimal tricuspid regurgitation, an eccentric jet, or a very large jet. This lack of reliability may be particularly problematic in HIV-infected patients, and a low PASP on echo is not adequate enough to excluded the diagnosis of PAH (**Fig. 4**). In a study of Doppler echocardiography, estimates of PASP were inaccurate in 19.7% of cases, and 1 in 3 patients with HIV-PAH was missed.[40]

Other echo findings such as RV enlargement, hypertrophy and systolic dysfunction, right atrial enlargement, characteristic pulmonic valve motion, and spectral Doppler characteristics should be considered when evaluating patients for possible PAH.[41] Left ventricular systolic function and clinically relevant valvular disease should be excluded by echocardiography.

The gold standard for hemodynamic evaluation remains invasive assessment with PAC[42]; if echocardiography supports a possible diagnosis of PAH, PAC is mandatory before initiation of any PAH-specific therapy. To minimize complications and optimize data collection, PAC should be performed by a clinician with expertise in hemodynamic assessment and diagnostic evaluation of patients with PH. Maneuvers to exclude occult left-sided diastolic dysfunction, such as fluid challenge or exercise, may be performed in patients with risk factors (left atrial enlargement, left ventricular hypertrophy, diabetes, or hypertension). Acute vasodilator challenge may be performed during right heart catheterization; however, few patients with HIV-PAH who have a positive acute vasodilator response will have long-term responses to calcium-channel blockers.[43]

Before considering treatment for PAH, other causes of PH such as lung disease, valvular or left heart disease, chronic thromboembolic disease, and sleep apnea should be excluded as per guideline recommendations.[44] Other diseases associated with PAH such as connective tissues disease, hemolytic disorders, portal hypertension, and congenital heart disease should be excluded because the approach to management and prognosis may be affected.

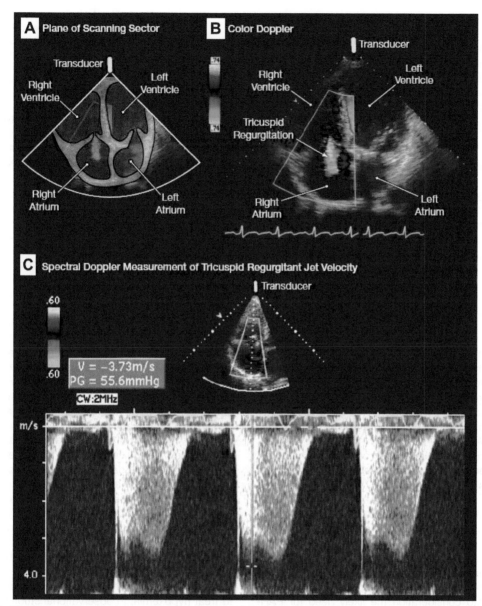

Fig. 3. (*A*) Plane of scanning sector. (*B*) Color Doppler demonstrating tricuspid regurgitation (*blue*). (*C*) Spectral Doppler measurement of tricuspid regurgitant jet velocity for the estimation of pulmonary artery systolic pressure, demonstrating a peak tricuspid regurgitant jet velocity of approximately 3.7 m/s. Sampling of the peak tricuspid regurgitant jet velocity is used to estimate the RV to right atrial systolic pressure gradient (55.6 mm Hg in the figure) with the use of the modified Bernoulli equation (4 × [tricuspid regurgitant jet velocity]^2). Pulmonary artery systolic pressure is quantified by adding the Bernoulli-derived pressure gradient to an estimate of mean right atrial pressure. (See video at http://jama.com/cgi/content/full/299/3/324/DC1.) (*From* Barnett CF, Hsue PY, Machado RF. Pulmonary hypertension. JAMA 2008;299:326; with permission.)

TREATMENT
Antiretroviral Treatment

The effects of ART in HIV-PAH are controversial. Two retrospective studies have shown a reduced incidence of HIV-PAH since ART became available, suggesting that HIV-targeted treatment is beneficial.[8,45] A small French cohort reported that combination ART alone improved exercise tolerance as assessed by 6-minute walk (6MW) distance, but no change in hemodynamics was observed.[38] In animal models, protease inhibitors have been shown to reverse hypoxia-induced PH.[46] Data from the Swiss Cohort study showed

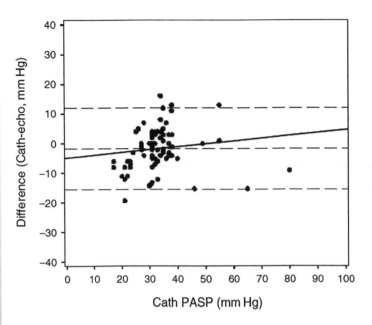

Fig. 4. Bland-Altman analysis demonstrating lack of agreement between the pulmonary artery systolic pressure estimated by Doppler echocardiogram and pulmonary artery systolic pressure (PASP) measured by right heart catheterization. (*From* Selby VN, Scherzer R, Barnett CF, et al. Doppler echocardiography does not accurately estimate pulmonary artery systolic pressure in HIV-infected patients. AIDS 2012;26:1968; with permission.)

that individuals with HIV-PAH diagnosed after 1995 had slightly improved survival compared with those diagnosed before this time, and a reciprocal relationship was noted between CD4 cell count and PAH incidence.[38] There have been no large prospective studies of the effects of ART on HIV-PAH.

Current guidelines recommend that all HIV-infected patients be treated with antiretroviral agents regardless of CD4 T-cell count and viral load,[47,48] so most patients diagnosed with HIV-PAH will already be on HIV therapy. In the authors' practice, antiretroviral therapy is started promptly in any individual newly diagnosed with HIV-PAH who was not previously on treatment. The choice of the initial antiretroviral regimen should be based on current guidelines; however, practitioners should take into consideration the likely need for PAH-specific therapies and relevant drug interactions.

Conventional Therapies

Initial treatment of patients with HIV-PAH will be determined by the severity of symptoms and hemodynamic compromise.[44] Few studies have specifically addressed the treatment of HIV-PAH, so approach to treatment is based on studies performed in patients with idiopathic or associated PAH. Many patients will be diagnosed in the outpatient setting; however, presentation with acute on chronic decompensated right heart failure associated with severe hypoperfusion or hypotension is not uncommon. Patients who present with decompensated right heart failure should be triaged to an intensive care unit and managed with a PAC to titrate vasopressors and inotropic agents, to restore perfusion accordingly. Hypoxemia can worsen pulmonary vasoconstriction and should be corrected with supplemental oxygen. Diuretic therapy should be instituted in patients with volume overload, and adjusted to achieve normal right-sided filling pressures. Despite few supportive data, digoxin may be considered in patients with acute right heart failure and for chronic management to reduce symptoms of heart failure. Because of the risk of hemodynamic decompensation with dihydropyridine calcium-channel blockers and β-blockers, digoxin is also used as a first-line agent in patients with atrial arrhythmias and HIV-PAH.

Long-term oxygen therapy should be continued to treat hypoxemia. In observational studies, survival is improved in PAH patients treated with warfarin, and current guidelines recommend titration to an international normalized ratio of 1.5 to 2.5.[44] Chronic digoxin therapy may be a useful adjunct to PAH-specific therapy.

Calcium-Channel Blockers

In several published reports, favorable long-term response to calcium-channel blockers has been limited to a minority of patients with idiopathic PAH.[49] A favorable response to acute vasodilator challenge or oral calcium-channel blockers has been reported in only a few patients with HIV-PAH.[36,38,43] As in all PAH patients, oral calcium-channel blockers should only be considered in those patients with a favorable response to acute vasodilator challenge, with careful long-term monitoring for signs of worsening PAH.

PAH-Specific Therapy

Retrospective cohort studies suggest that survival of patients treated with PAH-specific therapy in addition to ART is improved.[38] Because there are few well-designed trials for HIV-PAH, choice and timing of therapy are based on data from other trials of PAH.[50,51] Treatment of HIV-PAH is particularly challenging, owing to the potential for significant drug interactions and adverse effects. Safe initiation of PAH-specific therapy in a patient on ART requires planning and good communication with HIV specialists and pharmacists, as well as frequent patient follow-up to monitor for adverse effects and drug interactions.

Phosphodiesterase Inhibitors

Sildenafil and tadalafil function by inhibiting the metabolism of cyclic guanosine monophosphate, the second messenger that mediates the effects of nitric oxide, causing selective pulmonary vasodilation.[52] Sildenafil treatment in PAH improves exercise tolerance, and tadalafil improves exercise tolerance and reduces time to clinical worsening.[53] Data on the use of these agents in HIV-PAH is largely extrapolated from trials in PAH, but results from small series and case reports of HIV-PAH have been encouraging.[54,55] Ritonavir and other protease inhibitors are inhibitors of cytochrome P450 CYP3A4 and CYP 2C9, which are important in the metabolism of sildenafil and tadalafil. Marked increases in sildenafil levels have been observed during coadministration with indinavir,[56] saquinavir, and ritonavir,[57] and some guidelines consider this combination to be contraindicated. The clinical relevance of this interaction is unclear because increased sildenafil levels have not been associated with hypotension or adverse effects in pharmacokinetic studies,[57] and successful coadministration of ritonavir and sildenafil in HIV-PAH patients has been reported.[58] Tadalafil levels are less affected by ritonavir, and guidelines suggest only close monitoring if tadalafil therapy is initiated.

Endothelin Receptor Antagonists

Blockade of the endothelin receptor with bosentan (nonselective) or ambrisentan (selective) improves hemodynamics, exercise tolerance and prevents clinical worsening in patients with PAH. Bosentan was studied prospectively in 16 HIV-PAH patients in the prospective BREATHE-4 trial. After 16 weeks, NYHA FC improved by at least 1 class in 14

patients, cardiac index improved by 39%, mPAP decreased by 21%, and 6MW distance improved by 91 ± 60 m.[59] Another study examined long-term effects of bosentan in 59 patients after a median of 29 months of therapy, and showed short-term improvements in symptoms, exercise tolerance, and hemodynamic parameters.[60] In both studies, bosentan was well tolerated.

Ambrisentan has not been specifically studied in patients with HIV-PAH, but appears to have efficacy similar to that of bosentan.[61] Ambrisentan treatment is associated with a lower frequency of liver function test abnormalities. Monthly liver function testing is not mandatory, and pharmacokinetic studies suggest that there is no significant drug interaction with the protease inhibitor, ritonavir.[62–64]

Prostacyclin Analogues

Although no long-term trials in HIV-PAH patients have been performed, improvements in hemodynamics and exercise tolerance have been observed in small series of patients treated with catheter-based and inhaled prostanoid treatment. In one report, 6 patients with HIV-PAH were treated with intravenous epoprostenol for 12 to 47 months with improvements in NYHA FC. Acute improvements in mPAP, cardiac index, and PVR persisted at the time of repeat right heart catheterization.[43] Another observational study reported on 3 patients with severe HIV-PAH treated with 1 year of subcutaneous treprostinil. All patients had improvement in NYHA FC, increased 6MW distance by at least 75 m (baseline 313–500 m), and had improvement in hemodynamics determined by echocardiography.[65] Intravenous or subcutaneous treatment requires placement of an indwelling catheter, which may not be desirable in HIV-infected patients at risk for catheter-related infection and injection drug use.

Published experience in HIV-PAH with inhaled prostanoids is limited, but offers a desirable alternative delivery method. The effects of inhaled iloprost were reported in a study of 8 patients with severe HIV-PAH.[66] Hemodynamic effects following initial iloprost treatment improved, with a 31% reduction in PVR and a 21% increase in cardiac index. Treprostinil is another inhaled prostanoid with the advantage of reduced dosing frequency. HIV-PAH patients were included in the TRIUMPH study of treprostinil, which demonstrated improved exercise tolerance when treprostinil was added to baseline oral therapy.[67] The number of HIV-PAH patients, however, was too small for meaningful analysis.

Treat-to-Target Approach and Monitoring Effects of PAH-HIV Treatment

In the authors' practice, before initiation of PAH-specific therapy all patients undergo a thorough diagnostic evaluation, including right heart catheterization, to ensure that they meet criteria for a diagnosis of PAH and that other possible causes of PH or PAH are excluded. All patients undergo a baseline 6MW distance test to assess exercise tolerance, and this test is repeated at each subsequent clinic visit.[50,68] Conventional therapy with diuretics and oxygen are initiated, as well as warfarin if patients can comply with necessary monitoring. Treatment with either a phosphodiesterase inhibitor or an endothelin receptor antagonist is generally the first line. The choice of initial therapy is often dictated by concomitant ART therapy and the willingness and ability of the patient to follow up with necessary monthly monitoring for liver function test abnormalities, contraception, and pregnancy testing. Patients are closely followed in cooperation with the HIV clinic, and the initial therapy is titrated based on the patients' objective exercise tolerance and 6MW distance. The authors frequently initiate inhaled prostanoid, usually treprostinil, in patients who remain symptomatic despite maximal oral therapy or as a first-line agent in patients with severe symptoms at the time of presentation. Catheter-based therapies are avoided in this population, given the challenges of managing the therapy, risk of infection, and risk of the catheter being used for illicit drug administration (which is common in the authors' patient population). Despite the paucity of trials of combination therapy, a treat-to-target approach for patients with PAH has been advocated, with additional oral and inhaled therapies until patients' subjective and objective exercise tolerance improves to an acceptable level.

SUMMARY

The development of PAH in HIV-infected individuals is associated with high morbidity and mortality, and HIV-PAH may be an increasing problem as HIV-infected individuals survive longer. The pathogenesis of HIV-PAH is not completely understood, but HIV proteins, chronic immune activation, coinfections, or synergistic effects of other risk factors may be important. Physicians treating HIV-infected patients should monitor for symptoms of unexplained or new dyspnea, and patients should undergo an echocardiogram to estimate pulmonary artery pressures and to look for other signs of right heart dysfunction. A complete assessment including PAC is mandatory in confirming the diagnosis of HIV-PAH. PAH-specific therapy should be initiated by a physician with experience in managing PAH, in close collaboration with HIV specialists and pharmacists. An improved understanding of the pathogenesis of HIV-PAH is needed to inform the optimal approach to treatment.

REFERENCES

1. Deeks SG. HIV infection, inflammation, immunosenescence, and aging. Annu Rev Med 2011;62: 141–55.
2. Boccara F. Cardiovascular complications and atherosclerotic manifestations in the HIV-infected population: type, incidence and associated risk factors. AIDS 2008;22:S19–26. http://dx.doi.org/10.1097/01.aids.0000327512.76126.6e.
3. Tseng ZH, Secemsky EA, Dowdy D, et al. Sudden cardiac death in patients with human immunodeficiency virus infection. J Am Coll Cardiol 2012;59: 1891–6.
4. Hsue PY, Hunt PW, Wu Y, et al. Association of abacavir and impaired endothelial function in treated and suppressed HIV-infected patients. AIDS 2009;23: 2021–7.
5. Barnett CF, Hsue PY, Machado RF. Pulmonary hypertension. JAMA 2008;299:324–31.
6. Simonneau G, Galie N, Rubin LJ, et al. Clinical classification of pulmonary hypertension. J Am Coll Cardiol 2004;43:5S–12S.
7. WHO/UNAIDS. Global report: UNAIDS report on the global AIDS epidemic 2012. Geneva (Switzerland): WHO/UNAIDS; 2012. Available at: http://www.aidsinfo.unaids.org.
8. Zuber JP, Calmy A, Evison JM, et al. Pulmonary arterial hypertension related to HIV infection: improved hemodynamics and survival associated with antiretroviral therapy. Clin Infect Dis 2004;38:1178–85.
9. Kim KK, Factor SM. Membranoproliferative glomerulonephritis and plexogenic pulmonary arteriopathy in a homosexual man with acquired immunodeficiency syndrome. Hum Pathol 1987;18: 1293–6.
10. Speich R, Jenni R, Opravil M, et al. Primary pulmonary hypertension in HIV infection. Chest 1991;100: 1268–71.
11. Sitbon O, Lascoux-Combe C, Delfraissy JF, et al. Prevalence of HIV-related pulmonary arterial hypertension in the current antiretroviral therapy era. Am J Respir Crit Care Med 2008;177:108–13.
12. Hsue PY, Deeks SG, Farah HH, et al. Role of HIV and human herpesvirus-8 infection in pulmonary arterial hypertension. AIDS 2008;22:825–33.
13. Mondy KE, Gottdiener J, Overton ET, et al. High prevalence of echocardiographic abnormalities among HIV-infected persons in the era of highly

active antiretroviral therapy. Clin Infect Dis 2011;52: 378–86.

14. Quezada M, Martin-Carbonero L, Soriano V, et al. Prevalence and risk factors associated with pulmonary hypertension in HIV-infected patients on regular follow-up. AIDS 2012;26:1387–92.

15. Mehta NJ, Khan IA, Mehta RN, et al. HIV-Related pulmonary hypertension: analytic review of 131 cases. Chest 2000;118:1133–41.

16. Hsue PY, Hunt PW, Ho JE, et al. Impact of HIV infection on diastolic function and left ventricular mass. Circ Heart Fail 2010;3:132–9.

17. Kanmogne GD, Primeaux C, Grammas P. Induction of apoptosis and endothelin-1 secretion in primary human lung endothelial cells by HIV-1 gp120 proteins. Biochem Biophys Res Commun 2005; 333:1107.

18. Humbert M, Monti G, Fartoukh M, et al. Platelet-derived growth factor expression in primary pulmonary hypertension: comparison of HIV seropositive and HIV seronegative patients. Eur Respir J 1998; 11:554–9.

19. Mette SA, Palevsky HI, Pietra GG, et al. Primary pulmonary hypertension in association with human immunodeficiency virus infection. A possible viral etiology for some forms of hypertensive pulmonary arteriopathy. Am Rev Respir Dis 1992;145: 1196–200.

20. Marecki JC, Cool CD, Parr JE, et al. HIV-1 Nef is associated with complex pulmonary vascular lesions in SHIV-nef-infected macaques. Am J Respir Crit Care Med 2006;174:437–45.

21. George MP, Champion HC, Simon M, et al. Physiologic changes in a non-human primate model of HIV-associated pulmonary arterial hypertension. Am J Respir Cell Mol Biol 2013;48:374–81.

22. Almodovar S, Knight R, Allshouse AA, et al. Human immunodeficiency virus nef signature sequences are associated with pulmonary hypertension. AIDS Res Hum Retroviruses 2012;28:607–18.

23. Caldwell RL, Gadipatti R, Lane KB, et al. HIV-1 TAT represses transcription of the bone morphogenic protein receptor-2 in U937 monocytic cells. J Leukoc Biol 2006;79:192–201.

24. Fauci AS, Pantaleo G, Stanley S, et al. Immunopathogenic mechanisms of HIV infection. Ann Intern Med 1996;124:654–63.

25. Morse JH, Barst RJ, Itescu S, et al. Primary pulmonary hypertension in HIV infection: an outcome determined by particular HLA class II alleles. Am J Respir Crit Care Med 1996;153:1299–301.

26. Hsue PY, Deeks SG, Hunt PW. Immunologic basis of cardiovascular disease in HIV-infected adults. J Infect Dis 2012;205(Suppl 3):S375–82.

27. Morris A, Gingo MR, George MP, et al. Cardiopulmonary function in individuals with HIV infection in the antiretroviral therapy era. AIDS 2012;26:731–40.

28. Ascherl G, Hohenadl C, Schatz O, et al. Infection with human immunodeficiency virus-1 increases expression of vascular endothelial cell growth factor in T cells: implications for acquired immunodeficiency syndrome-associated vasculopathy. Blood 1999;93:4232–41.

29. Cool CD, Rai PR, Yeager ME, et al. Expression of human herpesvirus 8 in primary pulmonary hypertension. N Engl J Med 2003;349:1113–22.

30. Chang Y, Cesarman E, Pessin MS, et al. Identification of herpesvirus-like DNA sequences in AIDS-associated Kaposi's sarcoma. Science 1994;266: 1865–9.

31. Martin JN, Ganem DE, Osmond DH, et al. Sexual transmission and the natural history of human herpesvirus 8 infection. N Engl J Med 1998;338: 948–54.

32. Montani D, Marcelin AG, Sitbon O, et al. Human herpes virus 8 in HIV and non-HIV infected patients with pulmonary arterial hypertension in France. AIDS 2005;19:1239–40.

33. Nicastri E, Vizza CD, Carletti F, et al. Human herpesvirus 8 and pulmonary hypertension. Emerg Infect Dis 2005;11:1480–2.

34. George MP, Champion HC, Gladwin MT, et al. Injection drug use as a "second hit" in the pathogenesis of HIV-associated pulmonary hypertension. Am J Respir Crit Care Med 2012;185:1144–6.

35. Spikes L, Dalvi P, Tawfik O, et al. Enhanced pulmonary arteriopathy in simian immunodeficiency virus-infected macaques exposed to morphine. Am J Respir Crit Care Med 2012;185:1235–43.

36. Opravil M, Pechere M, Speich R, et al. HIV-associated primary pulmonary hypertension. A case control study. Swiss HIV Cohort Study. Am J Respir Crit Care Med 1997;155:990–5.

37. Petitpretz P, Brenot F, Azarian R, et al. Pulmonary hypertension in patients with human immunodeficiency virus infection. Comparison with primary pulmonary hypertension. Circulation 1994;89: 2722–7.

38. Degano B, Guillaume M, Savale L, et al. HIV-associated pulmonary arterial hypertension: survival and prognostic factors in the modern therapeutic era. AIDS 2010;24:67–75.

39. McGoon M, Gutterman D, Steen V, et al. Screening, early detection, and diagnosis of pulmonary arterial hypertension. ACCP evidence-based clinical practice guidelines. Chest 2004;126:14S–34S.

40. Selby VN, Scherzer R, Barnett CF, et al. Doppler echocardiography does not accurately estimate pulmonary artery systolic pressure in HIV-infected patients. AIDS 2012;26:1967–9.

41. Raymond RJ, Hinderliter AL, Willis PW IV, et al. Echocardiographic predictors of adverse outcomes in primary pulmonary hypertension. J Am Coll Cardiol 2002;39:1214–9.

42. Champion HC, Michelakis ED, Hassoun PM, et al. Comprehensive invasive and noninvasive approach to the right ventricle–pulmonary circulation unit: state of the art and clinical and research implications. Circulation 2009;120:992–1007.

43. Aguilar RV, Farber HW. Epoprostenol (prostacyclin) therapy in HIV-associated pulmonary hypertension. Am J Respir Crit Care Med 2000;162: 1846–50.

44. McLaughlin VV, Archer SL, Badesch DB, et al. ACCF/AHA 2009 Expert Consensus Document on Pulmonary Hypertension. A report of the American College of Cardiology Foundation Task Force on Expert Consensus Documents and the American Heart Association Developed in collaboration with the American College of Chest Physicians; American Thoracic Society, Inc.; and the Pulmonary Hypertension Association. J Am Coll Cardiol 2009; 53:1573–619.

45. Pugliese A, Isnardi D, Saini A, et al. Impact of highly active antiretroviral therapy in HIV-positive patients with cardiac involvement. J Infect 2000; 40:282–4.

46. Gary-Bobo G, Houssaini A, Amsellem V, et al. Effects of HIV protease inhibitors on progression of monocrotaline- and hypoxia-induced pulmonary hypertension in rats. Circulation 2010;122:1937–47.

47. Panel on Antiretroviral Guidelines for Adults and Adolescents. Guidelines for the use of antiretroviral agents in HIV-1-infected adults and adolescents. Department of Health and Human Services. Available at: http://aidsinfo.nih.gov/contentfiles/lvguidelines/AdultandAdolescentGL.pdf.

48. Thompson MA, Aberg JA, Hoy JF, et al. Antiretroviral treatment of adult HIV infection: 2012 recommendations of the international antiviral society—USA panel. JAMA 2012;308:387–402.

49. Sitbon O, Humbert M, Jaïs X, et al. Long-term response to calcium channel blockers in idiopathic pulmonary arterial hypertension. Circulation 2005; 111:3105–11.

50. Galiè N, Hoeper MM, Humbert M, et al. Guidelines for the diagnosis and treatment of pulmonary hypertension. Eur Heart J 2009;30:2493–537.

51. Galiè N, Rubin LJ, Hoeper MM, et al. Treatment of patients with mildly symptomatic pulmonary arterial hypertension with bosentan (EARLY study): a double-blind, randomised controlled trial. Lancet 2008;371:2093–100.

52. Barnett CF, Machado RF. Sildenafil in the treatment of pulmonary hypertension. Vasc Health Risk Manag 2006;2:411–22.

53. Galiè N, Brundage BH, Ghofrani HA, et al. Tadalafil therapy for pulmonary arterial hypertension. Circulation 2009;119:2894–903.

54. Ieong MH. Noninfectious pulmonary complications of HIV. Clin Pulm Med 2006;13:194–202.

55. Schumacher YO, Zdebik A, Huonker M, et al. Sildenafil in HIV-related pulmonary hypertension. AIDS 2001;15:1747–8.

56. Merry C, Barry MG, Ryan M, et al. Interaction of sildenafil and indinavir when co-administered to HIV-positive patients. AIDS 1999;13:101–7.

57. Muirhead GJ, Wulff MB, Fielding A, et al. Pharmacokinetic interactions between sildenafil and saquinavir/ritonavir. Br J Clin Pharmacol 2000;50: 99–107.

58. Chinello P, Cicalini S, Pichini S, et al. Sildenafil plasma concentrations in two HIV patients with pulmonary hypertension treated with ritonavir-boosted protease inhibitors. Curr HIV Res 2012;10: 162–4.

59. Sitbon O, Gressin V, Speich R, et al. Bosentan for the treatment of human immunodeficiency virus-associated pulmonary arterial hypertension. Am J Respir Crit Care Med 2004;170:1212–7.

60. Degano B, Yaici A, Le Pavec J, et al. Long-term effects of bosentan in patients with HIV-associated pulmonary arterial hypertension. Eur Respir J 2009;33:92–8.

61. Galiè N, Olschewski H, Oudiz RJ, et al. Ambrisentan for the treatment of pulmonary arterial hypertension: results of the Ambrisentan in Pulmonary Arterial Hypertension, Randomized, Double-Blind, Placebo-Controlled, Multicenter, Efficacy (ARIES) Study 1 and 2. Circulation 2008;117:3010–9.

62. Venitz J, Zack J, Gillies H, et al. Clinical pharmacokinetics and drug-drug interactions of endothelin receptor antagonists in pulmonary arterial hypertension. J Clin Pharmacol 2012;52:1784–805.

63. Ben-Yehuda O, Pizzuti D, Brown A, et al. Long-term hepatic safety of ambrisentan in patients with pulmonary arterial hypertension. J Am Coll Cardiol 2012;60:80–1.

64. Gillies H, Wang X, Staehr P, et al. PAH therapy in HIV: lack drug-drug interaction between ambrisentan and ritonavir. Am J Respir Crit Care Med 2011; 183:A5913.

65. Cea-Calvo L, Escribano Subias P, Tello de Menesses R, et al. Treatment of HIV-associated pulmonary hypertension with treprostinil. Rev Esp Cardiol 2003;56:421–5 [in Spanish].

66. Ghofrani HA, Friese G, Discher T, et al. Inhaled iloprost is a potent acute pulmonary vasodilator in HIV-related severe pulmonary hypertension. Eur Respir J 2004;23:321–6.

67. McLaughlin VV, Benza RL, Rubin LJ, et al. Addition of inhaled treprostinil to oral therapy for pulmonary arterial hypertension: a randomized controlled clinical trial. J Am Coll Cardiol 2010; 55:1915–22.

68. Vachiéry JL, Yerly P, Huez S. How to detect disease progression in pulmonary arterial hypertension. Eur Respir Rev 2012;21:40–7.

Interstitial Lung Disease in HIV

Sarah R. Doffman, MB ChB, FRCP[a],*,
Robert F. Miller, MBBS, FRCP[b]

KEYWORDS

- HIV - Interstitial pneumonitis - Pulmonary fibrosis - Idiopathic lung disease - Antiretroviral therapy

KEY POINTS

- Interstitial lung diseases, such as nonspecific interstitial pneumonitis and lymphocytic interstitial pneumonitis, may be less frequent in the HIV-infected population since the introduction of antiretroviral therapy.
- Other interstitial lung diseases, such as sarcoidosis, may actually be increasing since the introduction of antiretroviral therapy, possibly from renewed immune function.
- Treatment of interstitial lung disease is similar to that in the HIV-uninfected population.
- Many of the interstitial lung diseases have nonspecific presentations and other conditions, such as infections and malignancy, should be ruled out.

INTRODUCTION

Early reports of the pulmonary complications of the acquired immune deficiency syndrome (AIDS) focused on opportunistic infections and malignancies such as Kaposi sarcoma.[1] It soon became apparent that other noninfectious complications were occurring, including non-Hodgkin's lymphoma and lymphocytic interstitial pneumonia.[2] It was subsequently established that there is a spectrum of lymphocytic infiltrative disorders, including nonspecific interstitial pneumonitis (NSIP) and lymphocytic interstitial pneumonitis (LIP), that were frequently described in HIV-infected adults in the pre–antiretroviral therapy (ART) era (reviewed in[3,4]).

With the advent of ART, these conditions are less commonly encountered by clinicians, possibly as a consequence of the effects of treatment on pulmonary immunology, resulting in prevention of development of symptomatic disease (see article in this issue by Homer Twigg). In contrast, sarcoidosis is increasingly recognized among HIV-infected patients in the current era and may represent an immune reconstitution phenomenon (reviewed in[5]). Reports of sarcoidosis in HIV-infected persons were uncommon in the pre-ART era. Other causes of pneumonitis, including cryptogenic organizing pneumonia and drug-induced hypersensitivity pneumonitis, have been infrequently encountered among adult HIV-infected persons, both before and after the introduction of ART.

This article reviews interstitial lung disease in HIV-infected adults.

SEROCONVERSION PNEUMONITIS

Presentation with a subacute pneumonitis, mimicking *Pneumocystis* pneumonia (PCP), has been described at presentation with "primary HIV-1 infection" (also known as HIV "seroconversion"[5]). Other features of primary HIV-1 infection, such as rash and/or a transaminitis, may also be present. Stigmata of immune suppression are notably absent, and the CD4+ T-lymphocyte count may be low or normal. Exclusion of PCP and other infectious agents as the cause is required to make

The authors have nothing to disclose.
[a] Department of Respiratory Medicine, Royal Sussex County Hospital, Brighton and Sussex University Hospitals NHS Trust, Eastern Road, Brighton BN2 5BE, UK; [b] Research Department of Infection and Population Health, University College London, Mortimer Market Centre off Capper Street, London WC1E 6JB, UK
* Corresponding author.
E-mail address: Sarah.doffman@bsuh.nhs.uk

Clin Chest Med 34 (2013) 293–306
http://dx.doi.org/10.1016/j.ccm.2013.01.012
0272-5231/13/$ – see front matter © 2013 Elsevier Inc. All rights reserved.

chestmed.theclinics.com

the diagnosis, as well as laboratory evidence of HIV seroconversion.

NONSPECIFIC INTERSTITIAL PNEUMONITIS

NSIP has been most frequently described in the pre-ART era and likely represents part of a spectrum of "lymphocytic" pulmonary syndromes in HIV-infected persons, which include follicular bronchiolitis/bronchitis, lymphocytic bronchiolitis, LIP, and diffuse infiltrative CD8+ lymphocytosis syndrome (DILS).[3,4,6,7] The incidence of NSIP among adult HIV-infected adults with respiratory symptoms in the pre-ART era was approximately 38%, but the true incidence may have been higher.[8]

The cause of NSIP is not yet fully elucidated. It is described less commonly in the literature since the advent of ART, supporting the hypothesis that it is a manifestation of a disordered pulmonary immune reaction to HIV itself. One proposed mechanism is an influx of immunocompetent cells in response to HIV infection with oligoclonal expansion of major histocompatibility complex–restricted CD8+ T lymphocytes, which attack HIV structural proteins and restrict infection of the surrounding pulmonary microenvironment. This theory is supported by the presence of a persistent lymphocytic alveolitis with strong cytotoxic T-cell response to HIV. Any impairment of this anti-HIV lysis may result in progression of alveolitis and risk of opportunistic infection.[9]

Sattler and colleagues[10] described 351 HIV-infected persons presenting with symptoms suggestive of PCP. NSIP was the most frequently encountered diagnosis, seen in 15 of 67 cases where PCP was excluded by bronchoscopy, bronchoscopic alveolar lavage (BAL), and/or transbronchial biopsy. Patients with NSIP had higher CD4+ T-lymphocyte counts than those with PCP (mean = 492 vs 57 cells/μl, respectively). The presence of HIV was demonstrated within alveolar macrophages or pneumocytes in 5 of 15, and HIV *gag* and *env* genes were detectable by PCR in 10 of 15 patients. HIV RNA has also been detected in a proportion of lung biopsy specimens from patients with NSIP.[7]

Several other viral pathogens have been proposed as causative in lymphocytic pulmonary syndromes. For example, animal studies demonstrate similar pulmonary histopathologic abnormalities to those seen in LIP and NSIP in sheep infected with ovine lentivirus.[11,12] Epstein-Barr virus, cytomegalovirus, and herpes simplex virus have all been implicated as causative in NSIP, but there is no supportive pathologic data from biopsy specimens.[8,10]

Clinical Features

NSIP is most commonly found in patients who present with clinical features compatible with PCP, such as dyspnea, fevers, and cough (**Table 1**). The duration of fever may be prolonged. There may be crackles audible on auscultation of the chest. NSIP can occur in asymptomatic HIV-infected individuals as well.[13]

Diagnosis

Blood tests

There is no diagnostic blood test for NSIP. The CD4+ T-lymphocyte count is usually lower than that seen in LIP (200 cells/μl) but may be in the normal range.

Arterial blood gases (ABG) may be normal or demonstrate varying degrees of hypoxemia and widening of the alveolar-arterial (A-a) gradient, comparable to findings in PCP. The ABG is not helpful in differentiating NSIP from opportunistic infections or other pulmonary diseases.

Radiology

The chest radiograph may be normal in up to 50% cases.[13] Where abnormal, there are 2 main patterns of disease: interstitial infiltrates (reticular or reticulonodular shadowing) (**Fig. 1**) or alveolar infiltrates (perihilar loss of radiolucency). Other findings, such as pleural effusion or adenopathy, are not usually seen. On high-resolution computed tomography (HRCT), NSIP can resemble a variety of other interstitial lung diseases and does not have a pathognomonic appearance (**Fig. 2**).

Features described in NSIP are as follows:

- Ground glass infiltrates (predominantly basal and may be extensive)
- Areas of consolidation
- Honeycombing is described, but is not a dominant feature

Pathology

NSIP is characterized by the presence of an interstitial infiltrate of lymphocytes, plasma cells, and macrophages. In severe cases, there may be extension of the infiltrate into alveolar septae. This inflammatory infiltrate is usually not as dense as that seen in LIP. There may be type II pneumocyte hyperplasia and alveolar interstitial edema. The lymphocytes often aggregate in a perivascular and peribronchiolar distribution. Many of these lymphocytes are mature CD20+ B cells. T lymphocytes (both CD4+ and CD8+) tend to be present in a more diffuse pattern.[6]

Table 1
Comparison of major clinicopathologic features of interstitial lung disease in HIV-infected adults

	Nonspecific Interstitial Pneumonitis (NSIP)	Lymphocytic Interstitial Pneumonia (LIP)	Cryptogenic Organizing Pneumonia (COP)	Hypersensitivity Pneumonitis (HP)	Sarcoid
Clinical features					
Dyspnea and cough	+/-	+	+	+	+/-
Fevers	+/-	+	+	-	+/-
Usual CD4 count (cells/μl)	<200 (may be normal)	>350	Any	Usually >350	>200
Radiology					
Chest radiograph	Interstitial or alveolar infiltrates / Normal in up to 50%	Reticular or nodular shadowing	Consolidation	May be normal or diffuse nodules	BHL +/- reticulo-nodular opacities
HRCT					
Ground glass opacification	Basal, may be prominent	Present	Present	Diffuse or patchy	Occasional diffuse
Consolidation	May be present	Not usually a feature	Dominant feature	Not usually a feature	May be present
Honeycombing	Rarely may be present	Present in advanced disease	Not usually a feature	Present in advanced disease	May be present if fibrotic disease
Other		Reticular and nodular shadowing	Cavitating nodules	Mosaic attenuation	Adenopathy and nodules on fissures
Histopathologic features					
Features	Interstitial infiltrates of lymphocytes, plasma cells, and macrophages	Interstitial infiltrates of polyclonal lymphocytes, some histiocytes, and plasma cells with extension into alveolar septae	Organizing pneumonia, intraluminal polyps of granulation tissue	Peribronchiolar lymphocytic infiltrates and variable fibrosis in chronic disease	Noncaseating granuloma
Granulomata	Not present	Occasionally reported	Not present	Present	Prominent
Treatment and prognosis	Usually self-limiting / Use of combination antiretroviral therapy (cART) may lead to improvement in lymphocytic alveolitis	May be stable without treatment / Some role for steroids and cART / Rarely progresses to respiratory failure	Responds rapidly to corticosteroids	May be self-limiting on removal of causative agent / May require corticosteroids	May spontaneously remit / May require steroids

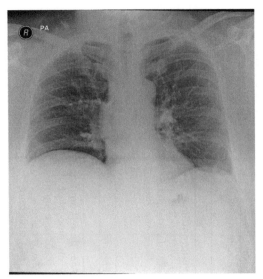

Fig. 1. Chest radiograph. Nonspecific interstitial pneumonitis.

Treatment

Most NSIP is self-limiting. The disease can remain stable for many years or regress spontaneously and does not require specific treatment, although in some cases, use of corticosteroids has been reported. Any clinical deterioration in patients with NSIP is often attributed to another complication of HIV infection, such as an opportunistic infection. Given the likelihood that NSIP is a disordered immune response to HIV itself, it seems likely that lymphocytic alveolitis may regress with institution of ART, although there is no biopsy evidence to support this hypothesis.

Diagnostic Dilemmas

NSIP in the HIV-uninfected population has varied and nonspecific clinical and radiologic features.[14]

In addition, in HIV-infected persons, NSIP has been described as an incidental finding on lung biopsy specimens, and its clinical significance remains uncertain in many cases.

LYMPHOCYTIC INTERSTITIAL PNEUMONIA AND DIFFUSE INFILTRATIVE CD8 LYMPHOCYTOSIS SYNDROME

LIP is more frequently described in HIV-infected infants, although it was also recognized in adults early in the AIDS pandemic.[1] In contrast to NSIP, where patients may be asymptomatic and have subclinical disease, LIP rarely presents without symptoms. Before the recognition of HIV/AIDS, it was predominantly a condition associated with rheumatologic or autoimmune disorders, such as primary Sjogrën syndrome, rheumatoid arthritis, systemic lupus erythematosis, and other diseases, including myasthenia gravis and chronic active hepatitis. In the context of HIV, LIP is more commonly seen in those of black African or Afro-Caribbean origin, particularly those from Haiti, although this finding may be because it is more frequently looked for in this population.

In DILS, an association with major histocompatibility complex antigens has been described with an increased frequency of HLA-DR5/DR6 in black individuals and HLA-DR7 in white individuals.[15,16] HIV has been detected by in situ hybridization in macrophages within germinal centers of lymphoid tissue, as in persistent generalized lymphadenopathy, and the amount of HIV detected seems to be proportional to the extent of lymphoid aggregates.[17] P24 antigen and antibody to HIV have also been detected in BAL fluid.[18,19] There is no evidence from lung biopsy in HIV-infected adults to support a role for cytomegalovirus or Epstein-Barr virus in the etiology of LIP.

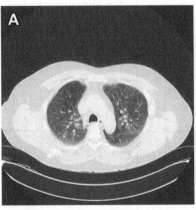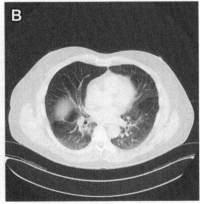

Fig. 2. (*A*) HRCT scan. Nonspecific interstitial pneumonitis, showing patchy "ground glass" infiltrates. (*B*) HRCT scan. Nonspecific interstitial pneumonitis, showing more extensive "ground glass" infiltrates.

Clinical Findings

Patients usually present with a nonproductive cough and progressive exertional dyspnea (see **Table 1**). Associated constitutional symptoms with fevers, weight loss, and fatigue are often prominent features.[20] Rarely, individuals may be asymptomatic but have abnormal radiologic findings.

Where LIP occurs as part of DILS, xerophthalmia and xerostomia may occur. Patients may also report abdominal discomfort caused by hepatosplenomegaly or discomfort after eating if lymphocytic gastritis is a feature. There may also be facial numbness or weakness caused by seventh cranial nerve palsy. Patients may complain of neck stiffness and headache if they have aseptic meningitis.

Examination Findings

Frequently, bibasilar fine crackles or rales may be audible on auscultation of the chest. The chest examination may also demonstrate wheezing.

In patients with DILS, there is also widespread lymphadenopathy, parotid gland enlargement, and salivary gland enlargement.[21] Hepatosplenomegaly commonly occurs. Several neurologic signs have been described: facial nerve palsy (unilateral or bilateral), signs of aseptic meningitis, and, rarely, peripheral motor neuropathy.[16,21]

Diagnosis

Blood tests

Biochemical tests are unhelpful in distinguishing from other causes of pulmonary disease. Serum lactate dehydrogenase may be elevated, but this finding is also seen in PCP. There is commonly a polyclonal gammopathy. The CD4+ T-lymphocyte count is usually within the normal range and not markedly reduced. A variable level of hypoxemia on arterial blood gases occurs, with widening of the A-a gradient. These findings are nonspecific and not helpful in differentiating the underlying cause.

Radiology

The chest radiograph demonstrates the following 3 main patterns of abnormality:

- The presence of fine reticulonodular opacities in a predominantly basal distribution (**Fig. 3**)
- A pattern resembling miliary tuberculosis with larger nodular opacities and reticular infiltrates
- More dense alveolar infiltration with a combination of micronodules and reticular shadowing

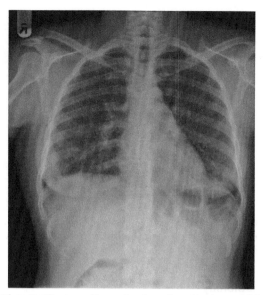

Fig. 3. Chest radiograph. Lymphocytic interstitial pneumonia, showing reticulonodular opacities.

HRCT demonstrates reticular shadowing, centrilobular nodules, and areas of ground glass opacification and interstitial infiltrates (**Fig. 4**A). There may also be evidence of fibrosis and honeycombing that is not visible on the chest radiograph. These changes may result from prolonged inflammation. Bronchiectasis resulting from chronic obstruction of respiratory bronchioles by lymphocytic infiltration may also be seen (see **Fig. 4**B). These features are not diagnostic of LIP, and other causes, such as hypersensitivity pneumonitis, tuberculosis, sarcoidosis, invasive fungal pneumonia, Kaposi sarcoma, and PCP, need to be excluded. In DILS, hepatosplenomegaly is evident on CT along with generalized adenopathy.

There is no role for radionuclide scanning with Gallium-67 in the diagnosis of LIP. Accelerated clearance of Technetium-99m diethylenetriamine penta-acetic acid has been described, but is nonspecific.

Pulmonary function tests

Commonly, there is a restrictive deficit on spirometry and the diffusion capacity is reduced (or occasionally normal). However, obstructive lung function is also described.

Bronchoscopy

BAL fluid demonstrates an abundance of lymphocytes, with a predominance of CD8+, CD44+ T lymphocytes. There is often a mild increase in eosinophils and alveolar macrophages. Viral, bacterial, and fungal pathogens and neoplastic cells should be undetectable.

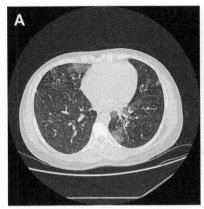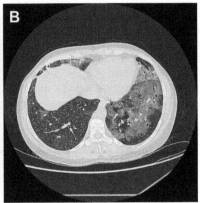

Fig. 4. (A) HRCT scan. Lymphocytic interstitial pneumonia, showing nodules and "ground glass" infiltrates. (B) HRCT scan. Lymphocytic interstitial pneumonia, showing extensive "ground glass" changes, as well as traction bronchiectasis.

Pathology

The diagnosis of LIP is based on characteristic histopathologic appearances and the exclusion of opportunistic infection. Open or video-assisted thoracoscopic (VATS) lung biopsy has a considerably higher yield than transbronchial biopsy. The macroscopic appearances of the lung may be normal. Histologic examination demonstrates the characteristic features of diffuse infiltrates of polyclonal lymphocytes, with occasional plasma cells and histiocytes. The infiltrate extends into alveolar septae along with alveolar aggregates of lymphocytic tissue, which may cause bronchiolitis and small airways plugging. Germinal centers are seen within lymphoid follicles. Hyperplasia of type II pneumocytes is commonly seen. There is no evidence of vasculitis or necrosis. Noncaseating granulomata have been described. Fibrosis may develop in more advanced cases. The main differentiating feature of LIP from NSIP is the extent and degree of lymphocytic infiltration and type II pneumocyte hyperplasia (see **Table 1**).

In DILS, biopsy of salivary and parotid glands demonstrates lymphoid follicles with germinal centers consisting of CD8+ T lymphocytes. There may be preserved architecture or interstitial fibrosis. Noncaseating granulomata are not a feature. Periportal CD8+ T-lymphocytic hepatitis occurs, as can lymphocytic gastric infiltration and thymic enlargement with massive lymphocyte accumulation.[16]

Diagnostic Dilemmas

Opportunistic infection must be excluded when considering a diagnosis of LIP, as the presentation of this condition is similar to that seen in several conditions, including PCP and mycobacterial disease.

Treatment

LIP rarely progresses to respiratory failure and death, particularly in the era of ART. In comparison to LIP in the non-HIV-infected population where prognosis is poor, disease can often be stable for many months without specific treatment. There is evidence for the role of corticosteroids in the treatment of LIP, with variable length of treatment.[15,22] In the case of DILS, more aggressive immunosuppression with chlorambucil has been described.[16]

Early studies reported a variable response to the introduction of zidovudine in the era before ART.[23,24] There are several case reports that suggest that commencement of ART can result in significant improvement of disease without the addition of corticosteroids.[25–27] A recent report describes treatment of LIP with rituximab in an HIV-uninfected adult with Sjögren syndrome,[28] but this treatment modality has not been evaluated in HIV-infected persons.

Lymphocytic Interstitial Pneumonia as Immune Reconstitution

A phenomenon of LIP presenting as an immune reconstitution inflammatory syndrome after commencing ART has been described in one patient.[29] After commencing ART, there was rapid development of a clinical syndrome suggestive of LIP. Opportunistic infection, including PCP, was excluded on BAL, but no lung biopsy was performed to confirm the diagnosis. The patient responded rapidly to corticosteroid treatment.

Complications

Cases of non-HIV LIP have demonstrated germinal center mutations similar to those found in a form of extranodal non-Hodgkin lymphoma (mucosa-associated lymphoid tissue [MALT] lymphoma).[30] BCL-6 gene mutations, found in HIV-associated LIP, are not implicated in the same mechanism of MALT lymphoma, and patients do not seem to progress to MALT lymphoma.[31]

FOLLICULAR BRONCHITIS/BRONCHIOLITIS

Follicular bronchitis/bronchiolitis has been described in rheumatologic conditions as well as in the setting of HIV infection. It represents a comparable disease process to LIP, but with more prominent peribronchiolar germinal centers causing compression of bronchioles and reduced expansion of lymphocytic infiltrate into the interstitium.[4] Clinical presentation and radiological appearances are indistinguishable from LIP and management is similar.

CRYPTOGENIC ORGANIZING PNEUMONIA

Formerly termed bronchiolitis obliterans-organizing pneumonia,[32] cryptogenic organizing pneumonia (COP) can occur in isolation as a separate disease entity or in association with another pulmonary disease, such as adenocarcinoma or PCP. It has been suggested that the incidence of COP has been underestimated as its presentation is similar to that of presumed (ie, empirically diagnosed) PCP, and concomitant corticosteroid use may result in resolution of disease without prior histopathologic confirmation of the presence of COP.[33] COP is most commonly described in patients with previously diagnosed HIV infection; however, there is one case report of COP being the presenting diagnosis of HIV infection.[34] COP as an immune reconstitution disease in association with PCP has been described at all levels of CD4+ T-lymphocyte count as a response to ART initiation.[35–37] Pneumocystis is usually detectable in BAL fluid/induced sputum, and clinical recovery occurs with PCP treatment and corticosteroids.

Clinical Findings

The presenting symptoms of COP are commonly dry nonproductive cough, fevers, weight loss, and exertional dyspnea, similar to those of respiratory infection. Symptom onset can range from acute (several days) to several months' duration.

Examination Findings

Bibasilar or diffuse crackles are audible on auscultation of the chest. Finger clubbing is not usually a feature.

Diagnosis

Blood tests

Inflammatory markers (C-reactive protein, erythrocyte sedimentation rate) are usually elevated. There may be a moderate neutrophilia. ABG demonstrates widening of the A-a gradient with arterial hypoxemia of varying severity.

Radiology

The chest radiograph demonstrates consolidation (either unilateral or bilateral) in a patchy distribution (**Fig. 5**). Presentation with reticulonodular opacities is also described.[34]

HRCT imaging shows that COP most commonly involves the lung bases and lower zones, with a combination of airspace consolidation (air bronchograms may be evident) and nodularity along bronchovascular bundles or larger cavitating nodules with patchy ground glass infiltrates (**Fig. 6**).

Pulmonary function tests

There is a restrictive lung defect with a reduced diffusing capacity for carbon monoxide in most patients. These findings are nonspecific.

Bronchoscopy

BAL fluid demonstrates a lymphocytosis with an increased percentage of CD8+ T lymphocytes. There is often a moderate increase in eosinophils and neutrophils. Viral, bacterial, and fungal pathogens are absent by staining and culture.

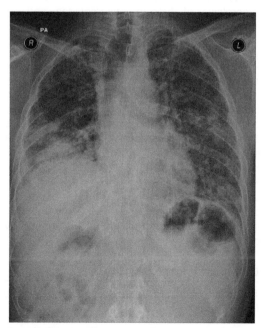

Fig. 5. Chest radiograph. Cryptogenic organizing pneumonia, showing patchy, bilateral consolidation.

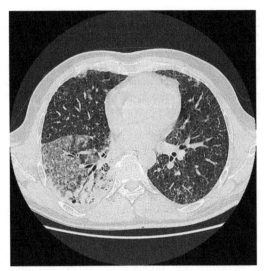

Fig. 6. HRCT scan. Cryptogenic organizing pneumonia, showing (on the *right*) evidence of patchy "ground glass" infiltrates, within which there is airspace consolidation, and air bronchograms.

Transbronchial biopsy may be diagnostic, but open or VATS lung biopsy is preferred.[38]

Pathology

The pathologic features of COP are of an organizing pneumonia that involves alveolar ducts and alveoli; additionally, there may be bronchiolar intraluminal polyps of granulation tissue. Varying degrees of interstitial infiltration can occur with hyperplasia of type II pneumocytes and an increase in foamy macrophages.

Treatment

Treatment with systemic corticosteroids usually results in a rapid and marked improvement; on occasion, high-dose intravenous methylprednisolone may be required. The usual dose is 1 mg/kg oral prednisolone, slowly tapering over several weeks (usually up to 3 months). COP in HIV behaves in a manner similar to that in non-HIV disease. However, caution is advised when using immunosuppressants in this population because of the increased risk of opportunistic infection, particularly those with advanced HIV disease.

Diagnostic Dilemmas

The main differential diagnoses include the following:

- Infection (specifically mycobacterial disease and opportunistic pathogens, including PCP)
- Lung adenocarcinoma (specifically the subtype formerly described as bronchoalveolar cell carcinoma)
- Hypersensitivity pneumonitis (secondary to drugs or other causes)
- Non-Hodgkin lymphoma
- Sarcoidosis

HYPERSENSITIVITY PNEUMONITIS

Hypersensitivity pneumonitis (HP) is well-described in the absence of HIV infection. It presents as either an acute, rapid-onset illness shortly after heavy exposure to a causative agent or as a subacute or chronic illness with gradual onset of exertional dyspnea, dry cough, fatigue, and weight loss generally in association with chronic lower level exposure to an allergen. Lymphocytic inflammation is a feature with a prominent CD8+ T-lymphocyte response in BAL fluid. Because the disease represents a disordered T-cell inflammatory response to an extrinsic allergen, in advanced HIV with relative depletion of both CD4+ and CD8+ lymphocytes, descriptions of HP before the ART era are absent. In the context of HIV infection, case reports largely refer to pneumonitis developing as an immune reconstitution phenomenon after commencement of ART[39] or with chronic allergen exposure.

HP due to drug-induced interstitial lung disease[40] has been described in HIV-infected persons receiving dapsone,[41] efavirenz,[42] and bleomycin.[43,44] Among the general population, drug-induced interstitial lung disease has been described in those receiving rifampicin,[45] isoniazid,[46] and ethambutol,[47] all of which are used for treating tuberculosis in HIV-infected persons.

Clinical Features

Frequently reported symptoms of HP include the following:

- Slowly progressive exertional dyspnea
- Nonproductive cough
- Weight loss
- Fatigue
- Rash

Examination Findings

Examination may be normal. Fine bibasilar end-inspiratory crackles can be present.

Diagnosis

Blood tests

The CD4+ T-lymphocyte count may vary. There may be a peripheral blood eosinophilia. Serum IgG antibodies (precipitins) for sensitizing organic allergens (eg, pigeon) may be tested for if known. A normal result serves only as a marker of exposure and is not diagnostic of HP. The causative agent may not be found.

Radiology

The chest radiograph may demonstrate the following:

- Normal
- Multiple diffuse nodules appearing as diffuse ground glass shadowing (**Fig. 7**).

HRCT The following are radiological features of HP:

- Diffuse or patchy ground glass opacification
- Widespread micronodular opacities (<5 mm diameter)
- Gas trapping, giving rise to the appearance of mosaic attenuation on expiratory films (differential diagnosis = obliterative bronchiolitis) (**Fig. 8**)
- In chronic disease, linear opacities, and fibrosis with honeycombing may occur

Pulmonary function tests

Spirometry demonstrates a restrictive defect of varying degrees of severity depending on the extent of disease. The diffusing capacity for carbon monoxide is usually reduced.

Bronchoscopy and lavage

BAL fluid often contains a predominance of lymphocytes. CD4+ and CD8+ T lymphocytes

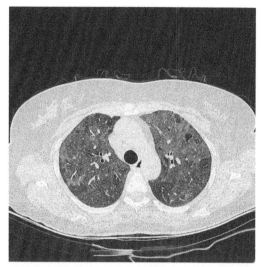

Fig. 8. HRCT scan. Hypersensitivity pneumonitis, showing widespread "ground glass" infiltrates and multiple areas of "mosaic attenuation."

usually occur in similar proportions to those in serum in HP with HIV infection. Eosinophils may be mildly increased.

Pathology

Typical features of HP are as follows:

- Peribronchiolar lymphocyte-dominant inflammatory infiltrates
- Non-necrotizing granulomata may be prominent
- In chronic HP fibrosis is also found

Treatment

With avoidance of the allergen or immediate discontinuation of the suspected causative drug, many patients improve without the need for corticosteroid immunosuppression. In the reported case of immune reconstitution inflammatory syndrome HP, the patient with bird-fancier's lung improved spontaneously on removal of the pets from her home.[39] In severe reactions, systemic treatment with corticosteroids may be required. In chronic disease, where fibrosis has developed (only described in HIV-uninfected HP), treatment may be more difficult. Allergen avoidance is the most important step, but prolonged steroid use may be necessary.

Diagnostic Dilemmas

The main differential diagnoses are as follows:

- Infection (particularly PCP and mycobacterial disease)

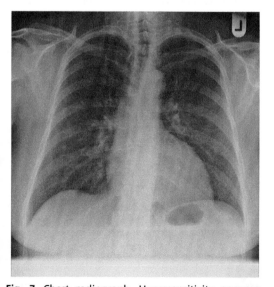

Fig. 7. Chest radiograph. Hypersensitivity pneumonitis, showing subtle bilateral peri-hilar "ground glass" opacities.

- Sarcoidosis
- In fibrotic HP, idiopathic pulmonary fibrosis and NSIP should be considered

SARCOIDOSIS

Sarcoidosis is a granulomatous multisystem disorder that affects the lungs as an isolated organ in approximately 50% of cases. The skin, liver, and eyes are the most common sites of disease outside of the lungs. It is more commonly seen in those of Afro-Caribbean and Scandinavian origin, with a female predominance. In the HIV-uninfected population, it is the second most common form of interstitial lung disease after idiopathic pulmonary fibrosis. Within the lungs, sarcoidosis can cause intrathoracic lymphadenopathy (stage I), lung parenchymal inflammation with mediastinal adenopathy (stage II), parenchymal inflammation with shrinkage of adenopathy (stage III), or fibrotic lung disease (stage IV).

Because patients with HIV frequently have either reduced circulating CD4+ T lymphocytes or dysfunctional T-cell-mediated immunity, the low incidence of sarcoidosis in the literature perhaps comes as no surprise. Nonnecrotizing granulomas in sarcoidosis are usually rich with CD4+ cells. As HIV becomes a more chronic disease with less impairment of cell-mediated immunity, it is likely that sarcoidosis will increase in incidence. Findings from a case series of coexistent sarcoidosis and HIV demonstrated CD4+ T-lymphocyte counts consistently greater than 200 cells/μL. The authors concluded that the development of sarcoidosis depends on an adequate absolute CD4+ T-lymphocyte count and, where counts are lower than 200 cells/μL, alternative infectious diagnoses, such as mycobacterial infection, should be considered.[48]

Case reports of coexistent sarcoidosis and HIV describe either an immune reconstitution phenomenon after commencing ART[48-50] or a recurrence of previous disease once HIV has been treated and the patient has achieved relative immunocompetence.[51,52] In the setting of HIV, it is extremely rare for sarcoidosis to present without either pulmonary involvement or mediastinal lymphadenopathy.

Clinical Findings

Patients may be asymptomatic. Commonly occurring symptoms are as follows:

- Cough— usually nonproductive
- Exertional dyspnea
- Fevers and night sweats may be a feature
- Symptoms related to extrapulmonary disease (anterior uveitis, granulomatous hepatitis, skin rashes, and lymphadenopathy)

Examination Findings

Physical examination is often normal. Bibasilar crackles can be heard on auscultation of the chest. Rash (papular or nodular skin lesions, lupus pernio, erythema nodosum) may be observed.

Diagnosis

Blood tests

CD4+ T-lymphocyte count is usually greater than 200 cells/μl. There may be mild anemia and a raised C-reactive protein or erythrocyte sedimentation rate. Serum angiotensin-converting enzyme levels are usually normal.

There is arterial hypoxemia in severe disease.

Radiology

Chest radiograph The chest radiograph may be normal in extrapulmonary involvement.

- Stage I: bilateral hilar adenopathy (BHL) (± right paratracheal adenopathy) (**Fig. 9**)
- Stage II: BHL and reticulonodular opacities (upper zone predominance less marked than in HIV-uninfected disease)
- Stage III: reticulonodular opacities in the absence of mediastinal adenopathy
- Stage IV: reticular opacification, small volume lungs, traction bronchiectasis, and fibrosis may be present

In disease in the HIV-uninfected population, sarcoidosis can mimic many other conditions on

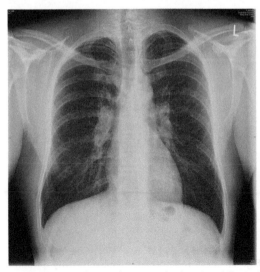

Fig. 9. Chest radiograph. Sarcoid, showing bilateral hilar lymphadenopathy.

HRCT examination, although there are some characteristic features. With coexistent HIV, the usual presentation is with bilateral interstitial shadowing or mediastinal adenopathy.

The following HRCT findings are all described in sarcoidosis:

- Hilar and mediastinal adenopathy
- Beading of fissures, alveolar septae, and bronchovascular bundles (**Fig. 10**)
- Subpleural and peribronchial nodules
- Diffuse ground glass infiltrates
- Consolidation with air bronchograms
- Traction bronchiectasis and honeycombing

Pulmonary function tests

There may be a restrictive lung defect, reduction in vital capacity, and reduced diffusing capacity for carbon monoxide. The vital capacity has most commonly been used in monitoring of disease, but it is recommended that lung function testing is repeated at regular intervals, and the indices that show most change are used to monitor for evidence of disease progression.

Bronchoscopy

BAL fluid shows a predominance of lymphocytes. Samples should be negative for neoplastic cells and mycobacterial and fungal culture. In suspected sarcoidosis in HIV-uninfected individuals, the yield from multiple transbronchial biopsies is high (up to 90%), but there is a risk of pneumothorax. Bronchial biopsies demonstrate nonnecrotizing granulomata in a significant proportion of patients (even in macroscopically normal airways)

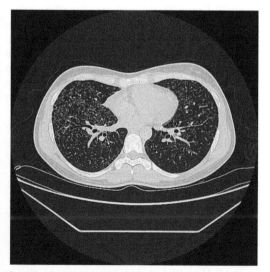

Fig. 10. HRCT scan. Sarcoid, showing multiple intrapulmonary nodules (more marked on the *right*) and fissural beading (more marked on the *left*).

and are safe. However, the diagnosis of sarcoid is not always obvious and therefore VATS or open lung biopsy may be required if another form of idiopathic interstitial pneumonia is suspected.

Endoscopic ultrasound-guided aspiration of mediastinal lymph nodes (either via bronchoscope or gastroscope) is useful for obtaining confirmation of granulomatous inflammation in the presence of negative mycobacterial culture.[53]

Pathology

The pathologic feature of sarcoidosis is the demonstration of nonnecrotizing granulomata in the absence of any microorganism or neoplasm, in the context of an appropriate clinical presentation. There is often some difficulty securing the diagnosis because there is considerable overlap between the symptoms and signs of sarcoidosis and features found in HIV (either because of disease, drug toxicity, or coexistent infection).

Treatment

As most cases of stage I, II, and III sarcoidosis spontaneously remit in HIV-uninfected persons, specific therapeutic intervention is often not required. If lung function is declining or if patients are highly symptomatic, systemic corticosteroids are indicated with starting doses of 0.5 mg/kg prednisolone per day recommended with a slow taper. Among HIV-infected patients who are taking a protease inhibitor, care should be taken with the dose of steroid, because this class of drugs partially block metabolism of corticosteroids, leading to an increased risk of Cushing syndrome. In addition, careful monitoring is warranted to avoid the risk of the patient developing an opportunistic infection while in receiving corticosteroids. The prognosis of sarcoidosis in HIV-infected persons seems to be comparable to that in the HIV-uninfected population.[52] Cessation of ART has not been required if sarcoidosis has presented as an immune reconstitution phenomenon.[52]

Diagnostic Dilemmas

Rigorous exclusion of opportunistic infections or neoplasm must be performed before settling on a diagnosis of sarcoidosis. Common differential diagnoses are as follows:

- Mycobacterial infection (tuberculosis, nontuberculous mycobacterial infection)
- Fungal infection: Cryptococcosis, histoplasmosis, PCP
- Toxoplasmosis
- Lymphoma
- Hypersensitivity pneumonitis

IDIOPATHIC PULMONARY FIBROSIS

Despite being the most common form of interstitial pneumonia in the HIV-uninfected population,[54] there are no reports of idiopathic pulmonary fibrosis in the context of HIV. It is possible that cases will occur with the advent of ART and with HIV becoming a disease of "chronicity."

SUMMARY

Among HIV-infected adults, a spectrum of noninfectious, nonmalignant lymphocytic infiltrative pulmonary disorders, including nonspecific interstitial pneumonitis and lymphocytic interstitial pneumonitis, were frequently described in the era before the introduction of ART. Following the introduction and uptake of ART, these conditions have been less commonly encountered by clinicians, possibly as a consequence of the effects of ART on pulmonary immunology, resulting in the prevention of the development of symptomatic disease. Reports of sarcoidosis among HIV-infected persons were uncommon in the pre-ART era; yet, by contrast, sarcoidosis is increasingly recognized in the post-ART era and may represent an immune reconstitution phenomenon. Other causes of pneumonitis, including cryptogenic organizing pneumonia and drug-induced hypersensitivity pneumonitis, are infrequently encountered among HIV-infected persons.

REFERENCES

1. Murray JF, Felton CP, Garay SM, et al. Pulmonary complications of the acquired immunodeficiency syndrome. Report of a National Heart, Lung, and Blood Institute workshop. N Engl J Med 1984;310: 1682–8.
2. Murray JF, Garay SM, Hopewell PC, et al. NHLBI workshop summary. Pulmonary complications of the acquired immunodeficiency syndrome: an update. Report of the second National Heart, Lung and Blood Institute workshop. Am Rev Respir Dis 1987;135:504–9.
3. Saukkonen JJ, Farber HW. Lymphocytic interstitial pneumonitis. In: Zumla A, Miller RF, Johnson MA, editors. AIDS and respiratory medicine. London: Chapman and Hall; 1996. p. 331–43.
4. Semple SJ. Non-neoplastic lymphoproliferative disorders. In: Semple SJ, Miller RF, editors. AIDS and the lung. Oxford (United Kingdom): Blackwell Science; 1997. p. 182–94.
5. Ong EL, Mandal BK. Primary HIV-1 infection associated with pneumonitis. Postgrad Med J 1991;67: 579–80.
6. Griffiths MH, Miller RF, Semple SJ. Interstitial pneumonitis in patients infected with the human immunodeficiency virus. Thorax 1995;50:1141–6.
7. Travis WD, Fox CH, Devaney KO, et al. Lymphoid pneumonitis in 50 adult patients infected with the human immunodeficiency virus: lymphocytic interstitial pneumonitis versus nonspecific interstitial pneumonitis. Hum Pathol 1992;23:529–41.
8. Suffredini AF, Ognibene FP, Lack EE, et al. Nonspecific interstitial pneumonitis: a common cause of pulmonary disease in the acquired immunodeficiency syndrome. Ann Intern Med 1987;107:7–13.
9. Benfield T. Non-infectious conditions in patients with human immunodeficiency virus infection. In: Spiro SG, Silvestri GA, Augusti A, editors. Clinical respiratory medicine. 4th edition. Philadelphia: Elsevier Science; 2012.
10. Sattler F, Nichols L, Hirano L, et al. Nonspecific interstitial pneumonitis mimicking Pneumocystis carinii pneumonia. Am J Respir Crit Care Med 1997;156: 912–7.
11. Thormar H. Maedi-visna virus and its relationship to human immunodeficiency virus. AIDS Rev 2005;7: 233–45.
12. Lairmore MD, Poulson JM, Adducci TA, et al. Lentivirus-induced lymphoproliferative disease. Comparative pathogenicity of phenotypically distinct ovine lentivirus strains. Am J Pathol 1988;130:80–90.
13. Ognibene FP, Masur H, Rogers P, et al. Nonspecific interstitial pneumonia without evidence of Pneumocystis carinii in asymptomatic patients infected with human immunodeficiency virus (HIV). Ann Intern Med 1988;109:874–9.
14. Hauber HP, Bittmann I, Kirsten D. Non-specific interstitial pneumonia (NSIP). Pneumologie 2011;65(8): 477–83 [in German].
15. Kazi S, Cohen PR, Williams F, et al. The diffuse infiltrative lymphocytosis syndrome. Clinical and immunogenetic features in 35 patients. AIDS 1996;10:385–91.
16. Itescu S, Brancato LJ, Buxbaum J, et al. A diffuse infiltrative CD8 lymphocytosis syndrome in human immunodeficiency virus (HIV) infection: a host immune response associated with HLA-DR5. Ann Intern Med 1990;112:3–10.
17. Montagnier L, Gruest J, Chamaret S, et al. Adaptation of lymphadenopathy associated virus (LAV) to replication in EBV-transformed B lymphoblastoid cell lines. Science 1984;225:63–6.
18. Linnemann CC Jr, Baughman RP, Frame PT, et al. Recovery of human immunodeficiency virus and detection of p24 antigen in bronchoalveolar lavage fluid from adult patients with AIDS. Chest 1989;96:64–7.
19. Teirstein AS, Rosen MJ. Lymphocytic interstitial pneumonia. Clin Chest Med 1988;9:467–71.
20. Das S, Miller RF. Lymphocytic interstitial pneumonitis in HIV-infected adults. Sex Transm Infect 2003;79: 88–93.

21. Basu D, Williams FM, Ahn CW, et al. Changing spectrum of the diffuse infiltrative lymphocytosis syndrome. Arthritis Rheum 2006;55:466–72.

22. Solal-Celigny P, Couderc LJ, Herman D, et al. Lymphoid interstitial pneumonitis in acquired immunodeficiency syndrome-related complex. Am Rev Respir Dis 1985;131:956–60.

23. Bach MC. Zidovudine for lymphocytic interstitial pneumonia associated with AIDS. Lancet 1987; 2:796.

24. Lin RY, Gruber PJ, Saunders R, et al. Lymphocytic interstitial pneumonitis in adult HIV infection. N Y State J Med 1988;88:273–6.

25. Scarborough M, Lishman S, Shaw P, et al. Lymphocytic interstitial pneumonitis in an HIV-infected adult: response to antiretroviral therapy. Int J STD AIDS 2000;11:119–22.

26. Innes AL, Huang L, Nishimura SL. Resolution of lymphocytic interstitial pneumonitis in an HIV-infected adult after treatment with HAART. Sex Transm Infect 2004;80:417–8.

27. Ripamonti D, Rizzi M, Maggiolo F, et al. Resolution of lymphocytic interstitial pneumonia in a human immunodeficiency virus-infected adult following the start of highly active antiretroviral therapy. Scand J Infect Dis 2003;35:348–51.

28. Swartz MA, Vivino FB. Dramatic reversal of lymphocytic interstitial pneumonitis in Sjogren's syndrome with rituximab. J Clin Rheumatol 2011;17(8):454.

29. Ingiliz P, Appenrodt B, Gruenhage F, et al. Lymphoid pneumonitis as an immune reconstitution inflammatory syndrome in a patient with CD4 cell recovery after HAART initiation. HIV Med 2006;7:411–4.

30. Kurosu K, Weiden MD, Takiguchi Y, et al. BCL-6 mutations in pulmonary lymphoproliferative disorders: demonstration of an aberrant immunological reaction in HIV-related lymphoid interstitial pneumonia. J Immunother 2004;172:7116–22.

31. Isaacson P, Wright DH. Malignant lymphoma of mucosa-associated lymphoid tissue. A distinctive type of B-cell lymphoma. Cancer 1983;52:1410–6.

32. American Thoracic Society, European Respiratory Society. American Thoracic Society/European respiratory Society International Multidisciplinary Consensus Classification of the idiopathic interstitial pneumonias. Am J Respir Crit Care Med 2002;165:277–304.

33. Joseph J, Harley RA, Frye MD. Bronchiolitis obliterans with organizing pneumonia in AIDS. N Engl J Med 1995;332:273.

34. Khater FJ, Moorman JP, Myers JW, et al. Bronchiolitis obliterans organizing pneumonia as a manifestation of AIDS: case report and literature review. J Infect 2004;49:159–64.

35. Mori S, Polatino S, Estrada YM. Pneumocystis-associated organizing pneumonia as a manifestation of immune reconstitution inflammatory syndrome in an HIV-infected individual with a normal CD4+ T-cell count following antiretroviral therapy. Int J STD AIDS 2009;20:662–5.

36. Godoy MC, Silva CI, Ellis J, et al. Organizing pneumonia as a manifestation of Pneumocystis jiroveci immune reconstitution syndrome in HIV-positive patients: report of 2 cases. J Thorac Imaging 2008;23:39–43.

37. Takahashi T, Nakamura T, Iwamoto A. Reconstitution of immune responses to Pneumocystis carinii pneumonia in patients with HIV infection who receive highly active antiretroviral therapy. Res Commun Mol Pathol Pharmacol 2002;112:59–67.

38. Miller RF, Pugsley WB, Griffiths MH. Open lung biopsy for investigation of acute respiratory episodes in patients with HIV infection and AIDS. Genitourin Med 1995;71:280–5.

39. Morris AM, Nishimura S, Huang L. Subacute hypersensitivity pneumonitis in an HIV-infected patient receiving antiretroviral therapy. Thorax 2000;55: 625–7.

40. Matsuno O. Drug-induced interstitial lung disease: mechanisms and best diagnostic approaches. Respir Res 2012;13:39.

41. Tobin-D'Angelo MJ, Hoteit MA, Brown KV, et al. Dapsone-induced hypersensitivity pneumonitis mimicking Pneumocystis carinii pneumonia in a patient with AIDS. Am J Med Sci 2004;327:163–5.

42. Behrens GM, Stoll M, Schmidt RE. Pulmonary hypersensitivity reaction induced by efavirenz. Lancet 2001;357:1503–4.

43. Denton AS, Simpson JK, Hallam M, et al. Effects on pulmonary function of two regimens of chemotherapy for AIDS-related Kaposi's sarcoma. Clin Oncol 1996;8:48–50.

44. Ezzat HM, Cheung MC, Hicks LK, et al. Incidence, predictors and significance of severe toxicity in patients with human immunodeficiency virus-associated Hodgkin lymphoma. Leuk Lymphoma 2012;53(12):2390–6.

45. Kunichika N, Miyahara N, Kotani K, et al. Pneumonitis induced by rifampicin. Thorax 2002;57:1000–1.

46. Endo T, Saito T, Nakayama M, et al. A case of isoniazid-induced pneumonitis. Nihon Kokyuki Gakkai Zasshi 1998;36:100–5.

47. Takami A, Nakao S, Asakura H, et al. Pneumonitis and eosinophilia induced by ethambutol. J Allergy Clin Immunol 1997;100:712–3.

48. Morris DG, Jasmer RM, Huang L, et al. Sarcoidosis following HIV infection: evidence for CD4+ lymphocyte dependence. Chest 2003;124:929–35.

49. Naccache JM, Antoine M, Wislez M, et al. Sarcoid-like pulmonary disorder in human immunodeficiency virus-infected patients receiving antiretroviral therapy. Am J Respir Crit Care Med 1999;159: 2009–13.

50. Mirmirani P, Maurer TA, Herndier B, et al. Sarcoidosis in a patient with AIDS: a manifestation of

immune restoration syndrome. J Am Acad Dermatol 1999;41:285–6.

51. Lenner R, Bregman Z, Teirstein AS, et al. Recurrent pulmonary sarcoidosis in HIV-infected patients receiving highly active antiretroviral therapy. Chest 2001;119(3):978–81.

52. Booth HL, Miller RF. Human immunodeficiency virus infection. In: Mitchell D, Wells AU, Spiro SG, et al, editors. Sarcoidosis. London: Hodder Arnold; 2012. p. 345–56.

53. Navani N, Booth HL, Kocjan G, et al. Combination of endobronchial ultrasound-guided transbronchial needle aspiration with standard bronchoscopic techniques for the diagnosis of stage I and stage II pulmonary sarcoidosis. Respirology 2011;16:467–72.

54. Raghu G, Collard HR, Egan JJ, et al. An official ATS/ERS/JRS/ALAT statement: idiopathic pulmonary fibrosis: evidence-based guidelines for diagnosis and management. Am J Respir Crit Care Med 2011;183:788–824.

Critical Care of Persons Infected with the Human Immunodeficiency Virus

Anuradha Ganesan, MBBS, MPH[a],*, Henry Masur, MD[b]

KEYWORDS

- ICU • HIV • AIDS • Antiretroviral therapy

KEY POINTS

- In the current antiretroviral therapy (ART) era, the spectrum of illnesses that necessitate admissions to an intensive care unit (ICU) in persons infected with the human immunodeficiency virus (HIV) has shifted; non-AIDS events account for more than half of all ICU admissions in the United States. AIDS-related opportunistic infections remain an important cause of admissions in newly diagnosed individuals and those not on ART.
- Noninfectious complications of HIV/AIDS, such as accelerated atherosclerotic cardiovascular disease and malignancies, must be retained in the differential while evaluating the critically ill patient infected with HIV.
- Immune reconstitution inflammatory syndrome associated with ART initiation and ART-related toxicities may necessitate ICU admission and should be recognized.
- ART should rarely be initiated in the ICU. For patients who are receiving ART, therapy should be continued in most patients who are likely to absorb oral medications, but such decisions and strategies should be developed with an expert.

INTRODUCTION

Individuals infected with the human immunodeficiency virus (HIV) who are admitted to the intensive care unit (ICU) can be grouped into 3 distinct populations. The first group includes individuals admitted to the ICU with an AIDS-related opportunistic infection (OI) such as *Pneumocystis jirovecii* pneumonia (PCP). Antiretroviral therapy (ART) has had a dramatic effect in reducing the incidence of OIs for those patients who have access to care and who are adherent to therapy. However, in the United States, only about 20% of patients are well controlled virologically.[1] The others are unaware of their HIV status, do not have access to care, or are not successfully controlled because

Acknowledgement: Supported by the Infectious Disease Clinical Research Program (IDCRP), a Department of Defense (DoD) program executed through the Uniformed Services University of the Health Sciences. This project has been funded in whole, or in part with federal funds from the National Institute of Allergy and Infectious Diseases, National Institutes of Health (NIH), under Inter-Agency Agreement Y1-AI-5072.

Disclaimer: The content of this publication is the sole responsibility of the authors and does not necessarily reflect the views or policies of the National Institutes of Health or the Department of Health and Human Services, the DoD, or the Departments of the Army, Navy, or Air Force. Mention of trade names, commercial products, or organizations does not imply endorsement by the U.S. Government.

[a] Department of Medicine, Division of Infectious Diseases, Walter Reed National Military Medical Center, Uniformed Services University of the Health Sciences, 8901, Wisconsin Avenue, Building 7, Room 1416, Bethesda, MD 20889, USA; [b] Critical Care Medicine Department, NIH Clinical Center, 10 Center Drive, Bethesda, MD 20892, USA

* Corresponding author.
E-mail address: Anuradha.ganesan.civ@health.mil

Clin Chest Med 34 (2013) 307–323
http://dx.doi.org/10.1016/j.ccm.2013.01.011
0272-5231/13/$ – see front matter

chestmed.theclinics.com

of adherence challenges or other issues. Thus, many hospitals continue to see OIs, especially in the 12 US cities that are home to 50% of the total HIV population.[2] Intensivists must be well versed in the management of AIDS-related OIs. The second group is those who are immunologically reconstituted but receive care in the ICU for a non-HIV-related condition such as complications of elective surgery, trauma-related admissions, pancreatitis, and gastrointestinal bleeding. Unique challenges faced in this group relate to the management of ART in the ICU, which requires knowledge about how to administer ART to preserve antiretroviral efficacy, the recognition of ART-related toxicities, and a critical understanding of the potential for drug-drug interactions with ICU medications. The third group is those admitted to the ICU for noninfectious complications of HIV/AIDS that are related to the enhanced inflammatory condition observed in patients infected with HIV.[3] Accelerated atherosclerotic cardiovascular and cerebrovascular disease and renal, hepatic, and neurocognitive disorders should be recognized as possibly HIV-related, as should solid tumors and hematologic malignant neoplastic diseases that were not traditionally linked to HIV/AIDS. In this review, recent advances in our understanding of immune reconstitution inflammatory syndrome (IRIS) are highlighted, management of some OIs is discussed, and the challenges of managing ART in the ICU are addressed.

THE STATE OF HIV INFECTION IN THE UNITED STATES

Although potent ART has been available since 1996, it is estimated that only 1 in 5 persons infected with HIV in the United States is receiving effective therapy and has an undetectable viral load.[1] In the United States, between 22% and 52% of individuals infected with HIV report ART use at ICU admission (**Table 1**).[4–10] Hence, not unexpectedly, even in the current ART era, 21% to 44% of all ICU admissions are caused by an AIDS-related illness (see **Table 1**).[5,8,9]

San Francisco General Hospital (SFGH) has carefully assessed their ICU admissions over the past 2 decades.[8–11] At SFGH, admissions to the ICU have declined,[9] and the spectrum of diseases that necessitate ICU admissions has shifted.[8–10] More than 60% of the admissions in the current ART era are attributed to a non-AIDS-related diagnosis.[8,9] Compared with the earliest ART era, in-hospital survival has significantly improved; although this finding could represent a shift in patient demographics, it more likely relates to the shift from AIDS-related to AIDS-unrelated diagnoses in

a city in which HIV services are highly developed. However, in more recent years (2005–2009), in-hospital mortality seems to have plateaued.[9]

SURVIVAL

In the combination ART era in the United States, between 56% and 71% of patients infected with HIV survive their stay in the ICU and are discharged alive from the hospital.[4–10] Similar rates (43%–80%) have been reported from Europe (see **Table 1**).[12–20] Survival rates clearly reflect the patient population being served: hospitals serving patients infected with HIV who present with OIs have higher mortality. In Brazil, where a high fraction of ICU admissions are HIV/AIDS-related, only a third survived their hospitalization.[21] Similarly, in other parts of the world where AIDS-related admissions predominate, mortality is higher.[22,23]

In the United States and Great Britain, short-term outcomes for patients infected with HIV and uninfected patients admitted to the ICU seem similar.[6,12,15] A 2007 British study reported similar survival rates among adult patients infected with HIV and uninfected adult patients admitted to a London ICU for a general medical condition of 65% and 68%, respectively.[15] In a US study that examined patients with acute lung injury, survivors infected with HIV and uninfected survivors spent similar number of days in the ICU (median length of stay: 12 vs 15 days) and in the hospital (median length of stay: 29 vs 25 days). ICU and hospital mortality were also comparable between the 2 groups, with 56% of the individuals infected with HIV and 61% of uninfected individuals surviving their hospitalization.[6]

ART use seems to positively affect long-term survival.[9,14,24] The effect of ART on short-term outcomes is mixed, with some studies showing improved outcomes with ART use, whereas others have failed to show a benefit.[8,10,12] **Table 1** and **Fig. 1** detail overall survival rates and survival by ART use.

SPECTRUM OF DISEASES NECESSITATING ICU ADMISSION

Respiratory failure remains the most common reason for ICU admissions for patients infected with HIV, accounting for 30% to 40% of all ICU admissions.[4,7,8,10,12,14,15,19] However, the proportion of ICU admissions related to respiratory failure has been decreasing. In a series from San Francisco, ICU admissions related to respiratory distress declined from 52% in 2000 to 34% in 2004.[8]

The cause of respiratory failure varies according to ART use. Although overall rates of respiratory failure caused by PCP have declined, among untreated individuals, PCP remains the leading cause of respiratory failure.[7,8,10,12] Streptococcus pneumoniae is also a common cause of pneumonia and respiratory failure.[13] Tuberculosis (TB) and fungal diseases are not common causes in most parts of the United States, unless there is an unusual demographic. Some pathogens that can cause substantial pulmonary morbidity in other populations, such as cytomegalovirus (CMV), atypical mycobacteria, or herpes simplex virus (HSV), are uncommon causes of clinically significant pulmonary disease among individuals infected with HIV.[13] Among ART-treated individuals, respiratory failure is often caused by complications associated with entities common in the general population, such as cardiogenic pulmonary edema, chronic obstructive pulmonary disease, community-acquired pneumonia, or adult respiratory distress syndrome caused by sepsis or trauma.[8,13] Sepsis accounts for between 15% and 30% of all ICU admissions for persons infected with HIV.[7,8,14,23] The causes of sepsis mirror the general population. Neurologic problems, such as AIDS-related cryptococcal meningitis (CM) and AIDS-unrelated events such as intracranial hemorrhage, account for 12% to 26% of all ICU admissions.[4,8,10,12,14,19] About half of the ICU admissions are now non-AIDS-related.[7-10,12,24] Non-AIDS admissions are varied in their cause and include admissions for gastrointestinal bleeding, cardiac disorders, metabolic complications, or those that follow elective surgery and trauma. The epidemiology and demographics of such patients mirror the HIV-uninfected populations.

RESPIRATORY DISTRESS

Intensivists need to clearly understand the relationship of recent CD4 count to the likely cause of respiratory disease. Although CD4 counts are not absolute indicators of susceptibility, in HIV disease they are extremely sensitive and specific markers for susceptibility to opportunistic pathogens. For example, PCP is more likely at a CD4 count less than 200 cells/μL compared with patients with higher CD4 counts.[25]

Patients admitted to the ICU with severe respiratory failure and HIV/AIDS are often assumed to have an infectious cause and are treated accordingly, yet intensivists must be vigilant to recognize noninfectious causes, many of which are similar to the HIV-uninfected population.[6,13] Patients infected with HIV are not any less susceptible than the general population to non-OIs such as influenza, respiratory syncytial virus, atypical pneumonias, exacerbations of chronic obstructive lung disease, asthma, ischemic cardiac disease, or to the occurrence of pulmonary emboli. Some noninfectious entities may occur more frequently in patients infected with HIV, such as congestive heart failure related to accelerated ischemic heart disease despite apparently adequate HIV viral suppression, or AIDS-related or ostensibly non-AIDS-related malignant neoplasms.[26,27]

Pulmonary Kaposi sarcoma (KS) and lymphoma are well recognized to occur with enhanced frequency among patients infected with HIV and can be confused with infectious processes when they occur in the lungs. KS can present as diffuse infiltrates, and the disease is often more subacute than typical bacterial or viral pneumonias. Patients may not have apparent cutaneous lesions.[28] Classically, pulmonary KS has been associated with bloody pleural effusions, but many patients do not have these effusions. The diagnosis can be established by visualizing endobronchial lesions and ruling out concurrent infections. Pulmonary KS is generally treated with systemic chemotherapy such as liposomal doxorubicin. Pulmonary lymphoma is often but not invariably associated with mediastinal adenopathy and extrapulmonary disease, but biopsy is required to establish this as the cause of pulmonary dysfunction, and concurrent infection must be ruled out.

Primary effusion cell lymphoma (PEL) is closely associated with HIV/AIDS. This unusual lymphoproliferative disorder is etiologically linked to human herpes virus 8.[29] Classic PEL originates in the serosal surface and can involve the pleura, pericardium, and peritoneum. Patients present with dyspnea, and radiographic imaging shows the presence of pleural/pericardial effusions usually without any accompanying parenychymal findings. The pleural fluid is exudative and shows the presence of malignant cells. Although a variety of approaches have been attempted, treatment of PEL is not highly effective.

When patients infected with HIV are admitted to the ICU with respiratory compromise or failure, the strategic management approach is not dramatically different from HIV-uninfected patients. In each population, there is an urgency to obtain a specific diagnosis so that therapy can be directed and not overly broad. If the patient seems to have an infectious process after blood cultures are obtained, and the patient can produce sputum, a conventional battery of stains, cultures, and molecular tests should be performed to assess the cause. If this strategy does not yield a pathogen, bronchoalveolar lavage usually suffices to identify the most likely bacterial, fungal, viral, and mycobacterial pathogens. Patients infected with

Table 1
Outcomes and characteristics of critically ill persons infected with HIV admitted to the ICU

Reference	Year Studied	Sample Size	Overall ICU/Hospital Survival (%)	Survival in ART Treated (%)	Survival in ART Untreated (%)	AIDS-Related Admission (%)	Newly Diagnosed HIV Infection at Hospitalization (%)	% on ART at ICU/Hospital Admission
United States								
Morris et al, 2002[10]	1996–1999	295	71[a]	80[a]	69[a,b]	37	5.6	25
Khouli et al, 2005[4]	1997–1999	259	70/61	51/56	49/44	60	NA	48
Narasimhan et al, 2004[7,c]	2001	53	71[a]	71[a]	49[a,b,d]	33	NA	52
Powell et al, 2009[8,e]	2000–2004	281	69[a]	70[a]	67[a]	21	NA	33
Mendez-Tellez et al, 2010[6,f]	2004–2007	66	59/56	60[a]	54[a]	NA	9	38
Greenberg et al, 2012[5,e,g]	2006–2009	120	58[a]	64[a]	55[a]	44	11	22
Yoon et al, 2011[9]	2005–2009	219	68[a]	NA	NA	24.8	NA	51
Europe								
Casalino et al, 2004[14]	1995–1996	196	77[e]	80[d,e]	73[d,e]	58	42	3
	1997–1999	230				37	40	28
Vincent et al, 2004[18]	1995–1996	189	74[e]	75[d,e]	73[d,e]	55	20	3
	1998–2000	236				50	28	50
Palacios et al, 2006[17]	1990–1996	17	33[a]	60[a]	40[a]	47[h]	35	NA
	1997–2003	49	43[a]			61[h]	31	31

Study	Years	N						
Dickson et al, 2007[15]	1999–2005	102	76/66	78/67	75/66	67[h]	27	37
Barbier et al, 2009[13,f]	1996–2006	147	88/80	70[a]	85[a]	50	29	29
Van Lelyveld et al, 2011[20]	1990–1996	47	53/40	65/45	71/61	55	16	0
	1996–2002	42	59/45			52	8	26
	2003–2008	38	79/66			47	15	47
Morquin et al, 2012[19]	1997–2008	98	63/47	61[e]	63[e]	26	8	45
Adlakha et al, 2011[12]	1999–2005	102	79/72	87/80[b]	75/67[b]	67[h]	27	37
	2006–2009	90				34[h]	10	60
Asia and South America								
Vargaz-Infante et al, 2007[22]	1986–1993	16	13[e]	Not applicable	13[e]	94	25	0
	1993–1996	22	29[e]	Not applicable	29[e]	76	48	0
	1996–2006	53	57[e]	NA	NA	77	26	28
Croda et al, 2009[21]	1996–2006	278	45/33	47[e]	42[e]	81	38	45
Chiang et al, 2011[23]	2001–2010	135	63/51	NA	NA	NA	44	36

Abbreviation: NA, data not available.
[a] Survival to hospital discharge.
[b] *P* value significant.
[c] Compared precombination and postcombination ART patients: compared 65 admissions between 1991 and 1992 with 63 admissions in the combination ART era (2001).
[d] Precombination and postcombination ART eras were compared.
[e] ICU survival.
[f] All admissions in this series were for acute lung injury.
[g] All admissions in this series were for a diagnosis of sepsis.
[h] HIV-related but not necessarily AIDS-related admissions.

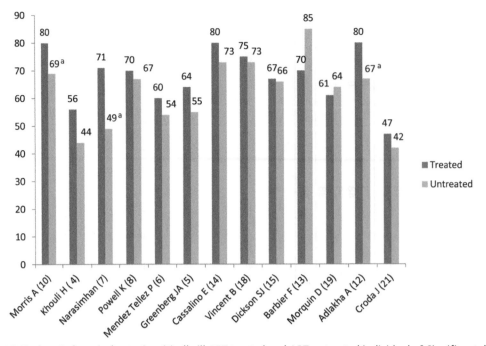

Fig. 1. ICU/in-hospital survival rates in critically ill ART-treated and ART-untreated individuals. [a] Significant differences were observed by ART use.

HIV have a wider differential diagnosis such that additional tests for pathogens such as *Pneumocystis*, *Histoplasma*, and *Mycobacterium tuberculosis* must be added depending on the clinical presentation and the epidemiology of the patient.

When there is suspicion of a noninfectious process in patients with HIV/AIDS, the diagnostic approach needs to focus on modalities that detect the cardiac, neoplastic, embolic, or other processes that might be involved. Similarly, in terms of empiric therapy, the approaches should follow the options discussed in the accompanying article on evaluation of respiratory disease in HIV/AIDS elsewhere in this issue by Laurence Huang.

Intensivists need to be cognizant of the possibility that patients infected with HIV may need to be placed in respiratory isolation. TB is a consideration depending on patient demographics and exposures. Among patients infected with HIV residing in the United States without obvious exposure, TB is surprisingly rare. Most cases among patients infected with HIV occur in those coming from endemic areas who reactivate their TB in the United States.[30] However, the principle remains that respiratory isolation should be carefully considered for all patients with HIV/AIDS admitted to the ICU with apparent respiratory infection. For a more detailed review on specific pneumonias and respiratory disorders, the reader is referred to other articles elsewhere in this issue.

SEPSIS

When patients infected with HIV or uninfected patients present with distributive shock, sepsis is the most likely explanation. However, in approaching such patients, intensivists need to consider HIV-related syndromes that may masquerade as sepsis, such as IRIS.

In the combination ART era, sepsis-related admissions seem to be increasing.[8,14] In a French study,[14] the relative proportion of patients who had sepsis listed as the main indication for their ICU admission increased from 3% in the precombination ART era to 22.6% in the postcombination ART era. The cause, diagnosis, and management of sepsis in patients with HIV do not differ substantially from other patient populations with similar non-HIV-related risk factors. Patients infected with HIV who are intravenous drug abusers or who have indwelling intravascular catheters develop infections caused by *Staphylococcus epidermidis*, *Staphylococcus aureus*, or gram-negative bacillary sepsis just as HIV-uninfected patients do.[5] Patients who are admitted to the ICU with non-HIV-related problems such as pneumonia, urosepsis, biliary complications, or diverticulitis, for example, develop the complications expected by the anatomy and microbiology of their disease.

Patients infected with HIV are predisposed to some causes of bacterial sepsis. In the United

States, the introduction of ART has resulted in declines in the rates of invasive pneumococcal disease; nevertheless, the risk of invasive pneumococcal infection remains substantially higher in individuals when compared with uninfected individuals.[31] Although *Streptococcus pneumoniae* is most common in patients infected with HIV with CD4 counts less than 100 cells/μL, pneumococcal pneumonia and pneumococcal sepsis occur with enhanced frequency, and perhaps with enhanced severity, at every CD4 count stratum. Fungi are also occasional causes of sepsis in patients with HIV infection.[5] *Cryptococcus* and histoplasma are important causes of fungemia, especially in patients with CD4 counts less than 100 cells/μL. Not all patients with cryptococcal sepsis have obvious clinical signs of meningitis. Histoplasma is especially common in certain geographic areas in the United States such as the midwest.[32] Although mucosal disease caused by *Candida* is common in patients infected with HIV, invasive disease is unusual unless there is concurrent intravenous drug abuse or an indwelling intravenous catheter.

There are reported cases of distributive shock in patients infected with HIV caused by *Pneumocystis*, CMV, varicella zoster, HSV, *Bartonella*, *Rhodococcus*, acute HIV infection, and many other organisms.[5] However, such causes of sepsis are unusual, and they are usually suggested by the presence of other typical manifestations such as skin lesions (*Bartonella*, zoster, or HSV), pneumonia (*Rhodococcus*), or specific end-organ damage (CMV).

The management of sepsis for patients with HIV infection should not differ from principles followed for HIV-uninfected patients. The use of fluids, pressors, and antibiotics should follow guidelines for surviving sepsis.[33] Whether patients with HIV infection are more likely to benefit from steroid supplementation than HIV-uninfected patients is unknown. Steroids seem to improve the responsiveness of HIV-uninfected patients to sepsis-related fluid resuscitation.[33] However, their use in the general population remains controversial, because their administration has not been shown to have survival benefit.[34]

As described later, other entities specific to HIV/AIDS can present as shock, including distributive shock. These entities include: (1) abacavir hypersensitivity reactions, which present with fever and rash, and are rare in the era of HLA testing[35] (2) lactic acidosis/hepatic steatosis, which is also unusual in this era because the major offending drugs (ie, DDI, D4T, and DDC) are rarely used[36]; (3) IRIS, which occurs in the days or months after initial ART is started (discussed in further detail later)[37]; (4) multicentric Castleman disease, which

is usually more subacute than bacterial or fungal sepsis.[38] but can present with a picture that resembles a systemic inflammatory response syndrome characterized by high fevers and cytopenias accompanied by lymphadenopathy, weight loss, and high circulating human herpesvirus 8 levels.[38]

NEUROLOGIC COMPLICATIONS

Neurologic issues are often cited as the primary reason for an ICU admission in individuals infected with HIV.[8,10,14,19] Neurologic complications can result from OIs such as toxoplasma encephalitis (TE), CM, or IRIS, or may be related to conditions that are unrelated to the underlying HIV status such as seizures related to alcohol withdrawal, community-acquired bacterial meningitis, viral encephalitis, or trauma.[39]

For HIV-related OIs, the most common presenting syndromes are meningitis, space-occupying lesions with or without seizures, and nonfocal cognitive decline. For each syndrome, knowledge of the most recent CD4 count, recent exposures, and concurrent medications (especially those recently started) help considerably in narrowing the differential diagnosis. The evaluation of stroke syndromes does not differ between patients infected with HIV and uninfected patients. However, clinicians should be aware that patients infected with HIV on ART, even if well controlled, seem to develop accelerated atherosclerosis.[40,41] Thus, relatively young patients not usually considered to be stroke candidates may present with thrombotic or embolic strokes.[40,41] Focal neurologic defects are often caused by mass lesions that are easily apparent on contrast-enhanced computed tomography scan or magnetic resonance imaging (MRI). In patients with CD4 counts less than 100 cells/μL, the major differential diagnosis is toxoplasmosis versus lymphoma.[42] The radiologic image does not definitively distinguish one from the other, although certain features such as the presence of multiple ring enhancing lesions favor TE.[43] Patients who are seronegative for toxoplasma are unlikely to have central nervous system (CNS) toxoplasmosis, although commercial laboratories may use relatively insensitive enzyme-linked immunosorbent assay tests that give false-negative results in patients who have low titers.[42,44] Those receiving and adhering to PCP prophylaxis are also unlikely to have TE.[45] If there is no contraindication to lumbar puncture (LP), a cerebrospinal fluid (CSF) analysis can be helpful. A positive CSF Epstein-Barr virus (EBV) polymerase chain reaction (PCR) test or CSF toxoplasma PCR is suggestive of a diagnosis of primary CNS lymphoma and TE, respectively.[46]

However, there is considerable variability in how these tests are performed, and neither the EBV nor the toxoplasma PCR in CSF should be considered a 100% sensitive or specific test.[47,48]

For patients with CD4 counts less than 100 cells and space-occupying lesions, most experts empirically treat for 2 weeks with 1 of the recommended antitoxoplasma regimens (sulfadiazine-pyrimethamine, clindamycin-pyrimethamine, or sulfamethoxazole-trimethoprim). If there is a clinical and radiologic response at 2 weeks, a full course of therapy is completed and the diagnosis is presumed to be toxoplasmosis. If there is no convincing response by both radiologic and clinical parameters, a brain biopsy is indicated. For patients who present with a CD4 count greater than 100 cells, the likelihood of toxoplasmosis is remote. Thus, such patients usually proceed directly to biopsy, unless some other test is considered definitive, such as a serum cryptococcal antigen titer. Interpretation of such tests is not straightforward. The advice of an expert should be sought in these cases. Other entities can present as mass lesions, but are less common. TB is always a consideration, although it is uncommon in native-born residents of the United States who have not had an identified exposure. Fungal infections (Cryptococcus, Histoplasma, Coccidioides) should also be considered in the appropriate epidemiologic setting. Non–HIV-related processes such as bacterial brain abscesses and primary and metastatic tumors should also be included in the diagnostic possibilities.

Patients with HIV/AIDS can develop meningitis caused by common community-acquired pathogens such as Streptococcus pneumoniae. However, for patients infected with HIV with CD4 counts less than 100 cells/μL, CM is a more likely cause. CM is an indolent disease and often presents with fever and headache, but patients can become progressively obtunded over days or weeks as the disease progresses. This subacute process differs in tempo of presentation from the acute presentation of common bacterial and viral pathogens. Patients with CM may have an antecedent pneumonia or skin lesions that are suggestive of disseminated disease.

If there are no contraindications a LP should be performed on all patients with suspected CM. Approximately 20% of patients with CM have a normal CSF formula (ie, normal CSF cell count, protein, and glucose).[49] Thus, CM cannot be ruled out in patients with normal CSF chemistries and cell counts. The diagnosis is generally established by a positive CSF cryptococcal antigen test, which is highly sensitive and specific. Because the burden of organisms is high in patients with HIV

infection, the India ink test, serum cryptococcal antigen tests, and blood cultures are also positive in a high percentage of patients.[50]

The treatment of choice for CM is amphotericin B with or without flucytosine.[51] Lipid formulations of amphotericin B are efficacious and should be used in preference to conventional amphotericin B, especially in patients at risk for renal insufficiency. Fluconazole is used for therapy in many parts of the world, but is inferior to liposomal amphotericin in terms of efficacy and should not be the drug of first choice in the United States.[52]

Increased intracranial pressure should be managed aggressively. If the opening pressure is greater than 250 mm H_2O, CSF drainage is indicated until the pressure is less than 200 mm H_2O, or to 50% of the initial opening pressure.[51] LPs should be performed daily if CSF pressures are increased and until they normalize.[51] There is no indication to treat patients with CM with corticosteroids.

When patients present with progressive cognitive decline, 3 entities should receive primary consideration: progressive multifocal leucoencephalopathy (PML), HIV encephalopathy, and CMV encephalitis. PML is an OI caused by the polyoma virus (JC virus). PML manifests with focal neurologic signs and symptoms. The symptoms are often insidious in onset, with symptoms progressing over weeks. The neuroradiologic features of PML are distinct and help differentiate this condition from other conditions such as TE and CNS lymphoma.[53,54] The white matter lesions are usually hyperintense on T2-weighted imaging and hypointense on T1-weighted imaging. In the precombination ART era, the CSF PCR was often positive for JC virus DNA, but the predictive value of the CSF PCR has been reported to be lower in the postcombination ART era.[55,56] The only effective treatment of PML is ART.[50] HIV encephalopathy presents with progressive cognitive impairment over weeks or months, without the focal motor and sensory defects seen in PML. CNS imaging shows no enhancing lesions, but enlarged ventricles and cortical atrophy. The only effective therapy is ART, which may stabilize the progression or be associated with modest improvement in cognitive function. CMV encephalitis presents more acutely than HIV encephalopathy and is more likely to present with delirium, confusion, and focal neurologic signs and symptoms.[57] CNS imaging is characterized by periventricular enhancement without significant cortical atrophy.[58] The CSF may show lymphocyte or neutrophil predominance. The CSF PCR for CMV should be positive.[59] Therapy is not highly effective. Whether combination therapy with ganciclovir plus foscarnet is better than either ganciclovir or foscarnet alone is uncertain.[50]

RENAL INJURY

Compared with HIV-uninfected hospitalized patients, acute kidney injury (AKI) was documented in a significantly greater proportion of hospitalized patients infected with HIV, in the era before widespread use of effective ART, and also more recently (2.9% vs 1% in 1995 and 6% vs 2.7% in 2003).[60] Between 2000 and 2002, 1 center reported that acute renal disease occurred in 9.4% of ambulatory patients with HIV.[61] Both short-term and long-term mortality is higher among patients infected with HIV who develop AKI.[62]

Many of the causes of AKI in this patient population are no different from HIV-uninfected patients. Although prerenal causes (infections and sepsis, hypovolemia, cirrhosis) and acute tubular necrosis (ischemic or drug-induced) account for many of these cases,[61] intensivists should be aware of the following specific associations: (1) tenofovir, one of the most commonly used antiretroviral agents, can cause acute renal failure with or without associated Fanconi syndrome.[63] (2) crystalluria (both indinavir [rarely used any more] and atazanavir can cause renal crystals and acute renal failure[64]) (interstitial nephritis caused by indinavir has also been reported); (3) HIV-associated microangiopathy can cause acute or chronic renal dysfunction (this condition is uncommonly seen in patients on effective ART); (4) several drugs used to treat HIV-associated complications are associated with acute renal injury, such as amphotericin B, foscarnet, cidofovir, pentamidine, high-dose trimethoprim-sulfamethoxazole, and acyclovir.[61]

ART dosing may need to be modified in patients with AKI. Whereas protease inhibitors (PI), nonnucleoside reverse transcriptase inhibitors (NNRTIs), and integrase inhibitors do not need dose modifications in AKI, all nucleoside and nucleotide reverse transcriptase inhibitors (NRTI) except abacavir need their doses adjusted. Tenofovir should not be used in patients with an estimated glomerular filtration rate (GFR) less than 50 mL/min. DDI and D4T, although uncommonly used nowadays, should also be discontinued. AZT (zidovudine) should be discontinued in patients with an estimated GFR less than 10 mL/min. Because most fixed-dose combinations include tenofovir, they cannot be used in patients with estimated GFR less than 50 mL/min.

Hepatic Failure

Liver disease is the leading cause of death in some recent series of patients infected with HIV.[65,66]

Chronic viral hepatitis is a common coinfection in patients, and is an important cause of liver-related morbidity and mortality in this patient population.[65,67] Alcohol use is frequent in this population and also contributes to liver-related mortality.[67] Although previous studies suggest that the prolonged exposure to antiretrovirals increases the risk of liver-related deaths, a 2012 report suggests that liver-related death caused by ART-related toxicities in HIV-monoinfected patients is rare.[65,68] Intensivists should recognize some unique associations with HIV that may result in increases of liver-related enzymes. For patients who are not on ART, and who have relatively low CD4 counts, OIs of the liver are not common, but do occur. Disseminated fungal disease (Cryptococcus, Histoplasma, other yeasts and molds), toxoplasma, and mycobacteria can involve the liver. OIs in the gastrointestinal lumen, such as cryptosporidia and microsporidia, can gain access to the biliary and pancreatic ducts, causing cholecystitis, cholangitis, and pancreatitis. CMV can also cause either hepatitis or cholangiopathies. Neoplastic processes such as lymphoma and KS can occasionally invade the liver as well.

Drugs are a common cause of acute liver injury. Common offenders for patients with HIV are isoniazid, fluconazole, and trimethoprim-sulfamethoxazole. None of the antiretrovirals in common use has high rates of hepatotoxicity. The hepatic steatosis and lactic acidosis seen with DDI, DDC, and D4T are now rare, because these drugs are used so uncommonly.[69] Nevirapine-induced immune-mediated liver injury can be averted by avoiding nevirapine in women with a CD4 count greater than 250 cells/μL or in men with CD4 counts greater than 400 cells/μL.[70] Intensivists should also be aware that patients starting ART who are hepatitis B antigen–positive or PCR-positive may develop a severe flare of their hepatitis. This reactivation of hepatitis B is likely caused by the suddenly enhanced immunologic function induced by ART. Discontinuation of drugs with activity against hepatitis B virus (HBV) such as tenofovir or lamivudine or emtricitabine can lead to flares in the underlying hepatitis B and severe liver failure.[71] Hence, discontinuation of ART with anti-HBV activity should be avoided in hepatitis B coinfected individuals.

ADMINISTRATION OF ART IN THE ICU
Continuation of ART for Admitted Patients Who Have Been on Stable Regimen

The administration of ART in the ICU is not easy to accomplish. Almost all antiretroviral drugs are available only in oral formulations (only zidovudine

Table 2
Common drug-drug interactions observed in the ICU setting

Drug-Drug Interactions of Commonly Used PIs and NNRTIs[a]	Notes
Proton-pump inhibitors (PPI) Both atazanavir (ATV) and rilpivirine require a low gastric pH for their absorption. Concomitant use of PPI reduces levels of both drugs	Rilpivirine: should not be used with PPI Unboosted ATV: should not be used with PPI Boosted ATV: boosted ATV and a PPI should be used only in PI-naive patients. PPIs should be avoided in PI-experienced patients who are receiving boosted ATV. The PPI dose should not exceed the equivalent of 20 mg omeprazole, and the 2 drugs should be administered at least 12 h apart
Warfarin ATV ± r: ↑ warfarin possible LPV/r: ↓ warfarin possible DRV/r: ↓ warfarin Efavirenz: ↑/↓ levels of warfarin Etravirine: ↑ warfarin possible Rilpivirine: no interactions identified	Monitor international normalized ratio closely when stopping or starting these drugs, and adjust warfarin dose accordingly
Anticonvulsants Carbamazepine ATZ/r, LPV/r: may ↓ PI levels substantially DRV/r: carbamazepine area under curve ↑ 45%; DRV: no significant change Efavirenz: carbamazepine and efavirenz levels ↓ when used concomitantly Etravirine: ↓ carbamazepine and ↓ etravirine possible Rilpivirine: ↓ rilpivirine possible	Consider alternative anticonvulsants when used with ATZ/r or LPV/r; if they are used together, anticonvulsant levels should be monitored When used with DRV/r, monitor anticonvulsant levels and adjust dose accordingly When using efavirenz, monitor anticonvulsant levels and use alternative anticonvulsants if possible Do not coadminister etravirine or rilpivirine with carbamazepine
Phenobarbital May ↓ all PI levels substantially	Consider alternative anticonvulsants with all PIs and efavirenz or monitor levels of both drugs and assess virologic response Do not coadminister with the NNRTIs etravirine and rilpivirine
Phenytoin ATV/r, LPV/r, DRV/r: ↓ phenytoin possible ↓ PI possible Efavirenz: ↓ efavirenz and ↓ phenytoin possible Etravirine: ↓ phenytoin and ↓ etravirine possible Rilpivirine: ↓ rilpivirine possible	Consider alternative anticonvulsants with all PIs and efavirenz. If used together monitor anticonvulsant levels and assess virologic response Do not coadminister with etravirine and rilpivirine
Dexamethasone ↓ PI levels possible Efavirenz: ↓ efavirenz Etravirine: ↓ etravirine Rilpivirine: significant ↓	Systemic dexamethasone should be used with caution with all PIs, efavirenz, and etravirine and an alternative corticosteroid should be considered for long-term use More than a single dose of dexamethasone should not be administered to patients on rilpivirine
Fluticasone ↑ fluticasone levels with all ritonavir-boosted PIs and decreases in cortisol levels	Coadministration can result in adrenal insufficiency and Cushing syndrome. Do not coadminister unless the benefits outweigh the risks

(continued on next page)

Table 2
(continued)

Drug-Drug Interactions of Commonly Used PIs and NNRTIs[a]	Notes
Benzodiazepines ↑ levels of alprazolam, diazepam, triazolam, and midazolam with PIs. These drugs should not be coadministered with PIs Efavirenz: should not be coadministered with oral midazolam, triazolam	Consider use of oxazepam, temazepam, and lorazepam; these benzodiazepines are metabolized through non-CYP450 pathways and there is less potential for interaction
Salmeterol ↑ salmeterol levels possible with all PIs	Do not coadminister with all PIs because of potential increased risk of salmeterol-associated cardiovascular events, including QT prolongation, palpitations, and sinus tachycardia

Abbreviations: ATV, atazanavir; DRV, darunavir; LPV, lopinavir; PPI, proton pump inhibitor; r, ritonavir.

[a] The following boosted PIs are discussed: atazanavir, darunavir, lopinavir. NNRTIs discussed include rilpivirine, efavirenz, and etravirine.

Adapted from Panel on Antiretroviral Guidelines for Adults and Adolescents. Guidelines for the use of antiretroviral agents in HIV-1-infected adults and adolescents. Department of Health and Human Services. Available at: http://aidsinfo.nih.gov/contentfiles/lvguidelines/AdultandAdolescentGL.pdf. Accessed September 9, 2012.

and enfuvirtide are available for parenteral administration). Patients in the ICU often have disrupted gastrointestinal motility. Administration of antiretroviral drugs to patients with uncertain gastrointestinal absorption may lead to suboptimal drug serum levels, which can lead to drug resistance and complicate future options. Drug levels may also be altered by drug interactions related to the urgent administration of drugs in the ICU. Stopping drugs safely to minimize the effects on ART efficacy requires sophisticated knowledge of drug pharmacokinetics. Although it may be safer to stop ART in the ICU, there are immunologic disadvantages related to HIV management to stopping drugs even for a short period. Moreover, for certain subpopulations of patients, such as those with hepatitis B infection, stopping antiretroviral drugs that are also active against HBV can lead to life-threatening flares of previously suppressed infection.[71] The decision to continue or discontinue ART depends on why the patient was admitted to the ICU, the severity of the acute illness, and multiple other factors that must be individualized for each patient.

Initiating ART in the ICU

ART is infrequently initiated in the ICU setting. For ART to be effective, patients need to be committed to adhering to lifelong therapy, a decision that is difficult to arrive at in the setting of an acute illness. The regimen must be appropriate for the patient's individual health status, and renal and hepatic function, which may also be difficult to predict in the ICU. Drug interactions must also be carefully considered, and it is often unclear what medical regimen the patient will receive on hospital discharge. Thus, initiating therapy in the ICU is fraught with hazards. For patients who are admitted to the ICU with a non-AIDS-related illness, there is no urgency to start ART in terms of days or even a few weeks.

For patients in the non-ICU setting receiving care for HIV/AIDS-related OIs, there is a growing body of literature[72] suggesting that early initiation of ART (ie, within 2 weeks of initiating OI therapy) is preferable to late initiation of ART. Numerous studies (conducted in both resource-rich and resource-constrained environments) have reported a survival benefit among patients initiating ART early.[73–76] The greatest benefits were observed in those with CD4 counts less than 50 cells/μL, the same group with the greatest risk of IRIS.[73,75] Exceptions seem to be patients undergoing treatment of Cryptococcal and TB meningitis; in these patients, the data do not support early initiation of ART, and early initiation of ART seems to be harmful in patients with CM.[77,78]

Several features of these studies reduce their generalizability to an ICU population. These studies generally excluded patients who were critically ill, and none included patients who required mechanical ventilation. Thus, the relevance of study conclusions for patients in the ICU is suspect. Given these challenges, the decision to initiate or discontinue ART in a critically ill patient should

Table 3
Life-threatening ART toxicities

Life-Threatening Toxicity	Drugs	Comment
Hypersensitivity syndrome	Abacavir and nevirapine have been primarily associated with this syndrome Rare cases have been reported in patients using raltegravir	Abacavir hypersensitivity syndrome often presents with fever and rash. The syndrome can mimic sepsis. The syndrome usually occurs within the first 6 weeks of initiating abacavir in individuals who are HLAB5701 positive. Screening for the presence of HLAB5701 is recommended in all patients initiating abacavir. Abacavir should be avoided in HLAB5701-positive individuals Nevirapine hypersensitivity presents with rash and hepatotoxicity. Risk is greater in women and highest in the first few months of starting treatment. Nevirapine should be avoided in ART-naive women with a CD4 count greater than 250 cells/μL or in men with a CD4 count greater than 400 cells/μL
Rapidly ascending paralysis	Stavudine	Mimics Guillain-Barré syndrome
Lactic acidosis	All nucleoside reverse transcriptase inhibitors; D4T>DDI>AZT>tenofovir and abacavir	Lactic acidosis has been reported with all NRTIs, especially with D4T, DDI, and AZT. Usually presents with lactate levels >5 mmol/L. The syndrome is often insidious, presenting with nonspecific signs and symptoms. Modest increases in liver function tests (<10 times the upper limit of normal) often accompany this condition. Rapidly progressive forms of the disease can occur and present with respiratory distress. The offending ART should be discontinued
AKI	Tenofovir, atazanavir, indinavir	Atazanavir and indinavir are associated with urolithiasis, whereas tenofovir-related AKI is often accompanied by evidence of tubular injury

(continued on next page)

Table 3
(continued)

Life-Threatening Toxicity	Drugs	Comment
Fanconi syndrome	Tenofovir	Fanconi syndrome is characterized by proximal tubular proteinuria, aminoaciduria, phosphaturia, and glycosuria. It is often reversible with discontinuation of tenofovir
Rhabdomyolysis and creatinine phosphokinase increase	Raltegravir and AZT	5%–13% of patients who are on a raltegravir-based regimen have increased creatinine phosphokinase levels, although clinically significant myopathy and rhabdomyolysis are rare. Cardiomyopathy has not been reported with raltegravir use AZT use has been associated with rare cases of cardiomyopathy
Stevens-Johnson syndrome and toxic epidermal necrolysis	NNRTI: highest incidence with nevirapine PI: darunavir, fosamprenavir, atazanavir	Darunavir and fosamprenavir have a sulfonamide moiety and should be used with caution in patients with known sulfonamide allergies
Hepatotoxicity	Primarily reported with the following agents PI: tipranavir NRTI: DDI, D4T, ZDV NNRTI: nevirapine	DDI and D4T especially when used in combination are associated with hepatic steatosis Long-term DDI use has been linked to noncirrhotic portal hypertension
Pancreatitis	DDI, D4T	Especially in patients receiving a combination of DDI and D4T

Adapted from Panel on Antiretroviral Guidelines for Adults and Adolescents. Guidelines for the use of antiretroviral agents in HIV-1-infected adults and adolescents. Department of Health and Human Services. Available at: http://aidsinfo.nih.gov/contentfiles/lvguidelines/AdultandAdolescentGL.pdf. Accessed September 9, 2012.

not be taken lightly and expert consultation with an infectious diseases specialist should be sought when initiating ART in a critically ill patient.

CHALLENGES ASSOCIATED WITH THE CONTINUATION/INITIATION OF ART
Drug Interactions

Whereas drug interactions are infrequent with NRTI, they occur commonly with NNRTIs and with PIs. Neither maraviroc (a C-C chemokine receptor type 5 inhibitor) nor raltegravir (an integrase inhibitor) significantly affects the levels of other drugs. **Table 2**

summarizes some commonly observed drug-drug interactions.

IRIS

In about 10% to 40% of individuals infected with HIV, the introduction of ART is associated with paradoxic worsening of signs and symptoms. This phenomenon can be life-threatening, and is referred to as IRIS. IRIS represents an exaggerated inflammatory response commonly to an infectious agent and is caused by the recovery of pathogen-specific T-cell responses. This syndrome occurs most often in the first few days or weeks after initial ART is started, and most typically occurs in patients with very low CD4 counts (<100 cells/μL) and high HIV viral burdens.[37,79] Manifestations may include fever, myalgias, and other nonspecific signs of inflammation. Patients may also present, although more infrequently, with life-threatening pulmonary dysfunction, vision-threatening retinitis, meningitis, or distributive shock, depending on which opportunistic pathogens are latent or subclinically active. There is no clinical or laboratory test that distinguishes IRIS from an infectious or neoplastic process, or from a drug toxicity. IRIS is a diagnosis of exclusion, and thus most patients must be managed as if they have an acute infectious process until appropriate tests and clinical monitoring make such diagnoses unlikely.

The overall mortality associated with any type of IRIS is estimated to be 5% but varies according to the patient's baseline immunologic and virologic status and the specific opportunistic pathogen involved.[80] Whereas nearly 21% of those with CM-associated IRIS died, the risk of death in patients diagnosed with TB IRIS was significantly lower, at about 3.5%.[80] IRIS that is not severe should be managed symptomatically with nonsteroidal antiinflammatory agents while continuing ART. Severe IRIS symptoms can be treated with prednisone or methylprednisone at a dose of 1 mg/kg, with a gradual taper after 1 to 2 weeks.

Life-Threatening ART-Related Toxicities

Life-threatening ART-related toxicities include hypersensitivity reactions, lactic acidosis, severe hepatitis, and acute renal failure. These toxicities and the offending drugs are summarized in **Table 3**.

SUMMARY

Critical care of the patient infected with HIV is not dissimilar from HIV-uninfected patients. The differential diagnosis must take into account the patient's immune status (ie, CD4 counts). At CD4 counts less than 200 cells/μL, OI, AIDS-defining malignancies should be considered, and at higher CD4 counts, the differential is similar to that in an uninfected patient. IRIS, unique ART-related toxicities, such as abacavir-induced hypersensitivity reaction, should be considered in the differential. In general, the use of ART in the ICU requires a nuanced approach, and whenever possible ART should be initiated in consultation with an HIV specialist.

REFERENCES

1. Gardner EM, McLees MP, Steiner JF, et al. The spectrum of engagement in HIV care and its relevance to test-and-treat strategies for prevention of HIV infection. Clin Infect Dis 2011;52:793–800.
2. Hall HI, Espinoza L, Benbow N, et al. Epidemiology of HIV infection in large urban areas in the United States. PLoS One 2010;5:e12756.
3. Neuhaus J, Jacobs DR Jr, Baker JV, et al. Markers of inflammation, coagulation, and renal function are elevated in adults with HIV infection. J Infect Dis 2010;201:1788–95.
4. Khouli H, Afrasiabi A, Shibli M, et al. Outcome of critically ill human immunodeficiency virus-infected patients in the era of highly active antiretroviral therapy. J Intensive Care Med 2005;20:327–33.
5. Greenberg JA, Lennox JL, Martin GS. Outcomes for critically ill patients with HIV and severe sepsis in the era of highly active antiretroviral therapy. J Crit Care 2012;27:51–7.
6. Mendez-Tellez PA, Damluji A, Ammerman D, et al. Human immunodeficiency virus infection and hospital mortality in acute lung injury patients. Crit Care Med 2010;38:1530–5.
7. Narasimhan M, Posner AJ, DePalo VA, et al. Intensive care in patients with HIV infection in the era of highly active antiretroviral therapy. Chest 2004;125:1800–4.
8. Powell K, Davis JL, Morris AM, et al. Survival for patients with HIV admitted to the ICU continues to improve in the current era of combination antiretroviral therapy. Chest 2009;135:11–7.
9. Yoon C, Weir D, Greene M, et al. Have we plateaued? Outcomes of HIV-infected patients admitted to the intensive care unit in the combined antiretroviral therapy era. American Thoracic Society (ATS) 2011 International Conference. 2011. Denver (Colorado), May 13–19, 2011.
10. Morris A, Creasman J, Turner J, et al. Intensive care of human immunodeficiency virus-infected patients during the era of highly active antiretroviral therapy. Am J Respir Crit Care Med 2002;166:262–7.
11. Nickas G, Wachter RM. Outcomes of intensive care for patients with human immunodeficiency virus infection. Arch Intern Med 2000;160:541–7.
12. Adlakha A, Pavlou M, Walker DA, et al. Survival of HIV-infected patients admitted to the intensive care unit in the era of highly active antiretroviral therapy. Int J STD AIDS 2011;22:498–504.
13. Barbier F, Coquet I, Legriel S, et al. Etiologies and outcome of acute respiratory failure in HIV-infected patients. Intensive Care Med 2009;35:1678–86.
14. Casalino E, Wolff M, Ravaud P, et al. Impact of HAART advent on admission patterns and survival in HIV-infected patients admitted to an intensive care unit. AIDS 2004;18:1429–33.

15. Dickson SJ, Batson S, Copas AJ, et al. Survival of HIV-infected patients in the intensive care unit in the era of highly active antiretroviral therapy. Thorax 2007;62:964–8.

16. Nuesch R, Geigy N, Schaedler E, et al. Effect of highly active antiretroviral therapy on hospitalization characteristics of HIV-infected patients. Eur J Clin Microbiol Infect Dis 2002;21:684–7.

17. Palacios R, Hidalgo A, Reina C, et al. Effect of antiretroviral therapy on admissions of HIV-infected patients to an intensive care unit. HIV Med 2006;7:193–6.

18. Vincent B, Timsit JF, Auburtin M, et al. Characteristics and outcomes of HIV-infected patients in the ICU: impact of the highly active antiretroviral treatment era. Intensive Care Med 2004;30:859–66.

19. Morquin D, Le Moing V, Mura T, et al. Short- and long-term outcomes of HIV-infected patients admitted to the intensive care unit: impact of antiretroviral therapy and immunovirological status. Ann Intensive Care 2012;2:25.

20. van Lelyveld SF, Wind CM, Mudrikova T, et al. Short- and long-term outcome of HIV-infected patients admitted to the intensive care unit. Eur J Clin Microbiol Infect Dis 2011;30:1085–93.

21. Croda J, Croda MG, Neves A, et al. Benefit of antiretroviral therapy on survival of human immunodeficiency virus-infected patients admitted to an intensive care unit. Crit Care Med 2009;37:1605–11.

22. Vargas-Infante YA, Guerrero ML, Ruiz-Palacios GM, et al. Improving outcome of human immunodeficiency virus-infected patients in a Mexican intensive care unit. Arch Med Res 2007;38:827–33.

23. Chiang HH, Hung CC, Lee CM, et al. Admissions to intensive care unit of HIV-infected patients in the era of highly active antiretroviral therapy: etiology and prognostic factors. Crit Care 2011;15:R202.

24. Akgun KM, Huang L, Morris A, et al. Critical illness in HIV-infected patients in the era of combination antiretroviral therapy. Proc Am Thorac Soc 2011;8:301–7.

25. Phair J, Munoz A, Detels R, et al. The risk of Pneumocystis carinii pneumonia among men infected with human immunodeficiency virus type 1. Multicenter AIDS Cohort Study Group. N Engl J Med 1990;322:161–5.

26. Butt AA, Chang CC, Kuller L, et al. Risk of heart failure with human immunodeficiency virus in the absence of prior diagnosis of coronary heart disease. Arch Intern Med 2011;171:737–43.

27. Triant VA. HIV infection and coronary heart disease: an intersection of epidemics. J Infect Dis 2012;205(Suppl 3):S355–61.

28. Aboulafia DM. The epidemiologic, pathologic, and clinical features of AIDS-associated pulmonary Kaposi's sarcoma. Chest 2000;117:1128–45.

29. Nador RG, Cesarman E, Chadburn A, et al. Primary effusion lymphoma: a distinct clinicopathologic entity associated with the Kaposi's sarcoma-associated herpes virus. Blood 1996;88:645–56.

30. CDC. Reported tuberculosis in the United States, 2011. Atlanta (GA): US Department of Health and Human Services, CDC; 2012. Available at: http://www.cdc.gov/tb/publications/factsheets/statistics/TBTrends.htm. Accessed November 6, 2012.

31. Heffernan RT, Barrett NL, Gallagher KM, et al. Declining incidence of invasive Streptococcus pneumoniae infections among persons with AIDS in an era of highly active antiretroviral therapy, 1995-2000. J Infect Dis 2005;191:2038–45.

32. Kauffman CA. Histoplasmosis. Clin Chest Med 2009;30:217–25, v.

33. Dellinger RP, Levy MM, Carlet JM, et al. Surviving Sepsis Campaign: international guidelines for management of severe sepsis and septic shock: 2008. Crit Care Med 2008;36:296–327.

34. Casserly B, Gerlach H, Phillips GS, et al. Low-dose steroids in adult septic shock: results of the Surviving Sepsis Campaign. Intensive Care Med 2012;38:1946–54.

35. Hetherington S, McGuirk S, Powell G, et al. Hypersensitivity reactions during therapy with the nucleoside reverse transcriptase inhibitor abacavir. Clin Ther 2001;23:1603–14.

36. Carr A. Lactic acidemia in infection with human immunodeficiency virus. Clin Infect Dis 2003;36:S96–100.

37. French MA. Immune reconstitution inflammatory syndrome: immune restoration disease 20 years on. Med J Aust 2012;196:318–21.

38. Stebbing J, Pantanowitz L, Dayyani F, et al. HIV-associated multicentric Castleman's disease. Am J Hematol 2008;83:498–503.

39. Ho EL, Jay CA. Altered mental status in HIV-infected patients. Emerg Med Clin North Am 2010;28:311–23 [Table of Contents].

40. Ovbiagele B, Nath A. Increasing incidence of ischemic stroke in patients with HIV infection. Neurology 2011;76:444–50.

41. Benjamin LA, Bryer A, Emsley HC, et al. HIV infection and stroke: current perspectives and future directions. Lancet Neurol 2012;11:878–90.

42. Luft BJ, Remington JS. Toxoplasmic encephalitis in AIDS. Clin Infect Dis 1992;15:211–22.

43. Ciricillo SF, Rosenblum ML. Use of CT and MR imaging to distinguish intracranial lesions and to define the need for biopsy in AIDS patients. J Neurosurg 1990;73:720–4.

44. Montoya JG. Laboratory diagnosis of Toxoplasma gondii infection and toxoplasmosis. J Infect Dis 2002;185(Suppl 1):S73–82.

45. Abgrall S, Rabaud C, Costagliola D. Incidence and risk factors for toxoplasmic encephalitis in human immunodeficiency virus-infected patients before and during the highly active antiretroviral therapy era. Clin Infect Dis 2001;33:1747–55.

46. Bossolasco S, Cinque P, Ponzoni M, et al. Epstein-Barr virus DNA load in cerebrospinal fluid and plasma of patients with AIDS-related lymphoma. J Neurovirol 2002;8:432–8.

47. Hirsch HH, Meylan PR, Zimmerli W, et al. HIV-1-infected patients with focal neurologic signs: diagnostic role of PCR for Toxoplasma gondii, Epstein-Barr virus, and JC virus. Clin Microbiol Infect 1998;4:577–84.

48. Mikita K, Maeda T, Ono T, et al. The utility of cerebrospinal fluid for the molecular diagnosis of toxoplasmic encephalitis. Diagn Microbiol Infect Dis 2012;75(2):155–9.

49. Rozenbaum R, Goncalves AJ. Clinical epidemiological study of 171 cases of cryptococcosis. Clin Infect Dis 1994;18:369–80.

50. Kaplan JE, Benson C, Holmes KH, et al. Guidelines for prevention and treatment of opportunistic infections in HIV-infected adults and adolescents: recommendations from CDC, the National Institutes of Health, and the HIV Medicine Association of the Infectious Diseases Society of America. MMWR Recomm Rep 2009;58:1–207 [quiz: CE1-4].

51. Perfect JR, Dismukes WE, Dromer F, et al. Clinical practice guidelines for the management of cryptococcal disease: 2010 update by the Infectious Diseases Society of America. Clin Infect Dis 2010; 50:291–322.

52. Bicanic T, Meintjes G, Wood R, et al. Fungal burden, early fungicidal activity, and outcome in cryptococcal meningitis in antiretroviral-naive or antiretroviral-experienced patients treated with amphotericin B or fluconazole. Clin Infect Dis 2007;45:76–80.

53. Whiteman ML, Post MJ, Berger JR, et al. Progressive multifocal leukoencephalopathy in 47 HIV-seropositive patients: neuroimaging with clinical and pathologic correlation. Radiology 1993;187:233–40.

54. Skiest DJ. Focal neurological disease in patients with acquired immunodeficiency syndrome. Clin Infect Dis 2002;34:103–15.

55. Cinque P, Scarpellini P, Vago L, et al. Diagnosis of central nervous system complications in HIV-infected patients: cerebrospinal fluid analysis by the polymerase chain reaction. AIDS 1997;11:1–17.

56. Marzocchetti A, Di Giambenedetto S, Cingolani A, et al. Reduced rate of diagnostic positive detection of JC virus DNA in cerebrospinal fluid in cases of suspected progressive multifocal leukoencephalopathy in the era of potent antiretroviral therapy. J Clin Microbiol 2005;43:4175–7.

57. Holland NR, Power C, Mathews VP, et al. Cytomegalovirus encephalitis in acquired immunodeficiency syndrome (AIDS). Neurology 1994;44:507–14.

58. McCutchan JA. Clinical impact of cytomegalovirus infections of the nervous system in patients with AIDS. Clin Infect Dis 1995;21(Suppl 2):S196–201.

59. Wolf DG, Spector SA. Diagnosis of human cytomegalovirus central nervous system disease in AIDS patients by DNA amplification from cerebrospinal fluid. J Infect Dis 1992;166:1412–5.

60. Wyatt CM, Arons RR, Klotman PE, et al. Acute renal failure in hospitalized patients with HIV: risk factors and impact on in-hospital mortality. AIDS 2006;20: 561–5.

61. Franceschini N, Napravnik S, Eron JJ Jr, et al. Incidence and etiology of acute renal failure among ambulatory HIV-infected patients. Kidney Int 2005;67:1526–31.

62. Choi AI, Li Y, Parikh C, et al. Long-term clinical consequences of acute kidney injury in the HIV-infected. Kidney Int 2010;78:478–85.

63. Verhelst D, Monge M, Meynard JL, et al. Fanconi syndrome and renal failure induced by tenofovir: a first case report. Am J Kidney Dis 2002;40:1331–3.

64. Chang HR, Pella PM. Atazanavir urolithiasis. N Engl J Med 2006;355:2158–9.

65. Weber R, Sabin CA, Friis-Moller N, et al. Liver-related deaths in persons infected with the human immunodeficiency virus: the D:A:D study. Arch Intern Med 2006;166:1632–41.

66. Smith C, Sabin CA, Lundgren JD, et al. Factors associated with specific causes of death amongst HIV-positive individuals in the D:A:D study. AIDS 2010;24:1537–48.

67. Rosenthal E, Salmon-Ceron D, Lewden C, et al. Liver-related deaths in HIV-infected patients between 1995 and 2005 in the French GERMIVIC Joint Study Group Network (Mortavic 2005 study in collaboration with the Mortalité 2005 survey, ANRS EN19). HIV Med 2009;10:282–9.

68. Kovari H, Sabin CA, Ledergerber B, et al. Antiretroviral drug-related liver mortality among HIV-positive persons in the absence of HBV or hepatitis C virus coinfection: the data collection on adverse events of anti-HIV drugs study. Clin Infect Dis 2012. [Epub ahead of print].

69. Kovari H, Weber R. Influence of antiretroviral therapy on liver disease. Curr Opin HIV AIDS 2011;6:272–7.

70. Panel on Antiretroviral Guidelines for Adults and Adolescents. Guidelines for the use of antiretroviral agents in HIV-1-infected adults and adolescents. Department of Health and Human Services. Available at: http://aidsinfo.nih.gov/contentfiles/lvguidelines/AdultandAdolescentGL.pdf. Accessed September 9, 2012.

71. Bellini C, Keiser O, Chave JP, et al. Liver enzyme elevation after lamivudine withdrawal in HIV-hepatitis B virus co-infected patients: the Swiss HIV Cohort Study. HIV Med 2009;10:12–8.

72. Grant PM, Zolopa AR. When to start ART in the setting of acute AIDS-related opportunistic infections: the time is now! Curr HIV/AIDS Rep 2012;9: 251–8.

73. Abdool Karim SS, Naidoo K, Grobler A, et al. Integration of antiretroviral therapy with tuberculosis treatment. N Engl J Med 2011;365:1492–501.

74. Blanc FX, Sok T, Laureillard D, et al. Earlier versus later start of antiretroviral therapy in HIV-infected adults with tuberculosis. N Engl J Med 2011;365:1471–81.

75. Havlir DV, Kendall MA, Ive P, et al. Timing of antiretroviral therapy for HIV-1 infection and tuberculosis. N Engl J Med 2011;365:1482–91.

76. Zolopa A, Andersen J, Powderly W, et al. Early antiretroviral therapy reduces AIDS progression/death in individuals with acute opportunistic infections: a multicenter randomized strategy trial. PLoS One 2009;4:e5575.

77. Makadzange AT, Ndhlovu CE, Takarinda K, et al. Early versus delayed initiation of antiretroviral therapy for concurrent HIV infection and cryptococcal meningitis in sub-Saharan Africa. Clin Infect Dis 2010;50:1532–8.

78. Torok ME, Yen NT, Chau TT, et al. Timing of initiation of antiretroviral therapy in human immunodeficiency virus (HIV)-associated tuberculous meningitis. Clin Infect Dis 2011;52:1374–83.

79. Lawn SD, Meintjes G. Pathogenesis and prevention of immune reconstitution disease during antiretroviral therapy. Expert Rev Anti Infect Ther 2011;9: 415–30.

80. Muller M, Wandel S, Colebunders R, et al. Immune reconstitution inflammatory syndrome in patients starting antiretroviral therapy for HIV infection: a systematic review and meta-analysis. Lancet Infect Dis 2010;10(4):251–61.

Future Directions
Lung Aging, Inflammation, and Human Immunodeficiency Virus

Meghan Fitzpatrick, MD[a], Kristina Crothers, MD[b],
Alison Morris, MD, MS[c],*

KEYWORDS

- Human immunodeficiency virus • Chronic obstructive pulmonary disease • Pulmonary hypertension
- Immune activation • Immune senescence • Inflammation

KEY POINTS

- Human immunodeficiency virus (HIV) is now a chronic disease among persons treated with highly active combination antiretroviral therapy and is frequently complicated by comorbid age-related conditions. Pulmonary comorbidities of chronic HIV are increasingly recognized.
- Chronic obstructive pulmonary disease (COPD) and pulmonary hypertension (PH) are both present at increased frequency among persons infected with HIV.
- Sustained HIV-associated systemic inflammation may result in accelerated cellular senescence with cardiopulmonary end-organ injury, thus contributing to COPD and pulmonary vascular disease.

BACKGROUND AND INTRODUCTION

Because of the success of combination antiretroviral therapy (ART) in restoring immune function, there have been marked declines in mortality from HIV infection in individuals with access to treatment.[1] As a result, more than 30% of the HIV-infected population in the United States is currently older than 50 years, with 50% expected to be over the age of 50 by the year 2020.[2] Unfortunately, these gains in longevity have been accompanied by a growing burden of age-related diseases, attributable to both natural aging and a recently described potential for HIV to cause accelerated cellular senescence.[3,4]

Diseases traditionally associated with aging have been identified in several organ systems (including renal, neurologic, and cardiac) at unexpected prevalence in cohorts of midlife HIV-infected individuals,[4–8] and similar findings are being investigated in the pulmonary system. Because of its unique exposure to airborne pathogens and toxins, the damage from which may be enhanced by HIV infection, the lung and its circulation may be particularly sensitive to early presentation of chronic disease. Two lung diseases in particular, chronic obstructive pulmonary disease (COPD) and pulmonary hypertension (PH), are accelerated in HIV and may be linked to senescence.[9–21]

The prevalence of COPD increases with age and is associated with senescence in both the HIV-uninfected and HIV-infected populations.[11,22–27] The hypothesis that HIV-associated COPD occurs as a consequence of accelerated cellular aging is

Funding Sources: NIH; Fitzpatrick: F32HL114426; Crothers: R01HL090342; Morris: R01HL090339, U01HL098962, P01HL103455.
Conflict of Interest: None.
[a] Department of Medicine, University of Pittsburgh, 3459 Fifth Avenue, 628 Northwest, Pittsburgh, PA 15213, USA; [b] Department of Medicine, Harborview Medical Center, University of Washington, 325 9th Avenue, Campus Box 359762, Seattle, WA 98104, USA; [c] Departments of Medicine and Immunology, University of Pittsburgh, 3459 Fifth Avenue, 628 Northwest, Pittsburgh, PA 15213, USA
* Corresponding author.
E-mail address: morrisa@upmc.edu

chestmed.theclinics.com

particularly compelling because inflammatory dysfunction, a hallmark of HIV-associated senescence, plays a central role in the pathogenesis of COPD.[28]

PH is also a possible senescence-related complication of HIV. Although PH is not typically considered an age-dependent phenomenon in the general population, subsets of PH, including those secondary to left ventricular dysfunction[29] or COPD, are associated with increasing age; furthermore, a recent study suggests that COPD-associated PH is related to leukocyte and smooth muscle cellular senescence.[30] Although the pathogenesis of HIV-associated PH is poorly understood, current studies are evaluating the possible relationships among immune activation, aging, and the development of HIV-associated PH.

This article reviews the features of cellular senescence in relation to HIV and immune activation and examines the foundation of the hypothesis that senescence is associated with COPD and PH in persons with HIV. Recent advances in the understanding of the complex interplay between antigenic exposures, host immune response, and inflammation in both chronic HIV infection and chronic cardiopulmonary dysfunction are addressed. Ongoing studies continue to investigate links between these disease states; these relationships may be instrumental in developing effective prevention and treatment of pulmonary complications associated with chronic HIV infection.

HIV, IMMUNE ACTIVATION, AND AGING: THE IMMUNOSENESCENCE HYPOTHESIS

Cellular senescence is one of the central features of aging organ systems and is defined by the inability of a cell to undergo further division. Senescence can be induced either by direct insult to cells (eg, oxidative stress) or via replicative senescence, a phenomenon whereby repeated cell division results in proliferative arrest. The cells of the immune system, which are subject to frequent rounds of division via clonal expansion following antigenic exposures,[31] are particularly susceptible to replicative senescence. In the case of HIV infection, either HIV itself or the coinfections commonly associated with HIV (including cytomegalovirus [CMV][32] and hepatitis C[33,34]) drive repeated cycles of immune activation and T-cell proliferation. As a result of repeated triggering and expansion, the immune cells reach a replicative limit, characterized by loss of the costimulatory surface receptor CD28.[35] These senescent CD28^{null} T cells are dysfunctional; they are less able to clear infections, but contribute to

a persistent upregulation of the inflammatory response with increases in peripheral inflammatory cytokines.[36–38] This smoldering inflammation resulting from persistent immune activation and immune senescence characterizes the systemic milieu of chronic HIV infection.

During acute and chronic HIV infection, T cells demonstrate elements of immune cell aging, with features of both chronic senescence and activation.[39–41] An early study of T-cell response to HIV found that during acute infection, both HIV-specific CD8^{+} cells non HIV-specific CD8^{+} cells are highly activated (expressing the cellular activation marker CD38 and the proliferative marker Ki67). Although the percentage of activated cells dropped during chronic infection, paralleling the decrease in the viral load, the terminally differentiated "senescent" T-cell population (CD28^{null}) was markedly enriched in chronic infection, a phenomenon that was even more pronounced in the overall CD8^{+} population than in HIV-specific CD8^{+} cells.[41] Further studies of CD4^{+} and CD8^{+} cell phenotypes in persons with chronic HIV infection have demonstrated that abnormal immune activation persists even in individuals with sustained viral suppression on ART.[42,43]

This state of immune activation and senescence, provoked by chronic HIV and by the chronic viral and recurrent bacterial infections that frequently accompany it, has been linked to features of aging and disease in the cardiovascular system[44] and is suspected to be at play in other disease states. Nonimmune organs may sustain collateral damage caused by the systemic inflammatory milieu, either via circulating inflammatory cytokines or from more direct insults, when activation and senescent T cells are recruited to these organs at sites of injury or infection. Because of its vulnerability to repeated exposures to tobacco smoke, other environmental toxins, and microbes (via infection or colonization), the lung and its circulation may be at heightened risk to sustain damage from senescent and activated circulating immune cells. COPD and PH, which are seen at higher than expected prevalence in midlife HIV-infected persons, have been associated with systemic immune activation and inflammation in the non-HIV population, and are therefore of particular interest.

COPD: RELATIONSHIPS TO IMMUNE ACTIVATION AND SENESCENCE

COPD is common in the HIV-uninfected population and is the fourth leading cause of mortality in the United States.[45] This disease typically presents in the sixth decade of life or later, but in the

HIV population, it is often diagnosed at a younger age. Investigators have reported severe emphysema in HIV-infected persons in their thirties,[13] and studies of COPD in HIV-infected cohorts have found a mean age of those with COPD to range from 40 to 50 years.[15] Studies have found a prevalence of 20% to 60% of physiologic measures of COPD in HIV-infected persons[12,14,15,17] in comparison with 7% reported in the general population.[46] In general, most ART-era studies of HIV-infected persons show a high overall prevalence of airflow obstruction, ranging from 8% to 21%,[12,14,15,17] despite the relatively young age of the HIV-infected participants. While HIV-infected persons do have particularly high exposure to pulmonary risk factors (most notably cigarette smoking[12,47])

that likely interact with other factors to contribute to chronic respiratory illness, these data provide epidemiologic support for the hypothesis that the lung may be another end-organ affected by senescence in HIV.

Molecular data examining immune-mediated inflammatory pulmonary cell damage and resultant accelerated alveolar epithelial cell senescence also support the role of aging in HIV COPD (**Fig. 1**). Recent advances in COPD have shown that the disease is not driven by one mechanism, but is a syndrome that is precipitated by multiple insults which may act individually or in concert to cause irreversible damage to the airways or alveoli.[48,49] Immune-mediated inflammatory pulmonary cell damage and resultant

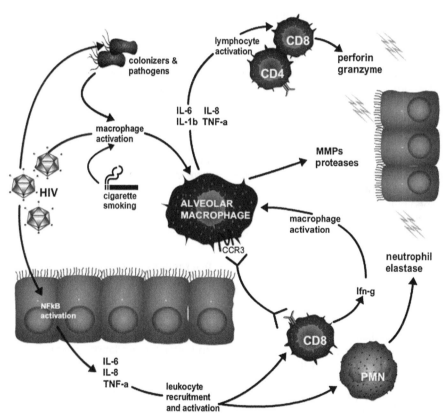

Fig. 1. Theoretical framework of development of HIV-associated chronic obstructive pulmonary disease (COPD). HIV-associated immune deficiency allows for a high burden of microbial infection and colonization; both HIV virions and other microbes lead to macrophage activation. In addition to releasing matrix metalloproteinases, activated alveolar macrophages express inflammatory cytokines that activate local CD4+ and CD8+ lymphocytes. Moreover, activated macrophages express the cytokine receptor CCR3, encouraging trafficking of CD8+ T cells from the circulation. Activated CD8+ cells (which are likely to be senescent in the setting of chronic HIV infections) elaborate interferon-γ, which leads to amplification of macrophage activation. HIV directly activates nuclear factor κB in alveolar epithelial cells, leading to expression of inflammatory cytokines, further driving leukocyte recruitment and activation. Recruited and activated immune cells may cause local pulmonary damage (ie, COPD) and epithelial cell senescence via the expression of proteases, perforin, granzyme, and neutrophil elastase. CCR, chemokine receptor; IFN, interferon; IL, interleukin; MMP, matrix metalloproteinase; NF, nuclear factor; PMN, polymorphonuclear cells; TNF, tumor necrosis factor.

accelerated alveolar epithelial cell senescence may contribute to HIV COPD. Immune activation and senescence have not been directly investigated in HIV-associated COPD, but indirect links from studies of aging and inflammation in COPD in the HIV-uninfected population support a role for aging in HIV-associated COPD as well. The presence and severity of obstruction in COPD in the general population has been associated with increased systemic inflammatory cytokines, including high-sensitivity C-reactive protein, interleukin (IL)-6, and fibrinogen. Persistence of this systemic inflammatory phenotype predicts both COPD exacerbation rate and all-cause mortality.[50] A study specifically examining intracellular cytokine levels in circulating leukocytes and bronchoalveolar lavage cells found elevated interferon (IFN)-γ and tumor necrosis factor (TNF)-α within circulating CD8$^+$ cells and bronchoalveolar lavage CD8$^+$ and CD4$^+$ cells in persons with COPD.[51]

Whereas human studies of inflammation and COPD have been largely associative, animal and in vitro studies are able to investigate the directionality of the relationship. For example, researchers have determined that chronic systemic inflammation in a murine model results in pulmonary inflammation and senescent lung changes.[52] A recent murine study that induced chronic systemic inflammation via subcutaneous lipopolysaccharide (LPS) implant found that LPS-exposed mice developed pulmonary inflammatory changes (increased alveolar macrophages) and evidence for pulmonary cell DNA double-strand breaks, which are precursors of cellular apoptosis and senescence.[52] In turn, senescence of pulmonary epithelial cells may also lead to regional lung inflammation, creating a vicious cycle of local damage. Induction of an in vitro senescent phenotype in lung epithelial cells in culture leads to higher levels of proinflammatory nuclear factor (NF)-κB activation and also results in higher pulmonary epithelial production of the inflammatory cytokines IL-6, IL-8, and TNF-α. Ex vivo studies of lung-tissue explants established that type II epithelial cells from COPD patients demonstrate higher expression of the cellular senescence marker p16 and that senescent cells more frequently demonstrate a proinflammatory phenotype as measured by the presence of phosphorylated NF-κB.[53] These findings further bolster the supposition that chronic systemic inflammation may lead to the inflammatory and senescent changes of COPD.

In addition to data supporting inflammation and pulmonary cell senescence as possible drivers of COPD, several investigations have specifically addressed the contributions of immune senescence. A cross-sectional study examining the T-cell repertoire and inflammatory response in association with COPD found that higher senescent (CD28^{null}) circulating CD4$^+$ cell percentage correlated with lower forced expiratory volume in 1 second (FEV$_1$) percent-predicted and greater midflow obstruction.[25] Although some circulating inflammatory markers (IFN-γ, TNF-α, and IL-1β) were associated with better FEV$_1$ percent-predicted, when T cells in culture were activated, the cells from early-stage COPD secreted increased levels of IFN-γ and TNF-α, suggesting that local stimulation (eg, at the alveolar-capillary interface) of primed senescent cells may lead to enhanced release of these proinflammatory cytokines.[25] A cross-sectional assessment of the relationship between immune cell telomere length (whereby shorter telomeres may identify a more senescent cell phenotype) and lung function found that participants with COPD have shorter telomeres in circulating leukocytes than do healthy controls. In addition, telomere shortening was correlated with reduced activity of superoxide dismutase (a free radical scavenger that may provide protection from COPD).[54] A similar study found that circulating leukocyte telomere shortening was associated with COPD and that higher circulating levels of the inflammatory cytokine IL-6 were associated with both telomere attrition and the presence of COPD.[55] Given the immune dysfunction described in the previous section, any or all of these mechanisms are likely to play a role in the pathogenesis of HIV-associated COPD.

PULMONARY HYPERTENSION: RELATIONSHIPS TO IMMUNE ACTIVATION AND SENESCENCE

PH, like COPD, is described at increased frequency among persons with HIV. Both before and after the availability of combination ART, PH has been found at a prevalence of 0.5% among HIV-infected persons.[20,56] Further directed investigations assessing pulmonary artery pressures in current-era HIV-infected cohorts have found prevalence of echocardiographic markers of pulmonary hypertension ranging from 15.5% to 35%,[18,21,57] with potential risk factors including male sex,[20] injection drug use,[20] and a CD4$^+$ count of fewer than 200 cells/μL.[18,20] Animal models have supported the direct pathogenic role of HIV in the development of PH. For example, in a recently published study, simian immunodeficiency virus (SIV) and simian-human immunodeficiency virus (SHIV)-infected macaques developed echocardiographic and right heart catheterization findings of PH that were significantly worse when compared with uninfected controls.[58] Mechanisms underlying HIV-associated PH are a subject of ongoing investigation; potential contributors are covered in another article in this issue by Barnett and Hsue and in several previous review articles.[16,59,60] These potential contributors include enhanced production of growth factors also implicated in non-HIV PH (including platelet-derived growth factor and vascular endothelial growth factor) and virus-specific factors, namely *nef* and the viral envelope glycoprotein 120.

As with COPD, immune dysfunction, immune senescence, and constitutive cell (in this case, endothelial and pulmonary artery smooth muscle cell) senescence may play a role in development of HIV-associated PH. Studies of non-HIV PH have demonstrated mixed associations with inflammatory markers, but the data generally suggest that inflammation of some variety contributes to disease pathogenesis. Inflammatory infiltrates of mononuclear cells have been identified in the characteristic plexiform lesions of PH, and a recent study has demonstrated organized lymphoid structures in idiopathic PH.[61] Multiple markers of inflammation and immune dysfunction have been described in association with non-HIV PH and are summarized in depth in recent review articles.[59,62] In addition, there is potential evidence for inflammation-mediated senescence in non-HIV PH a study investigating markers of cell senescence in participants with COPD found that higher circulating IL-6 and shorter telomeres in circulating leukocytes correlate with increasing pulmonary artery pressures.[30]

The possible inflammatory and immunosenescent features of HIV-associated PH have only recently been investigated, but early data are promising. One study identified that circulating IL-8, IFN-γ, and activated T cells (CD8$^+$CD69$^+$) were associated with elevated pulmonary artery systolic pressure (PASP) and tricuspid regurgitant jet velocity (TRV), as was sputum IL-8.[18] Of interest, increasing PASP and TRV were independently associated with pulmonary function abnormalities, including worse spirometry and lower diffusing capacity for carbon monoxide. Of note, none of the participants required oxygen and none had severe COPD, arguing against preexisting hypoxemic lung disease as the cause of the elevated pulmonary artery (PA) pressures. In addition, elevated TRV was associated with serologic markers of poorly controlled HIV (CD4 <200 cells/µL or elevated HIV RNA levels), irrespective of ART use.[18] These findings suggest that systemic and/or pulmonary immune activation and resultant inflammation, which is worse in the setting of more

advanced HIV, may underlie both pulmonary dysfunction and elevated PA pressures in HIV-infected persons.

THE COMPLEX INTERPLAY AMONG HIV, IMMUNE ACTIVATION, AND PULMONARY DYSFUNCTION: FUTURE DIRECTIONS

While the accelerated pulmonary disease seen in HIV is in part related to traditional risk factors, the early and unusually prevalent presentations of disorders such as COPD and PH suggest a distinctive contribution of HIV that may involve unique mechanistic pathways (see **Fig. 1**). Senescent and activated T cells, which are commonly elevated even among virally suppressed persons, may contribute to lung and pulmonary circulatory damage either indirectly (via inflammatory cytokines expressed in the circulation) or directly, when they are recruited to the lung or its circulation in response to stimuli (including cigarette smoke, other inhaled toxins, or pulmonary microbes). There is also potential for cellular aging in the resident immune cells or constitutive cells of the lung and PA, either as a direct effect of HIV or as a result of inflammation caused by trafficking of dysregulated systemic immune cells. While these relationships remain speculative, current research directed at describing the associations between indicators of HIV-associated immune activation, immune senescence, epithelial and endothelial cell aging, and outcomes of pulmonary dysfunction is under way. Determining the roles of accelerated immune aging and chronic inflammation in HIV may eventually allow for effective directed interventions in this population.[63]

REFERENCES

1. Palella FJ Jr, Delaney KM, Moorman AC, et al. Declining morbidity and mortality among patients with advanced human immunodeficiency virus infection. HIV Outpatient Study Investigators. N Engl J Med 1998;338:853–60.
2. Hall HI, Song R, Rhodes P, et al. Estimation of HIV incidence in the United States. JAMA 2008;300:520–9.
3. Justice AC. HIV and aging: time for a new paradigm. Curr HIV/AIDS Rep 2010;7:69–76.
4. Effros RB, Fletcher CV, Gebo K, et al. Aging and infectious diseases: workshop on HIV infection and aging: what is known and future research directions. Clin Infect Dis 2008;47:542–53.
5. Clifford DB. HIV-associated neurocognitive disease continues in the antiretroviral era. Top HIV Med 2008;16:94–8.
6. Wand H, Calmy A, Carey DL, et al. Metabolic syndrome, cardiovascular disease and type 2

diabetes mellitus after initiation of antiretroviral therapy in HIV infection. AIDS 2007;21:2445–53.

7. Bozzette SA, Ake CF, Tam HK, et al. Cardiovascular and cerebrovascular events in patients treated for human immunodeficiency virus infection. N Engl J Med 2003;348:702–10.

8. Deeks SG. HIV infection, inflammation, immunosenescence, and aging. Annu Rev Med 2011;62: 141–55.

9. Crothers K. Chronic obstructive pulmonary disease in patients who have HIV infection. Clin Chest Med 2007;28:575–87, vi.

10. Crothers K, Butt AA, Gibert CL, et al. Increased COPD among HIV-positive compared to HIV-negative veterans. Chest 2006;130:1326–33.

11. Crothers K, Huang L, Goulet JL, et al. HIV infection and risk for incident pulmonary diseases in the combination antiretroviral therapy era. Am J Respir Crit Care Med 2011;183:388–95.

12. Cui Q, Carruthers S, McIvor A, et al. Effect of smoking on lung function, respiratory symptoms and respiratory diseases amongst HIV-positive subjects: a cross-sectional study. AIDS Res Ther 2010;7:6.

13. Diaz PT, King MA, Pacht ER, et al. Increased susceptibility to pulmonary emphysema among HIV-seropositive smokers. Ann Intern Med 2000; 132:369–72.

14. George MP, Kannass M, Huang L, et al. Respiratory symptoms and airway obstruction in HIV-infected subjects in the HAART era. PLoS One 2009;4:e6328.

15. Gingo MR, George MP, Kessinger CJ, et al. Pulmonary function abnormalities in HIV-infected patients during the current antiretroviral therapy era. Am J Respir Crit Care Med 2010;182:790–6.

16. Gingo MR, Morris A. Pathogenesis of HIV and the lung. Curr HIV/AIDS Rep 2012;10:42–50.

17. Hirani A, Cavallazzi R, Vasu T, et al. Prevalence of obstructive lung disease in HIV population: a cross sectional study. Respir Med 2011;105:1655–61.

18. Morris A, Gingo MR, George MP, et al. Cardiopulmonary function in individuals with HIV infection in the antiretroviral therapy era. AIDS 2012;26:731–40.

19. Petrache I, Diab K, Knox KS, et al. HIV-associated pulmonary emphysema: a review of the literature and inquiry into its mechanism. Thorax 2008;63: 463–9.

20. Sitbon O, Lascoux-Combe C, Delfraissy JF, et al. Prevalence of HIV-related pulmonary arterial hypertension in the current antiretroviral therapy era. Am J Respir Crit Care Med 2008;177:108–13.

21. Mondy KE, Gottdiener J, Overton ET, et al. High prevalence of echocardiographic abnormalities among HIV-infected persons in the era of highly active antiretroviral therapy. Clin Infect Dis 2011; 52:378–86.

22. Aoshiba K, Nagai A. Senescence hypothesis for the pathogenetic mechanism of chronic obstructive pulmonary disease. Proc Am Thorac Soc 2009;6: 596–601.

23. Ito K, Barnes PJ. COPD as a disease of accelerated lung aging. Chest 2009;135:173–80.

24. Karrasch S, Holz O, Jorres RA. Aging and induced senescence as factors in the pathogenesis of lung emphysema. Respir Med 2008;102:1215–30.

25. Lambers C, Hacker S, Posch M, et al. T cell senescence and contraction of T cell repertoire diversity in patients with chronic obstructive pulmonary disease. Clin Exp Immunol 2009;155:466–75.

26. MacNee W. Accelerated lung aging: a novel pathogenic mechanism of chronic obstructive pulmonary disease (COPD). Biochem Soc Trans 2009; 37:819–23.

27. Tsuji T, Aoshiba K, Nagai A. Alveolar cell senescence in patients with pulmonary emphysema. Am J Respir Crit Care Med 2006;174:886–93.

28. Gadgil A, Duncan SR. Role of T-lymphocytes and pro-inflammatory mediators in the pathogenesis of chronic obstructive pulmonary disease. Int J Chron Obstruct Pulmon Dis 2008;3:531–41.

29. Lam CS, Borlaug BA, Kane GC, et al. Age-associated increases in pulmonary artery systolic pressure in the general population. Circulation 2009;119: 2663–70.

30. Noureddine H, Gary-Bobo G, Alifano M, et al. Pulmonary artery smooth muscle cell senescence is a pathogenic mechanism for pulmonary hypertension in chronic lung disease. Circ Res 2011;109:543–53.

31. Karrer U, Sierro S, Wagner M, et al. Memory inflation: continuous accumulation of antiviral CD8+ T cells over time. J Immunol 2003;170:2022–9.

32. Hunt PW, Martin JN, Sinclair E, et al. Valganciclovir reduces T cell activation in HIV-infected individuals with incomplete CD4+ T cell recovery on antiretroviral therapy. J Infect Dis 2011;203:1474–83.

33. Kovacs A, Karim R, Mack WJ, et al. Activation of CD8 T cells predicts progression of HIV infection in women coinfected with hepatitis C virus. J Infect Dis 2010;201:823–34.

34. Sajadi MM, Pulijala R, Redfield RR, et al. Chronic immune activation and decreased CD4 cell counts associated with hepatitis C infection in HIV-1 natural viral suppressors. AIDS 2012;26:1879–84.

35. Effros RB. Loss of CD28 expression on T lymphocytes: a marker of replicative senescence. Dev Comp Immunol 1997;21:471–8.

36. Yi JS, Cox MA, Zajac AJ. T-cell exhaustion: characteristics, causes and conversion. Immunology 2010; 129:474–81.

37. Vallejo AN, Weyand CM, Goronzy JJ. T-cell senescence: a culprit of immune abnormalities in chronic inflammation and persistent infection. Trends Mol Med 2004;10:119–24.

38. Sansoni P, Vescovini R, Fagnoni F, et al. The immune system in extreme longevity. Exp Gerontol 2008;43: 61–5.

39. Cao W, Jamieson BD, Hultin LE, et al. Premature aging of T cells is associated with faster HIV-1 disease progression. J Acquir Immune Defic Syndr 2009;50:137–47.

40. Desai S, Landay A. Early immune senescence in HIV disease. Curr HIV/AIDS Rep 2010;7:4–10.

41. Appay V, Papagno L, Spina CA, et al. Dynamics of T cell responses in HIV infection. J Immunol 2002; 168:3660–6.

42. Valdez H, Connick E, Smith KY, et al. Limited immune restoration after 3 years' suppression of HIV-1 replication in patients with moderately advanced disease. AIDS 2002;16:1859–66.

43. Hunt PW, Martin JN, Sinclair E, et al. T cell activation is associated with lower CD4+ T cell gains in human immunodeficiency virus-infected patients with sustained viral suppression during antiretroviral therapy. J Infect Dis 2003;187:1534–43.

44. Kaplan RC, Sinclair E, Landay AL, et al. T cell activation and senescence predict subclinical carotid artery disease in HIV-infected women. J Infect Dis 2011;203:452–63.

45. Xu JQ, Kochanek K, Tejada-Vera B. Deaths: preliminary data for 2007. National Vital Statistics Reports. National Center for Health Statistics. 2009;58.

46. Mannino DM, Gagnon RC, Petty TL, et al. Obstructive lung disease and low lung function in adults in the United States: data from the National Health and Nutrition Examination Survey, 1988-1994. Arch Intern Med 2000;160:1683–9.

47. Niaura R, Shadel WG, Morrow K, et al. Human immunodeficiency virus infection, AIDS, and smoking cessation: the time is now. Clin Infect Dis 2000;31: 808–12.

48. Barnes PJ. Chronic obstructive pulmonary disease. N Engl J Med 2000;343:269–80.

49. Casanova C, de Torres JP, Aguirre-Jaime A, et al. The progression of chronic obstructive pulmonary disease is heterogeneous: the experience of the BODE cohort. Am J Respir Crit Care Med 2011; 184:1015–21.

50. Agusti A, Edwards LD, Rennard SI, et al. Persistent systemic inflammation is associated with poor clinical outcomes in COPD: a novel phenotype. PLoS One 2012;7:e37483.

51. Hodge G, Nairn J, Holmes M, et al. Increased intracellular T helper 1 proinflammatory cytokine production in peripheral blood, bronchoalveolar lavage and intraepithelial T cells of COPD subjects. Clin Exp Immunol 2007;150:22–9.

52. Arimura K, Aoshiba K, Tsuji T, et al. Chronic lowgrade systemic inflammation causes DNA damage in the lungs of mice. Lung 2012;190(6):613–20.

53. Tsuji T, Aoshiba K, Nagai A. Alveolar cell senescence exacerbates pulmonary inflammation in patients with chronic obstructive pulmonary disease. Respiration 2010;80:59–70.

54. Houben JM, Mercken EM, Ketelslegers HB, et al. Telomere shortening in chronic obstructive pulmonary disease. Respir Med 2009;103:230–6.

55. Savale L, Chaouat A, Bastuji-Garin S, et al. Shortened telomeres in circulating leukocytes of patients with chronic obstructive pulmonary disease. Am J Respir Crit Care Med 2009;179:566–71.

56. Speich R, Jenni R, Opravil M, et al. Primary pulmonary hypertension in HIV infection. Chest 1991;100: 1268–71.

57. Hsue PY, Deeks SG, Farah HH, et al. Role of HIV and human herpesvirus-8 infection in pulmonary arterial hypertension. AIDS 2008;22:825–33.

58. George MP, Champion HC, Simon M, et al. Physiologic changes in a non-human primate model of HIV-associated pulmonary arterial hypertension. Am J Respir Cell Mol Biol 2012. [Epub ahead of print].

59. Price LC, Wort SJ, Perros F, et al. Inflammation in pulmonary arterial hypertension. Chest 2012;141: 210–21.

60. Cicalini S, Almodovar S, Grilli E, et al. Pulmonary hypertension and human immunodeficiency virus infection: epidemiology, pathogenesis, and clinical approach. Clin Microbiol Infect 2011;17:25–33.

61. Perros F, Dorfmuller P, Montani D, et al. Pulmonary lymphoid neogenesis in idiopathic pulmonary arterial hypertension. Am J Respir Crit Care Med 2012; 185:311–21.

62. El Chami H, Hassoun PM. Immune and inflammatory mechanisms in pulmonary arterial hypertension. Prog Cardiovasc Dis 2012;55:218–28.

63. Plaeger SF, Collins BS, Musib R, et al. Immune activation in the pathogenesis of treated chronic HIV disease: a workshop summary. AIDS Res Hum Retroviruses 2012;28:469–77.

Index

Note: Page numbers of article titles are in **boldface** type.

Clin Chest Med 34 (2013) 333–340
http://dx.doi.org/10.1016/S0272-5231(13)00066-X
0272-5231/13/$ – see front matter © 2013 Elsevier Inc. All rights reserved.

chestmed.theclinics.com

Moving?

Make sure your subscription moves with you!

To notify us of your new address, find your **Clinics Account Number** (located on your mailing label above your name), and contact customer service at:

Email: journalscustomerservice-usa@elsevier.com

800-654-2452 (subscribers in the U.S. & Canada)
314-447-8871 (subscribers outside of the U.S. & Canada)

Fax number: 314-447-8029

Elsevier Health Sciences Division
Subscription Customer Service
3251 Riverport Lane
Maryland Heights, MO 63043

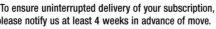

ELSEVIER

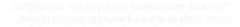

Printed and bound by CPI Group (UK) Ltd, Croydon, CR0 4YY

03/10/2024

01040346-0002